T0283405

THE COMPLETE GUIDE TO STRENGTH TRAINING METHODS

Keven **Arseneault**

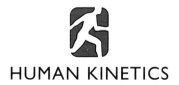

HUMAN KINETICS

Library of Congress Cataloging-in-Publication Data

Names: Arseneault, Keven, 1986- author.
Title: The complete guide to strength training methods / Keven Arseneault.
Other titles: Bible des stratégies et planifications d'entraînement.
  English
Description: Champaign, IL : Human Kinetics, [2024] | "This book is a
  revised edition of La Bible des Stratégies et Planifications
  D'Entraînement, published in 2020 by Éditions Amphora, Paris"-- Title
  page verso. | Includes bibliographical references.
Identifiers: LCCN 2022040637 (print) | LCCN 2022040638 (ebook) | ISBN
  9781718216693 (paperback) | ISBN 9781718216709 (epub) | ISBN
  9781718216716 (pdf)
Subjects: LCSH: Weight training. | Weight lifting. | Muscle strength. |
  BISAC: SPORTS & RECREATION / Bodybuilding & Weightlifting | SPORTS &
  RECREATION / Training
Classification: LCC GV546 .A7713 2024 (print) | LCC GV546 (ebook) | DDC
  613.7/13--dc23/eng/20220923
LC record available at https://lccn.loc.gov/2022040637
LC ebook record available at https://lccn.loc.gov/2022040638

ISBN: 978-1-7182-1669-3 (print)

This publication is written and published to provide accurate and authoritative information relevant to the subject matter presented. It is published and sold with the understanding that the author and publisher are not engaged in rendering legal, medical, or other professional services by reason of their authorship or publication of this work. If medical or other expert assistance is required, the services of a competent professional person should be sought.

This book is a revised edition of *La Bible des Stratégies et Planifications D'Entraînement*, published in 2020 by Éditions Amphora, Paris, www.ed-amphora.fr.

The web addresses cited in this text were current as of August 2022, unless otherwise noted.

Editors: Candice Roger, Amphora; Hannah Werner, Human Kinetics; **Copyeditor:** Heather Gauen Hutches; **Graphic Designers:** Lionel Rousseau, Amphora; Julie L. Denzer, Human Kinetics; **Cover Designer:** Keri Evans; **Cover Design Specialist:** Susan Rothermel Allen; **Photograph (cover):** Mike Kemp/Tetra images/Getty Images; **Photo Production Manager:** Jason Allen; **Printer:** Walsworth

Printed in the United States of America   10 9 8 7 6 5 4 3 2 1

The paper in this book was manufactured using responsible forestry methods.

Human Kinetics
1607 N. Market Street
Champaign, IL 61820
USA

United States and International
Website: **US.HumanKinetics.com**
Email: info@hkusa.com
Phone: 1-800-747-4457

Canada
Website: **Canada.HumanKinetics.com**
Email: info@hkcanada.com

E8860

CONTENTS

INTRODUCTION

This book is the result of more than 20 years of experience in the field of strength training. By 2009, I was working full time developing training programs as a kinesiologist. At the time, my range of techniques was very limited, and I found myself repeatedly using the same methods. I thought it was a shame that there was no book containing a large number of different training techniques to introduce more variety to my programs and help create new modifications for my clients. It was then that I decided to conduct a meta-analysis of training techniques I encountered in my university education, my favorite books, and other search methods. Before long, I had amassed a collection of more than 150 different techniques! It was the origin of this handbook of training techniques. (My research since has increased this number to include more than 230 different techniques in this text.)

To ensure its ease of use, I ranked the techniques by level of difficulty to help my clients progress using these methods. I then separated those that developed more muscular strength (intensification) from those that favored hypertrophy (accumulation). In this way, I gave myself more tools to stimulate and diversify my clients' training. However, because I never prescribe an exercise or method that I am unable to demonstrate, I could not yet use all of these new techniques with my clients. I had no tangible experience of their level of difficulty and had no way of knowing whether adjustments were necessary. Therefore, I began to incorporate these techniques into each new personal program in order to help me visualize the best exercises for each of these methods and to better educate my clients on their practical application.

Starting in 2010, my colleagues began to see the results of my research and asked to use the techniques I was practicing with my clients. I shared my document with them, which at the time was an enormous table listing all of the techniques, along with my notes on their characteristics. It was then that I realized the significance of what I had created. When I saw the enthusiasm of my clients and colleagues as they were testing these new techniques, it only confirmed the need for such a book to be released on the market. The more I spoke of this work in progress to my students and former kinesiology classmates, the more requests for copies I received. So I decided to turn my document into a book in order to improve the final presentation of the techniques and to share my comments on each of them after carefully testing them out.

It should be noted that I did not want to write a book laden with theories. This was not my main objective; I wanted to emphasize the more practical applications of these techniques. There are many well-designed books available on the theoretical aspects of muscle contraction, the effects of concentric versus eccentric versus isometric training, intra- or intermuscular coordination, the impact of submaximal or maximal training in terms of motor unit recruitment and fatigue, the use of training accessories, the advantages of structural versus functional modifications, and more. All of this information is essential to understand what is happening in your body, and I would suggest picking up books such as those found at the end of this volume to deepen your understanding of these topics.

However, before you begin reading this book, I do feel the need to cover certain important principles about factors that influence muscular strength. These principles are at the root of the development of the physical qualities targeted in this book, and I believe that introducing them will provide a solid foundation for understanding the effects of each type of training on your body.

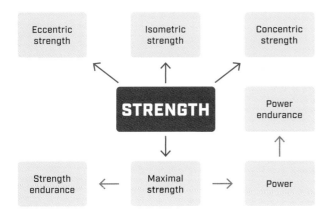

Factors That Influence Strength

The maximal strength of any level of athlete depends primarily on seven basic concepts that can be developed using the techniques in this book. Some of these concepts will be more or less targeted depending on the methods used. It is up to you to vary the use of techniques in order to maximize the development of your muscular strength.

1. **The recruitment of motor units.** The higher the load, the more motor units will be recruited to engage more muscle fibers in contraction according to the size principle, thus increasing the amount of force produced. The size principle, which is illustrated in the illustrations on page 6, states that motor units with a low activation threshold (slow-twitch, or smaller, fibers) are activated first, followed by motor units with a high activation threshold (fast-twitch, or bigger, fibers).

   The illustrations on page 6 show the differences between the recruitment of motor units (a) during submaximal exercise, (b) during exercise with repeated efforts from 13RM-30RM, (c) during exercise with repeated efforts from 6RM-12RM, (d) during exercise with maximum efforts from 1RM-5RM, and (e) during explosive exercise.

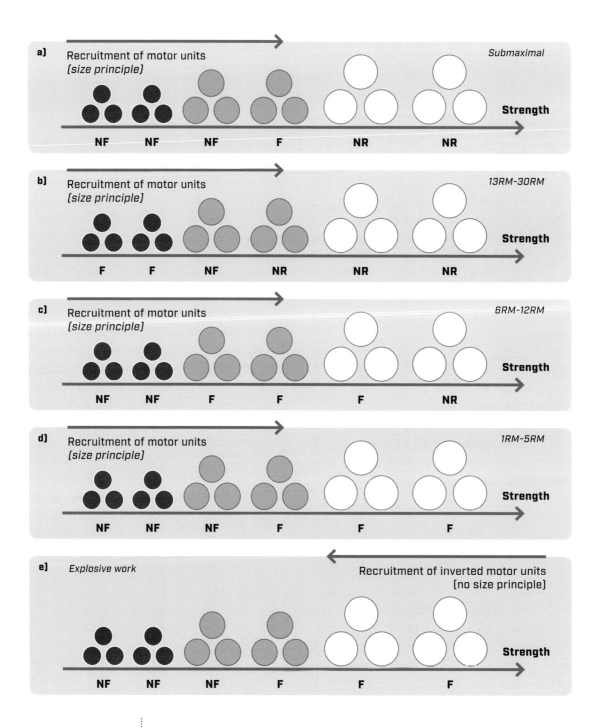

NF: Nonfatigued motor units that are recruited
F: Fatigued motor units that are recruited
NR: Nonrecruited motor units

If you remember only one thing from these illustrations, it should be this: *A fiber that is not fatigued is a fiber that is not trained.* Therefore, you will choose one of these examples to fatigue your fibers depending on the muscular qualities you are aiming to develop. If your goal is muscular hypertrophy, combine recruitments (b), (c), (d), and (e) to train muscle fibers of different thresholds and maximize overall development. You may also want to incorporate endurance exercises at the end of the session to fatigue your slow-twitch fibers (example b).

2. **The firing rate of motor units.** It is possible to improve the strength of a muscle without having to recruit more motor units. In fact, the size principle may be overcome when using explosive movements because muscle fibers must be recruited quickly and dynamically. A small number of muscle fibers will be recruited (mainly fast-twitch fibers), and a large amount of power will still be generated. In this way, the muscle can adapt to use the preferred motor units based on the characteristics of the movement and develop more strength despite the recruitment of fewer motor units (compared with a strength movement, for example).

3. **Motor unit synchronization.** During low-intensity exercise, recruitment is asynchronous, meaning that certain fibers are activated while others are deactivated. However, high-intensity exercise does not mean that motor unit synchronization is automatic: It must be developed. As this aspect improves, muscle fibers are recruited simultaneously. This is what is referred to as *intramuscular coordination* (the synchronization of fibers from the same muscle) and *intermuscular coordination* (the synchronization of fibers from agonist muscles).

4. **The stretch–shortening cycle of the muscle.** This is actually a plyometric movement that requires a concentric contraction preceded by a rapid eccentric contraction. By incorporating a rapid but controlled eccentric contraction in the last quarter of the movement before the concentric phase, we can teach the muscle to use stored elastic energy and promote the activation of the myotatic reflex, which recruits more fast-twitch fibers for strength gains. This optimizes overall muscle activation and can be a good strategy to use during each of your reps.

5. **Neuromuscular inhibition.** This refers to the inhibition of the Golgi tendon organs, which are receptors within the tendons that control the amount of force exerted on them. The more force exerted on a tendon that is not often exposed to this kind of tension, the more these receptors will fight against your brain to deactivate the muscle you are trying to contract. Using maximal and supramaximal loads will help reduce the involvement of these receptors and decrease this protective inhibition in order to maximize strength gains.

6. **The type of muscle fiber.** An athlete with a high percentage of fast-twitch (type II) muscle fibers in a muscle will gain more strength and power in that muscle over time than an athlete with a slower muscle type. This helps explain why some individuals progress more quickly than others, but unfortunately the muscle type encoded in an athlete's DNA cannot be modified using training techniques. You can give type II fibers certain characteristics typical of type I fibers and vice versa through training, but you will never be able to change their most basic features or the size of the motor neuron that innervates them. You will have to learn to work with your genetic makeup

to achieve the best results (e.g., someone with a lot of slow-twitch fibers in her legs will see better hypertrophy gains if her training program focuses on endurance work in this area).

7. **Muscular hypertrophy.** Increasing the cross-sectional area of a muscle will facilitate the expression of strength simply because there are more contractile elements in the muscle. It should be noted, however, that certain individuals have more muscle mass without necessarily having the muscular strength one would expect. This type of individual possesses great potential strength thanks to his existing mass, but his nervous system is incapable of recruiting all of its motor units. Strength training is therefore required to improve the first five elements mentioned earlier and to finally unlock this dormant strength.

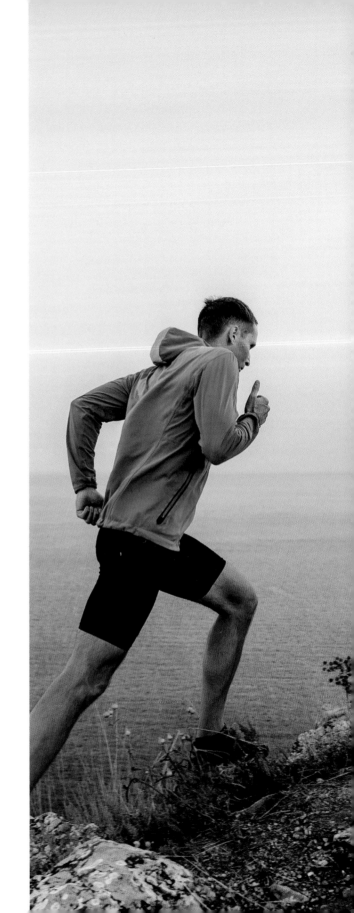

DETERMINING NEEDS

No matter your goal, you must figure out what your needs are before you start working out. If you want to gain muscle mass, the goal is simple. But if you want to improve your downhill skiing or your speed as a hockey player, you need to think a little more. The objective of this book is not to train you as a physical trainer—because other books do it very well—but to give you the tools to help you reflect on your needs. Then, once these have been determined, you can choose the appropriate training techniques according to the muscular or cardiovascular qualities to be developed. If you need to develop your anaerobic alactic, anaerobic lactic, or aerobic system, you can refer to the training techniques in chapter 1. Do you need better muscle strength? Apply the techniques from chapters 2, 4, and 5. Need to jump higher or farther? Integrate the techniques from chapter 6. Do you lack flexibility? Chapter 9 will have the techniques for you.

Appendix #1 is a priority for anyone who wishes to develop their physical capacity in any sport. It will tell you where to look for the right information in this book to meet your goals. Any physical trainer or kinesiologist will greatly appreciate this reference for their clients as well, whether they participate in amateur or professional sport. I suggest that you make photocopies of it in order to use it over and over again depending on your needs or those of your clients. It forces you to ask yourself questions before planning your training. As the old saying goes, "If you fail to plan, then you are planning to fail."

INTRODUCTORY PAGES

Chapters 1 to 9 begin with a training program overview. This is a page that summarizes the important elements to consider when you want to develop certain muscle qualities. For example, chapter 3 (Concentric Training: Hypertrophy) mainly presents training techniques that promote muscle mass gain. Therefore, the outline in chapter 3 describes what to consider when building a training program with this goal. Let's take a closer look.

For example, to gain muscle mass, you should opt for loads between 50% and 85% of your maximum and perform between 6 and 12 repetitions (or 15-50 seconds under tension) where each repetition should be accomplished with a concentric phase in maximum speed. Your training should end up with a maximum of 16 sets (e.g., a maximum of 4 exercises with 4 sets each) per muscle group. Between 12 and 16 sets per muscle group per session is ideal for gains in muscle hypertrophy.

The recovery time will vary from 30 seconds to 3 minutes depending on the training technique used. If you do 16 sets per muscle group, I suggest you limit yourself to 2 muscle groups per session, which will actually add up to 32 sets for your session. For two sessions that do not recruit the same muscle groups directly, you should rest 24-48 hours between workouts. For two sessions that target the same muscles, a 72-hour rest in between is preferable.

The beginning of each chapter includes such a summary of the prescriptions for each element when designing your workout. These guidelines, as well as all of the training techniques in each chapter, will help give you optimal results—whether you intend to develop your maximum strength, endurance, power, power endurance, or flexibility—and will help you avoid doing substandard training or, conversely, overtraining.

TRAINING TECHNIQUE DESCRIPTIONS

A training technique description is the textual and visual representation of a method. Each page provides a variety of information on the method's characteristics. You will learn how to apply the method, its effects on the development of muscular or cardiovascular qualities, and its advantages and disadvantages. Before we start learning about the techniques, let's take a look at how to read a training technique description (you can also find a blank training technique template in appendix #10 to record your own plans):

How Does It Work?
The text explains how to apply the technique in a clear and simple way.

Advantages and Disadvantages
This section lists the advantages and disadvantages of each training technique.

Perceived Effort
This rating shows the level of physical and mental difficulty felt when using the technique.

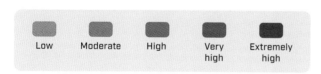

Effect on Hypertrophy
This rating shows the potential gains in muscular hypertrophy that can be achieved using the technique.

Effect on Strength and Power
This rating shows the potential gains in muscular strength or power that can be achieved using the technique.

Effect on Muscular Endurance
This rating shows the potential gains in muscular endurance that can be achieved using the technique.

Effect on Anaerobic Alactic System (chapter 1 only)
This rating shows the potential improvements in the anaerobic alactic system that can be achieved using the technique.

Effect on Anaerobic Lactic System (chapter 1 only)
This rating shows the potential improvements in the anaerobic lactic system that can be achieved using the technique.

Effect on Aerobic System (chapter 1 only)
This rating shows the potential improvements in the aerobic system that can be achieved using the technique.

Effect on Active Flexibility (chapter 9 only)
This rating shows the potential improvements in the active flexibility that can be achieved using the technique.

Effect on Passive Flexibility (chapter 9 only)
This rating shows the potential improvements in the passive flexibility that can be achieved using the technique.

Experience Required
These boxes represent the ideal number of years of intensive strength training experience you should have before attempting the method.

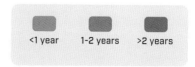

Accumulation Method

An accumulation method is a technique with a high training volume. Training volume refers to the total amount of activity performed during a workout. It is determined by two factors:

1. The duration of the workout
2. The distance covered (running) or the tonnage (resistance training) (tonnage = number of sets × number of reps × load)

The most common ways of increasing an athlete's training volume are by increasing the frequency of workouts, increasing the volume within a workout, or a combination of the two. This box is checked if the technique consists of performing a large number of reps with low to medium intensity. This is generally the case for strength endurance and hypertrophy techniques.

Strategies used to modify training volume include the following:

→ Increasing the duration of workouts (most common in endurance training)
→ Increasing the frequency of workouts (e.g., 1 vs. 2 workouts per day; 3 vs. 5 workouts per week)
→ Increasing the number of reps, sets, stations, or technical elements per workout
→ Increasing the distance covered or the duration of a rep or station

Intensification Method

An intensification method is a technique that has a high training intensity due to the loads used or the speed generated. In general, intensity varies as a function of neuromuscular activation. Thus, a higher intensity produced using heavier loads or maximal speed of movement will require higher neuromuscular activation. This is mainly true of maximal strength techniques, power techniques, and power endurance techniques.

If we want to assess the intensity of a strength training exercise, we must first determine its 1 repetition max (1RM, 100%). The closer to a 1RM, the higher the intensity of the exercise (e.g., a 6RM is more intense than an 8RM). For exercises with no load, such as running, we must determine maximum speed for comparison. For example, if an athlete runs a 100-meter sprint in 10 seconds, this corresponds to a running speed of 10 m/s (100%). If she later incorporates shorter distances in her workouts and manages to achieve a higher speed (e.g., 10.1 m/s), the intensity will be considered supramaximal.

The following table illustrates the relationship between intensity as a percentage of maximal performance, its classification, and its rating on a scale of 6.

Intensity zone	Percentage of maximal performance [%]	Intensity
6	>100	Supramaximal
5	90-100	Maximal
4	80-90	High
3	70-80	Moderate
2	50-70	Low
1	<50	Very low

Strategies used to modify the intensity of a workout include the following:

→ Increasing the velocity of a movement over a greater distance or increasing speed at agility stations
→ Increasing effort (e.g., resistance or load) during strength training
→ Increasing power output
→ Performing endurance, interval, and agility work at a higher heart rate

If hypertrophy is the objective, programs that incorporate more accumulation methods and those with more intensification methods should be alternated or used with a 2:1 ratio (2 accumulation programs for every 1 intensification program). You should never design a program with both high intensity and high training volume over an extended period of time—this is a sure path to overtraining! The exception is during a single feat of strength-speed endurance performed as part of a workout in order to develop very specific physical qualities.

Prescription Table

This section shows the prescription limitations of the technique in question to help guide you in its application. It includes the load or intensity; the number of reps, sets, and exercises to be performed per muscle group; and the suggested recovery time between sets or repetitions.

Practical Application

This section of the training technique description uses text, tables, and images to illustrate concrete examples that I often use in the gym to apply the technique. Other visual representations of the application of the method help to further improve understanding.

Trainer Tips

This is where I give you tips developed through my experimentation with each technique and my extensive experience to help you apply the method in question.

Training Strategies and Plans

This book contains both training strategies and plans. Training strategies are techniques that apply to an exercise—in other words, what to do now, in the very short term. Training plans, on the other hand, are techniques that can help you organize your training session, week, or month—in other words, what to do in the short to medium term. Each technique will therefore be identified with an S or a P in the upper right corner.

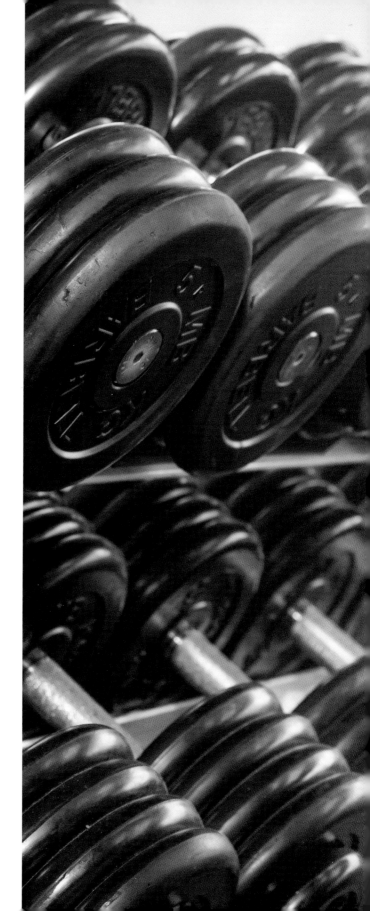

ACKNOWLEDGMENTS

I would like to thank all those whose participation helped make this project a reality—in particular, my wife, Marie-Maude, and my daughters, Lyvia and Maxym. These three girls have been there for my accomplishments and have endured my absence during those weeknights when I stayed at the office after work to write this book. Thank you to the women in my life.

I would like to acknowledge Christian Thibaudeau, Richard Chouinard, Noël Decloître, and Raymond Veillette, who served as my mentors in the field of fitness and physical preparation. You have done so much to fuel my passion for the profession.

Also, special thanks are dedicated to Human Kinetics and Amphora (who published the original French version of this book) for believing in my project and creating an amazing book for all trainers, kinesiologists, and strength training lovers.

I am very grateful to all of you.

PHOTO CREDITS

Pages 8, 16-17, 20: sportpoint/Adobestock; page 13: maxoidos/Adobestock; page 26: kegfire/Adobestock; page 27: coachwood/Adobestock; page 28: Prostock-studio/Adobestock; page 29: Carlos Die Ben R/Adobestock; page 30: robot Dean/Adobestock; page 33: baranq/Adobestock; page 41: chalabala/Adobestock; pages 42-43: Rido/Adobestock; pages 67 (left), 188 (right): Kzenon/Adobestock; pages 67 (right), 188 (right), 229 (left): Scvos/Adobestock; pages 82-83: bnenin/Adobestock; page 111: © Human Kinetics; pages 192-193, 195: Yakobchuk Olena/Adobestock; page 203: Fotos 593/ Adobestock; pages 204-205, 207: torsakh/Adobestock; pages 220-221, 223, 244-245, 247: Leika production/Adobestock; page 225: Paul/Adobestock; pages 226 (left), 249: matimix/Adobestock; page 226 (right): Phawat Topaisan/Adobestock; page 229 (middle and right): Mix and Match Studio/Adobestock; page 231: Maridav/Adobestock; pages 256-257, 259: torwaiphoto/Adobestock; pages 274-275, 278: deniskomarov/Adobestock; page 279: Drobot Dean/Adobestock; page 280: nazarovsergey/Adobestock; page 281 (left): moodboard/Adobestock; page 281 (right): undrey/Adobestock; pages 282, 306-307, 311: WavebreakmediaMicro/Adobestock; page 283: Robert Kneschke/Adobestock; pages 284-293: Gelpi/Adobestock; pages 294-295: dusanpetkovic1/Adobestock

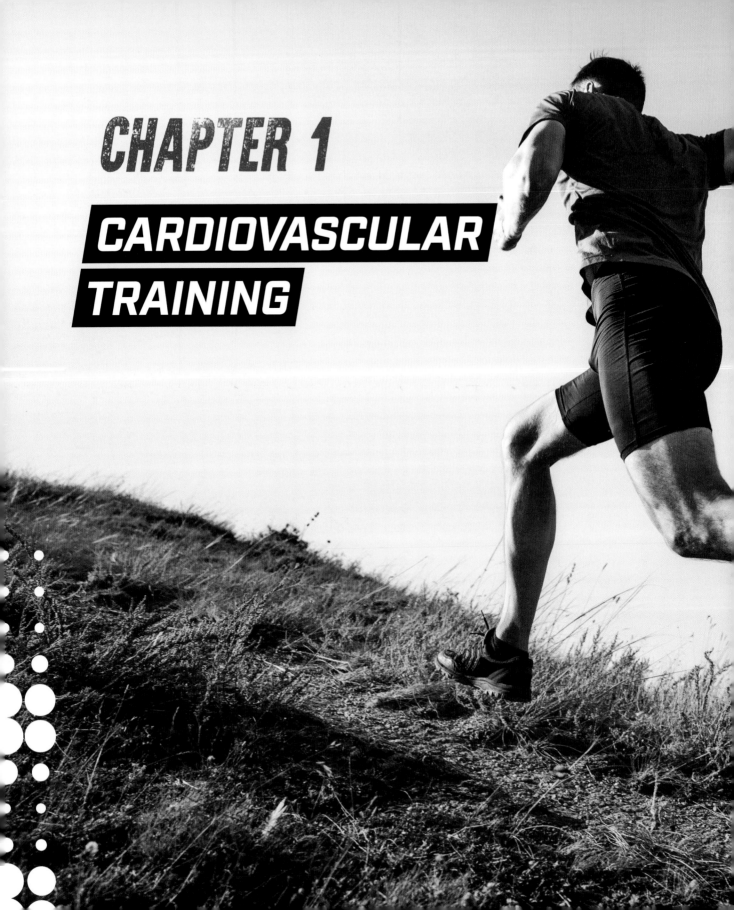

CHAPTER 1

CARDIOVASCULAR TRAINING

TRAINING PROGRAM

+ Intensity: **80%-100% (max speed [Smax]), 61%-125% (max aerobic speed [MAS])**

+ Number of repetitions: **2-8 (Smax), 3-12 (MAS)**

+ Sets per exercise: **1-6 (Smax), 2-6 (MAS)**

+ Rest between reps: **30-60 seconds (Smax), 10 seconds to 6 minutes (MAS)**

+ Rest between sets: **2-5 minutes**

+ Rest between workouts: **24-72 hours**

#1

CARDIOVASCULAR TRAINING

Athletic development—or simply improvement of cardiovascular health—requires developing a good cardiovascular system. This means developing adaptations in the lungs, heart, blood capillaries, and muscles through aerobic training in order to improve the body's oxygen supply during physical exertion. For this reason, many individuals jump on the first cardiovascular machine they see in the gym, such as the treadmill, elliptical, stationary bike, or rowing machine. Unfortunately, there is a big difference between using your cardiovascular system and developing it. To accomplish the latter, you will have to plan a training session in the same way that you will do for a strength training session—by choosing the exercises, the loads, the number of repetitions, and so on. Structuring each session helps to ensure achievement of the desired results. Randomly performing a cardiovascular workout will achieve mostly random results. This chapter will help you to structure your training by giving you the tools you need to plan your sessions for running, cycling, swimming, or other cardiovascular workouts.

Cardiovascular training can be divided into two main categories: aerobic training (with oxygen) and anaerobic training (without oxygen). These two systems seem quite distinct but are in fact intricately linked. Having a well-developed anaerobic system means it can effectively manage metabolic acidosis by buffering hydrogen ions (H+), a hallmark of anaerobic training. This means, for example, if you have aerobically trained for long distances and need to climb a very steep slope, your anaerobic system would support you in completing the climb without too much negative impact. Conversely, a poor anaerobic system would force you to walk half the hill in order to eliminate the excess H+ ions that would accumulate.

On the other hand, if you are going to perform in an anaerobic sport (usually events involving bursts of physical activity lasting 20-120 seconds), you will also need a very good aerobic cardiovascular system. Imagine two athletes who must perform in an event that requires a maximum aerobic speed (MAS) of 16 km/h (9.9 mph). (Note: This value can be determined by a cardiovascular test of $\dot{V}O_2$max.) One athlete has an MAS of 15 km/h (9.3 mph) and the other has an MAS of 17 km/h (10.5 mph). This means that for the first athlete, a run slower than 15 km/h will be aerobic in nature and consume oxygen, whereas a run faster than 15 km/h, after a certain distance, will be anaerobic and cause metabolic acidosis. For this athlete, the specific development of his anaerobic system will not be the most useful way to increase his performance in the event in question, although it may seem logical.

In fact, we are much more efficient at producing energy in the presence of oxygen. As a result, the athlete with an MAS of 17 km/h will find this task easier, because he will be working below his maximum oxygen uptake capacity. In other words, the more oxygen can be utilized during high-intensity physical activity, the better the performance will be. Thus, the first objective for our athlete with an MAS of 15 km/h will be to work as much as possible on his aerobic system in order to increase his MAS, and the second is to work his anaerobic lactic system a few weeks or months before the event.

The anaerobic system can be divided into four main elements that can be developed with training, followed by three that are unique to the aerobic system:

1. **Anaerobic alactic power (AAP):** A very short effort (0-7 seconds) characterized by the ability to regenerate adenosine triphosphate (ATP) quickly.

2. **Anaerobic alactic capacity (AAC):** A very short effort (8-20 seconds) characterized by maintaining AAP as long as possible.

3. **Anaerobic lactic power (ALP):** A short effort (21-45 seconds) characterized by the ability to buffer metabolic acidosis produced by the massive influx of lactate and H+ ions.

4. **Anaerobic lactic capacity (ALC):** A short effort (46-120 seconds) characterized by the ability to maintain ALP for as long as possible in order to constantly buffer the metabolic acidosis produced by the massive influx of lactate and H+ ions.

5. **Maximum aerobic power (MAP) or maximum aerobic speed (MAS):** The maximum rate at which oxygen can be used during a specified period (usually 2-8 minutes), typically during intense exercise. MAP or MAS therefore takes into account $\dot{V}O_2$max, but also the quality of the individual's technical efficiency in the event (e.g., running, swimming).

6. **Aerobic endurance limit (AEL):** The ability to train for several minutes at a high percentage of $\dot{V}O_2$max (80%-100%).

7. **Aerobic endurance (AE):** The ability to maintain a high percentage of MAP for several minutes or hours. It is also subdivided into aerobic endurance of short duration (2-8 minutes), medium duration (8-30 minutes), long duration (30-90 minutes), and very long duration (90 minutes and more).

For optimal progress, you should start by training your aerobic system, followed by your anaerobic alactic system and your anaerobic lactic system. General athletes could use the first annual training plan that follows, while specialized athletes could use the second annual training plan, either moving from left to center or right to center depending on the needs of these energy systems for their sport:

AE → AEL → MAP/MAS → AAP → AAC → ALP → ALC
AAP → AAC → ALP → ALC ← MAP/MAS ← AEL ← AE

Warming Up for Injury Prevention

Training the anaerobic system involves working at very high intensity (95%-100% of Smax). As a result, the muscle groups involved will be tasked with producing great force and power, increasing the risk of strain or injury. Under no circumstances should you start an anaerobic alactic or lactic workout without first completing a specific 15- to 20-minute warm-up. The warm-up should include joint mobilizations, agility and running technique sequences, concentric and eccentric contractions mainly targeting the hamstrings, accelerations, and progressive sprints. The sprinting warm-up in appendix #2 is a great warm-up sequence to do before this type of workout.

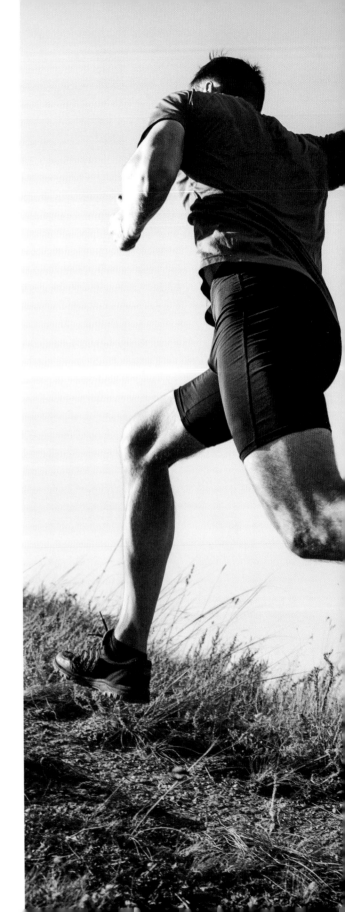

Technique #1

Perceived effort

▪▪▪▫▫

Effect on anaerobic alactic system

▪▪▪▪▫

Effect on anaerobic lactic system

▪▪▫▫▫

Effect on aerobic system

▪▫▫▫▫

Experience required

▪▪▫

☐ Accumulation method

☑ Intensification method

ANAEROBIC ALACTIC POWER

Ⓢ

HOW DOES IT WORK?

This method involves performing maximum linear sprints without changing direction. This technique is applied for distances of 60 meters or less or for an effort of 7 seconds or less. Recovery time between repetitions ranges from 16 to 20 times the exertion time.

ADVANTAGES

→ It is a suitable first step for all sports that require sprinting (e.g., soccer, American football, hockey).
→ It forms the basis of anaerobic alactic capacity.

DISADVANTAGES

→ It cannot be performed on a treadmill.
→ It requires a running track if the residential area is sloping.

PRESCRIPTION TABLE

Intensity (% of maximal speed)	Number of repetitions per set	Number of sets per exercise	Rest between repetitions	Rest between sets
95%-100%	2-8	2-4	1.5-2.5 minutes	5-10 minutes

THE FOLLOWING ARE EXAMPLES OF PROGRESSIVE ANAEROBIC ALACTIC POWER TRAINING SESSIONS:

→ 2 sets of 6 × 30-meter sprints, 90 seconds rest between repetitions, 5 minutes between sets
→ 3 sets of 5 × 30-meter sprints, 90 seconds rest between repetitions, 5 minutes between sets
→ 2 sets of 6 × 40-meter sprints, 2 minutes rest between repetitions, 6 minutes between sets
→ 3 sets of 5 × 40-meter sprints, 2 minutes rest between repetitions, 6 minutes between sets

Technique #2

Perceived effort

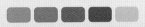

Effect on anaerobic alactic system

Effect on anaerobic lactic system

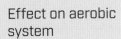

Effect on aerobic system

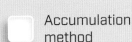

Experience required

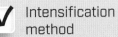

☐ Accumulation method

✓ Intensification method

Trainer Tips

For the development of anaerobic alactic capacity, you will need to train 2-3 times per week. A rest of 36 hours between sessions is sufficient. To maintain anaerobic alactic capacity, complete 1 session per week.

ANAEROBIC ALACTIC CAPACITY

HOW DOES IT WORK?

This method consists of performing maximum linear sprints without changing direction. This technique is applied for distances of 100-200 meters or for an effort of 15-30 seconds. The recovery time between repetitions varies from 12 to 16 times the exertion time.

ADVANTAGES

→ It is a suitable first step for all sports that require sprinting (e.g., soccer, American football, hockey).

→ It forms the basis of anaerobic lactic power.

DISADVANTAGES

→ It cannot be performed on a treadmill.

→ It requires a running track if the residential area is sloping.

PRESCRIPTION TABLE

Intensity [% of maximal speed]	Number of repetitions per set	Number of sets per exercise	Rest between repetitions	Rest between sets
80%-94%	3-4	2-3	3-4 minutes	6-12 minutes

THE FOLLOWING ARE EXAMPLES OF PROGRESSIVE ANAEROBIC ALACTIC CAPACITY TRAINING SESSIONS:

→ 2 sets of 3 × 100-meter sprints, 3 minutes rest between repetitions, 8 minutes between sets

→ 3 sets of 3 × 100-meter sprints, 3 minutes rest between repetitions, 8 minutes between sets

→ 2 sets of 3 × 150-meter sprints, 3 minutes rest between repetitions, 10 minutes between sets

→ 3 sets of 3 × 150-meter sprints, 3 minutes rest between repetitions, 10 minutes between sets

Technique #3

Perceived effort

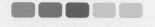

Effect on anaerobic alactic system

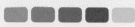

Effect on anaerobic lactic system

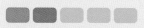

Effect on aerobic system

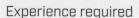

Experience required

☐ Accumulation method

☑ Intensification method

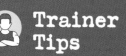

Trainer Tips

Ideally, you should calculate the volume of your workout so that it is between 15 and 24 repetitions in total. This technique can also be performed in competition with a training partner.

ACCELERATION

HOW DOES IT WORK?

This method is part of anaerobic alactic power training. It consists of performing accelerations (sprints) from a stationary position to maximum speed over a distance of 10-30 meters or an effort time of 2-4 seconds. You can also include more technical skills such as hurdles, cones, or beginning from a lying or kneeling position.

ADVANTAGES

→ It is suitable as a first step for all sports that require sprinting (e.g., soccer, American football, hockey).

→ It forms the basis of the ability to perform acceleration with changes of direction (technique #15).

DISADVANTAGES

→ Ideally, it requires a long, flat running surface such as an athletic track or synthetic turf.

→ If you perform this technique in competition with a training partner, it requires a third person to give the starting signal.

PRESCRIPTION TABLE

Intensity (% of maximal speed)	Number of repetitions per set	Number of sets per exercise	Rest between repetitions	Rest between sets
95%-100%	4-6	4-6	30-60 seconds	3-5 minutes

YOU MIGHT TRY SOME OF THE FOLLOWING STARTING POSITIONS BEFORE ACCELERATING:

→ Left or right knee on the ground

→ Lying on your stomach, hands under your chin

→ Abdominal plank position

→ Standing with your back to the start line

→ Making dynamic movements (e.g., quick butt taps) while waiting for the starting signal

→ Kneeling with your back to the start line

Technique #4

Perceived effort

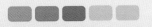

Effect on anaerobic alactic system

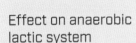

Effect on anaerobic lactic system

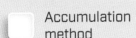

Effect on aerobic system

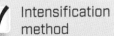

Experience required

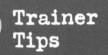

☐ Accumulation method

☑ Intensification method

Trainer Tips

Maximum speed can also be trained in athletes using sport-specific movement. For example, a boxer throwing quick punches into the air or a martial artist practicing fast kicks improves maximum speed.

Ⓢ

MAXIMUM SPEED (VELOCITY)

HOW DOES IT WORK?

This method develops maximum speed in cyclic movement (e.g., running). One of the most important points in sprinting is stride frequency (i.e., how often the feet touch the ground). The higher the stride frequency, the greater the maximum speed potential will be. This technique uses a distance of 40-100 meters or an effort time of 4-15 seconds. For the purposes of progression and variation, several pieces of equipment can be used during training to create overspeed such as elastic bands, bungee cords, or a suspended treadmill.

ADVANTAGES

→ It allows you to reach and train maximum running speed.

DISADVANTAGES

→ It requires a flat running surface, ideally an athletic track or synthetic turf.

PRESCRIPTION TABLE

Intensity (% of maximal speed)	Number of repetitions per set	Number of sets per exercise	Rest between repetitions	Rest between sets
100%-105%	4-6	4-6	1-3 minutes	3-5 minutes

A good way to quantify your maximum speed training is to get photoelectric sensors that will calculate your run time to hundredths of a second. To do this, prepare a 50-meter zone with sensors placed at 30 and 50 meters. You will accelerate for the first 30 meters in order to reach your maximum speed, which will be calculated for the final 20 meters.

Technique #5

Perceived effort

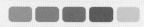

Effect on anaerobic alactic system

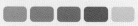

Effect on anaerobic lactic system

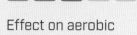

Effect on aerobic system

Experience required

☐ Accumulation method

☑ Intensification method

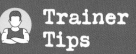
Trainer Tips

This technique is best used later in the training plan in order to have previously worked on power and anaerobic capacity.

SPEED ENDURANCE

HOW DOES IT WORK?

This technique improves the maintenance of maximum speed once reached. To improve speed endurance, you should use a distance or time 100%-120% the length of the targeted event.

ADVANTAGES

→ It improves your endurance over distances slightly longer than the event itself.

DISADVANTAGES

→ It may require an athletic track or artificial turf for running events because most fitness center treadmills cannot reach the top speeds of many athletes.

→ It requires a large body of water for swimming events, ideally a lake, because most pools are not long enough to maintain top speed without a rotation on the pool's wall.

PRESCRIPTION TABLE

Intensity (% of maximal speed)	Number of repetitions per set	Number of sets per exercise	Rest between repetitions	Rest between sets
95%-100%	2-8	1-3	2-7 minutes	5-10 minutes

THE FOLLOWING ARE EXAMPLES OF SPEED ENDURANCE TRAINING:

→ 100-meter sprint: 3 sets of 6 × 110-meter sprints, 4 minutes rest between repetitions, 8 minutes between sets

→ 50-meter swim: 3 sets of 5 × 60-meter sprints, 5 minutes rest between repetitions, 10 minutes between sets

Technique #6

Perceived effort

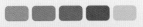

Effect on anaerobic alactic system

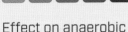

Effect on anaerobic lactic system

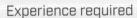

Effect on aerobic system

Experience required

☐ Accumulation method

☑ Intensification method

Trainer Tips

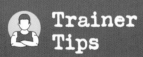

If you opt to use a parachute, have a partner hold it at your height during takeoff. This will help it catch the wind and prevent it from dragging on the ground and breaking. You can also use a harness and bungee cord for indoor workouts (if space allows).

SPRINTS WITH SLED, TIRE, OR PARACHUTE

(S)

HOW DOES IT WORK?

This method involves performing resisted accelerations over a distance of 15-20 meters with a harness or belt to which a sled, a tire, or a parachute is attached. The loads used for the sled and the tire can be light or heavy, depending on the muscle qualities being developed. A light weight may be an unloaded sled or a tire about 10% of your body weight and will allow you to maintain maximal speed quality. A heavy weight should be more than 10% of your body weight up to when the maximum speed cannot be maintained.

ADVANTAGES

→ If the loads used are light, it will improve the power of the sprint as well as the length of the strides.

→ If the loads used are heavy, it will improve takeoff power as well as the force applied during each stride.

DISADVANTAGES

→ It requires specific equipment (harness and tire, parachute, or sled).

→ It must be done on an exterior surface or in an indoor facility with a cement or turf floor.

PRESCRIPTION TABLE

Intensity (% of maximal speed)	Number of repetitions per set	Number of sets per exercise	Rest between repetitions	Rest between sets
95%-100%	4-6	4-6	2-3 minutes	3-5 minutes

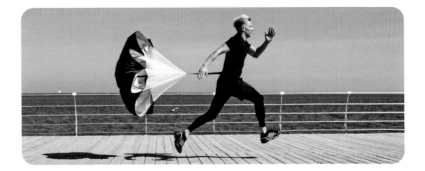

Technique #7

Perceived effort

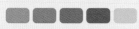

Effect on anaerobic alactic system

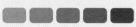

Effect on anaerobic lactic system

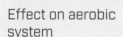

Effect on aerobic system

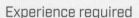

Experience required

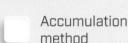

☐ Accumulation method

✓ Intensification method

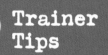

Trainer Tips

To ensure a smooth transition, the use of a harness with Velcro is ideal. This will allow you to remove the harness in the middle of the sprint without too much difficulty.

CONTRAST SPRINTS WITH SLED, TIRE, OR PARACHUTE

HOW DOES IT WORK?
This method consists of performing resisted accelerations over a distance of 10-20 meters with a harness or a belt to which a sled, tire, or parachute is attached, followed by a sprint at maximum speed over 10-20 meters without the overload (you will therefore have to detach the harness after the first sprint). The loads used with the sled or the tire must be light to maintain maximal speed quality (an unloaded sled or a tire about 10% of your body weight is ideal).

ADVANTAGES
→ It improves the length of takeoff strides and maximum stride frequency.
→ It increases the starting speed and the transition to maximum speed.

DISADVANTAGES
→ It requires specific equipment (harness and tire, parachute, or sled).
→ It must be done on an exterior surface or in an indoor facility with a cement or turf floor.

PRESCRIPTION TABLE

Intensity (% of maximal speed)	Number of repetitions per set	Number of sets per exercise	Rest between repetitions	Rest between sets
95%-100%	4-6	4-6	2-3 minutes	3-5 minutes

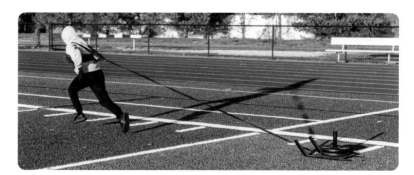

Technique #8

Perceived effort

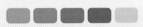

Effect on anaerobic alactic system

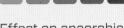

Effect on anaerobic lactic system

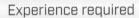

Effect on aerobic system

Experience required

☐ Accumulation method

☑ Intensification method

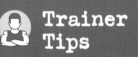

Trainer Tips

If you are training with a partner who has a higher maximum running speed than yours, link yourselves with a band a few meters in length, let your partner go 2 seconds before you, then accelerate. The tension put on the elastic by your partner while running will allow you to achieve overspeed.

ASSISTED OVERSPEED WITH BAND

Ⓢ

HOW DOES IT WORK?

This method consists of performing accelerations over 10-20 meters while wearing a harness attached to an elastic band of a length equal to the distance to be covered (between 10-20 meters). As a partner (or tree or other stable object) holds the other end of the elastic stretched taut (15-25 meters away), you will run toward your partner, releasing the tension of the rubber band. Your acceleration combined with this additional tension will create overspeed, which is a faster running speed than your usual rate.

ADVANTAGES

→ It improves stride frequency during acceleration.

→ It allows you to train and become comfortable with speeds higher than your maximum.

→ It improves balance and coordination needed at high speeds.

DISADVANTAGES

→ It requires a very long elastic band (10-20 meters), which is not usually found in standard training facilities.

→ It requires a partner (or other means) to hold the other end of the band.

PRESCRIPTION TABLE

Intensity (% of maximal speed)	Number of repetitions per set	Number of sets per exercise	Rest between repetitions	Rest between sets
95%-100%	4-6	4-6	2-3 minutes	3-5 minutes

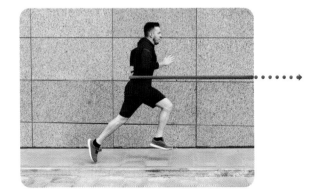

Technique #9

Perceived effort

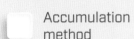

Effect on anaerobic alactic system

Effect on anaerobic lactic system

Effect on aerobic system

Experience required

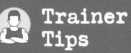

☐ Accumulation method

✓ Intensification method

Trainer Tips

This technique can also be accomplished with a Velcro harness attached to a rope. Your partner will hold the other end of the rope to create resistance. Then put on the Velcro harness and start running. You will have difficulty moving forward until the Velcro gives way and you can accelerate without the harness.

CONTRAST SPRINTS WITH A PARTNER

HOW DOES IT WORK?
This method consists of performing accelerations over 10-20 meters with a start resisted by a partner. You will start running explosively from a bent-over 45-degree angle while your partner uses her hands, a towel, or a rope to hold you back. After about 5 strides, your partner will let go.

ADVANTAGES
→ It allows you to produce more force during the resisted portion and helps you keep producing force when your partner releases you.
→ It improves the speed of transition from acceleration to top speed.
→ It improves stride frequency during acceleration.

DISADVANTAGES
→ It requires a training partner and a running track or a long stretch of turf in order to perform the accelerations.

PRESCRIPTION TABLE

Intensity (% of maximal speed)	Number of repetitions per set	Number of sets per exercise	Rest between repetitions	Rest between sets
95%-100%	4-6	4-6	2-3 minutes	3-5 minutes

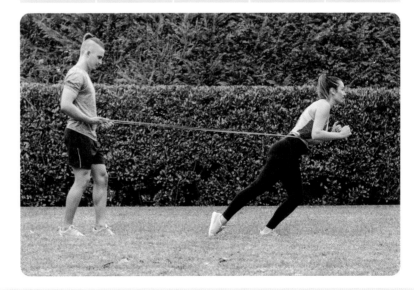

Technique #10

Perceived effort

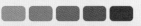

Effect on anaerobic alactic system

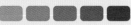

Effect on anaerobic lactic system

Effect on aerobic system

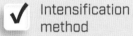

Experience required

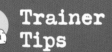

☐ Accumulation method

☑ Intensification method

Trainer Tips

During winter, you might try high-speed treadmill running at an incline of 15-20 degrees. This is not optimal because—unlike a natural run—the treadmill moves your leg back with each step, but it may help to maintain improvements in the off-season.

CLIMBING ACCELERATION

HOW DOES IT WORK?

This method consists of performing accelerations of 4-8 seconds on an inclined surface. You can run on a hill or on an outdoor track that slopes between 20 and 35 degrees. Count the number of strides and mark your place of arrival according to the chosen run time, then try to accomplish the distance with fewer strides in subsequent runs.

ADVANTAGES

→ It improves starting power.
→ It improves stride length during acceleration.

DISADVANTAGES

→ It requires a location with a steep enough slope to allow this type of training.

PRESCRIPTION TABLE

Intensity (% of maximal speed)	Number of repetitions per set	Number of sets per exercise	Rest between repetitions	Rest between sets
95%-100%	4-6	4-6	2-3 minutes	3-5 minutes

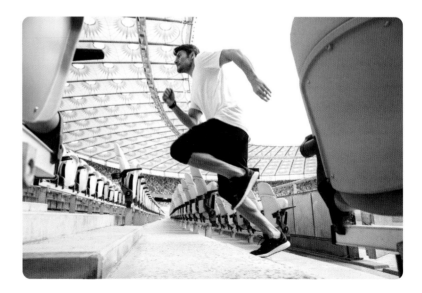

Technique #11

Perceived effort

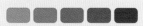

Effect on anaerobic alactic system

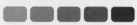

Effect on anaerobic lactic system

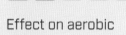

Effect on aerobic system

Experience required

 Accumulation method

☑ Intensification method

Trainer Tips

During winter, you might try high-speed treadmill running at an incline of 1-3 degrees. This is not optimal because—unlike a natural run—the treadmill moves your leg back with each step, but it may help to maintain improvements in the off-season.

CLIMBING MAXIMAL SPEED

HOW DOES IT WORK?

This method involves performing sprints for 15-30 seconds on a surface with an incline of 1-3 degrees. Because the aim is to improve maximum running speed, do not exceed 3 degrees of incline. Higher inclines are more suitable for developing the acceleration mechanics.

ADVANTAGES

→ It improves strength and power during the sprint.

→ It improves stride length.

DISADVANTAGES

→ It requires access to an adequately graded slope between 1 and 3 degrees. You may need to walk around your neighborhood to find a suitable space.

PRESCRIPTION TABLE

Intensity (% of maximal speed)	Number of repetitions per set	Number of sets per exercise	Rest between repetitions	Rest between sets
90%-94%	3-4	2-3	3-4 minutes	6-12 minutes

Technique #12

Perceived effort

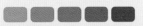

Effect on anaerobic alactic system

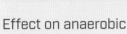

Effect on anaerobic lactic system

Effect on aerobic system

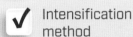

Experience required

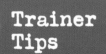

☐ Accumulation method

☑ Intensification method

Trainer Tips

Note that this technique unfortunately cannot be applied to indoor treadmill workouts, because the rapid transition between inclines is not possible—the mechanical transition on a treadmill from 15 degrees to a horizontal position can take up to 20 seconds.

CONTRAST CLIMBING MAXIMAL SPEED

(S)

HOW DOES IT WORK?

This method involves performing sprints on a slope of 15-20 degrees over a distance of 10-20 meters, then continuing for an additional distance of 15-25 meters on flat ground. The goal is for you to reach your near-maximum speed on the top of the hill, then shift to maximum speed on the level surface.

ADVANTAGES

→ It improves stride length and starting speed.
→ It improves the transition to maximum speed.

DISADVANTAGES

→ It requires access to a properly graded slope between 15 and 20 degrees that is followed by a level surface. You may need to explore your area to find a suitable space.

PRESCRIPTION TABLE

Intensity [% of maximal speed]	Number of repetitions per set	Number of sets per exercise	Rest between repetitions	Rest between sets
95%-100%	4-6	4-6	2-3 minutes	3-5 minutes

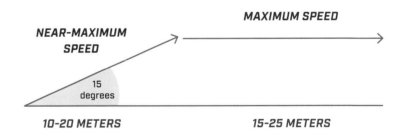

Technique #13

Perceived effort

▪▪▪▫▫

Effect on anaerobic alactic system

▪▪▪▪▫

Effect on anaerobic lactic system

▪▫▫▫▫

Effect on aerobic system

▪▫▫▫▫

Experience required

▪▪▫

☐ Accumulation method

☑ Intensification method

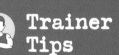

Trainer Tips

To prevent injury if you fall, first perform this type of run on a grassy surface instead of asphalt. Once you have mastered the correct posture and mechanics, you can then make the transition to a harder surface to allow you to reach your maximum speed.

MAXIMUM DOWNHILL SPEED

HOW DOES IT WORK?

This method involves performing sprints for 10-20 meters on a slope that declines between 3 and 7 degrees. The assistance of gravity creates overspeed, allowing an increase in stride frequency.

ADVANTAGES

→ It promotes proper top speed mechanics.

→ It increases stride frequency and maximum speed.

DISADVANTAGES

→ It requires access to an adequately graded slope between 3 and 7 degrees. You may need to walk around your neighborhood to find a suitable space.

→ The risk of falling is high in inexperienced individuals. Progression in the sprint speed is essential.

PRESCRIPTION TABLE

Intensity (% of maximal speed)	Number of repetitions per set	Number of sets per exercise	Rest between repetitions	Rest between sets
95%-100%	4-6	4-6	2-3 minutes	3-5 minutes

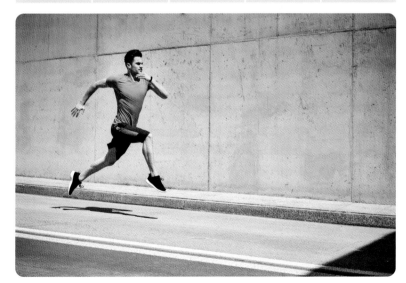

Technique #14

Perceived effort

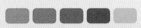

Effect on anaerobic alactic system

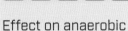

Effect on anaerobic lactic system

Effect on aerobic system

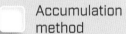

Experience required

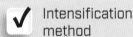

☐ Accumulation method

☑ Intensification method

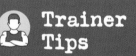

Trainer Tips

To prevent injury if you fall, first perform this type of run on a grassy surface instead of asphalt. Once you have mastered the correct posture and mechanics, you can then make the transition to a harder surface to allow you to reach your maximum speed.

CONTRAST MAXIMUM DOWNHILL SPEED

Ⓢ

HOW DOES IT WORK?

This method involves performing sprints on a slope of 3-5 degrees over a distance of 10-20 meters, then continuing for an additional distance of 10-15 meters on flat ground. The goal is for you to reach supramaximal speed at the bottom of the hill. The objective of this sprint is to try to maintain the supramaximal speed reached for 2-3 seconds once on flat ground.

ADVANTAGES

→ It increases stride frequency and maximum speed.
→ It allows you to work in overspeed without the need for specific equipment.

DISADVANTAGES

→ It requires access to a properly graded slope between 3 and 5 degrees that is followed by a level surface. You may need to explore your area to find a suitable space.

PRESCRIPTION TABLE

Intensity (% of maximal speed)	Number of repetitions per set	Number of sets per exercise	Rest between repetitions	Rest between sets
95%-100%	4-6	4-6	2-3 minutes	3-5 minutes

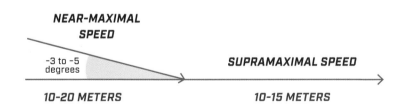

Technique #15

Perceived effort

■ ■ ■ ■ ☐

Effect on anaerobic alactic system

■ ■ ■ ■ ■

Effect on anaerobic lactic system

■ ■ ☐ ☐ ☐

Effect on aerobic system

■ ☐ ☐ ☐ ☐

Experience required

■ ■ ☐

☐ Accumulation method

✓ Intensification method

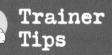

ACCELERATION WITH CHANGES OF DIRECTION

HOW DOES IT WORK?

This method consists of performing accelerations from a stationary position to maximum speed at various stations. Each station has a different difficulty level and must use different athletic skills.

ADVANTAGES

→ It is very representative of skills required in sports such as American football, soccer, and hockey.

→ It promotes team spirit.

→ It promotes competitiveness and self-improvement.

DISADVANTAGES

→ It requires a large field, such as an American football or soccer field, in order to perform the various stations.

PRESCRIPTION TABLE

Intensity (% of maximal speed)	Number of repetitions per set	Number of sets per exercise	Rest between repetitions	Rest between sets
95%-100%	6-8	2-4	2-3 minutes	4-5 minutes

EXAMPLES OF STATIONS

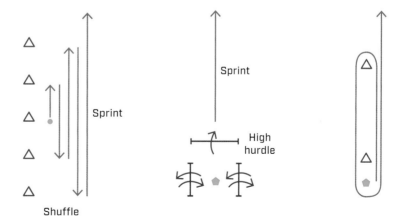

Technique #16

Perceived effort

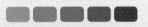

Effect on anaerobic alactic system

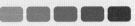

Effect on anaerobic lactic system

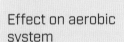

Effect on aerobic system

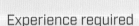

Experience required

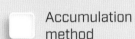

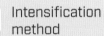

☐ Accumulation method

☑ Intensification method

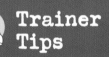

Trainer Tips

This type of training is very good for sports teams. Doubling your stations so that teams can compete against each other will motivate your athletes to give 100% effort.

CHANGE OF DIRECTION CONE DRILLS

Ⓢ

HOW DOES IT WORK?

This method consists of performing precise sequences of movements between cones at 6-8 different stations. Each station, lasting 5-10 seconds, will be completed with a cool-down of 30-60 seconds. When the stations are completed, rest 4-5 minutes. The stations are preferably practiced before starting the session.

ADVANTAGES

→ It allows you to work on strength, power, acceleration, deceleration, coordination, balance, agility, and changes of direction.
→ It includes fairly broad work on the physical qualities necessary for an athlete.

DISADVANTAGES

→ It requires the design and preparation of stations in advance.
→ It requires a very large surface of natural or synthetic grass (e.g., an American football field) in order to arrange the various stations.

PRESCRIPTION TABLE

Intensity [% of maximal speed]	Number of repetitions per set	Number of sets per exercise	Rest between repetitions	Rest between sets
95%-100%	6-8	2-4	30-60 seconds	4-5 minutes

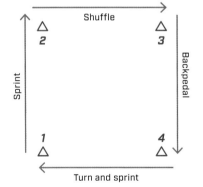

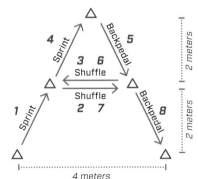

Technique #17

Perceived effort

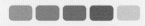

Effect on anaerobic alactic system

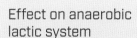

Effect on anaerobic lactic system

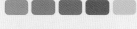

Effect on aerobic system

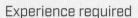

Experience required

☐ Accumulation method

✓ Intensification method

 Trainer Tips

This is a very demanding technique, but necessary to develop systemic anaerobic ability. I used this technique as part of the training for world FireFit champion Claude Bélanger.

ANAEROBIC LACTIC POWER   Ⓢ

HOW DOES IT WORK?

This technique consists of performing maximum linear sprints without changes of direction. This technique is applied for distances of 400 meters or less or for an effort of 20-50 seconds. The recovery time between repetitions varies from 5 to 8 times the exertion time.

ADVANTAGES

→ It develops tolerance to pain caused by the accumulation of lactic acid.

→ It is a prerequisite to working on anaerobic lactic capacity.

DISADVANTAGES

→ It usually requires a flat outdoor surface or athletic track, although athletes with less training experience may be able to use a treadmill.

PRESCRIPTION TABLE

Intensity (% of maximal speed)	Number of repetitions per set	Number of sets per exercise	Rest between repetitions	Rest between sets
85%-90%	2-10	1-2	1.5-7 minutes	5-10 minutes

THE FOLLOWING ARE EXAMPLES OF PROGRESSIVE ANAEROBIC LACTIC POWER TRAINING SESSIONS:

→ 6 × 30-second sprints, 2.5 minutes rest between repetitions

→ 2 sets of 5 × 30-second sprints, 2.5 minutes rest between repetitions, 5 minutes rest between sets

→ 5 × 45-second sprints, 3 minutes rest between repetitions

→ 2 sets of 4 × 45-second sprints, 3 minutes rest between repetitions, 6 minutes rest between sets

Technique #18

Perceived effort

Effect on anaerobic alactic system

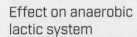

Effect on anaerobic lactic system

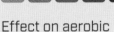

Effect on aerobic system

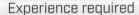

Experience required

 ✓ Accumulation method

✓ Intensification method

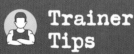

Trainer Tips

For the development of anaerobic lactic capacity, you will need to train 2-3 times per week. A rest of 36-48 hours between sessions is sufficient. To maintain anaerobic lactic capacity, complete 1 session per week.

ANAEROBIC LACTIC CAPACITY

HOW DOES IT WORK?

This method consists of performing maximum linear sprints without changes of direction. This technique is applied for distances of 400-800 meters or for an effort of 50-120 seconds. The recovery time between repetitions varies from 5 to 8 times the exertion time.

ADVANTAGES

→ It develops tolerance to pain caused by the accumulation of lactic acid.

DISADVANTAGES

→ It usually requires a flat outdoor surface or athletic track, although athletes with less training experience may be able to use a treadmill.

PRESCRIPTION TABLE

Intensity [% of maximal speed]	Number of repetitions per set	Number of sets per exercise	Rest between repetitions	Rest between sets
80%-85%	2-4	1-2	4-16 minutes	15-20 minutes

THE FOLLOWING ARE EXAMPLES OF PROGRESSIVE ANAEROBIC LACTIC CAPACITY TRAINING SESSIONS:

→ 4 × 60-second sprints, 5 minutes rest between repetitions
→ 2 sets of 3 × 60-second sprints, 5 minutes rest between repetitions, 15 minutes rest between sets
→ 2 × 90-second sprints, 6 minutes rest between repetitions
→ 2 sets of 2 × 90-second sprints, 6 minutes rest between repetitions, 18 minutes rest between sets

Technique #19

Perceived effort

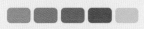

Effect on anaerobic alactic system

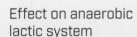

Effect on anaerobic lactic system

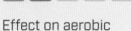

Effect on aerobic system

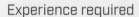

Experience required

✓ Accumulation method

☐ Intensification method

Trainer Tips

Appendix #4 will help you determine your running speed (in km/h) or the distance to cover (in meters) depending on the percentage to use. However, a $\dot{V}O_2$max test (running or cycling) is preferable so that you work with your actual maximum value. As an example, see the Mercier treadmill test in appendix #3.

MAXIMUM AEROBIC SPEED (MAS)

HOW DOES IT WORK?

This technique uses percentages varying between 90% and 125% of maximum aerobic speed (MAS) for running or maximum aerobic power (MAP) for cycling.[32] The goal is to work the $\dot{V}O_2$max with a higher working power than during continuous training and shorter exercise times. Work-to-rest ratios vary depending on the intensity of the exercise.

ADVANTAGES

→ It allows you to work on running mechanics at high speeds.

→ It allows you to work at a higher speed than during long tests.

DISADVANTAGES

→ It requires a maximum aerobic test in order to obtain your $\dot{V}O_2$max.

→ It requires a calculation of the distance to be covered or the speed to be used before the session.

TRAINING EXAMPLES

Medium intermittent:

1. **90%-95% MAS:** 6-7 repetitions × 1.5-4 minutes, 3-5 minutes rest between repetitions

Short intermittent (3-5 minutes rest between sets):

1. **95%-100% of MAS:** 2 sets of 3-4 repetitions × 60-90 seconds, 3-4.5 minutes rest between repetitions
2. **100%-105% of MAS:** 2 sets of 5-6 repetitions × 45-60 seconds, 1.5-3 minutes rest between repetitions
3. **105%-110% of MAS:** 2-3 sets of 5-6 repetitions × 30-45 seconds, 60-135 seconds rest between repetitions

Very short intermittent (2-3 minutes rest between sets):

1. **100% of MAS:** 2-4 sets of 6-8 repetitions × 30 seconds, 30 seconds rest between repetitions
2. **110% of MAS:** 2-4 sets of 6-10 repetitions × 20 seconds, 20 seconds rest between repetitions
3. **120% of MAS:** 3-5 sets of 6-10 repetitions × 15 seconds, 15 seconds rest between repetitions
4. **125% of MAS:** 4-6 sets of 8-12 repetitions × 10 seconds, 10 seconds rest between repetitions

Technique #20

Perceived effort

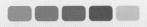

Effect on anaerobic alactic system

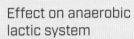

Effect on anaerobic lactic system

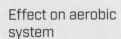

Effect on aerobic system

Experience required

✓ Accumulation method

☐ Intensification method

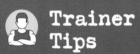

Trainer Tips

Limited aerobic endurance training is useful for anyone who plans to do a 5K, 10K, half-marathon, or marathon. It is also favorable for cyclic sports (e.g., cycling, kayaking) with events lasting 2-8 minutes.

LIMITED AEROBIC ENDURANCE

HOW DOES IT WORK?

Limited aerobic endurance training involves working between 71% and 90%[26] of your $\dot{V}O_2$max, which is generally lower than MAS training, but higher than long-term aerobic endurance training duration. The goal is to work on your ability to maintain a high percentage of your $\dot{V}O_2$max over long distances and durations.

ADVANTAGES

→ It improves the ability to last at intensities near your 100% ($\dot{V}O_2$max).

DISADVANTAGES

→ It requires a maximum aerobic test in order to obtain your $\dot{V}O_2$max.
→ It requires a calculation of the distance to be covered or the speed to be used before the session.

TRAINING EXAMPLES

1. **71%-80% of MAS:** 1 repetition of 18-90 minutes of effort (>5 kilometers). Aim for a target heart rate of 82% HRmax.
2. **81%-83% of MAS:** 1 repetition of 17-18 minutes of effort. Aim for a target heart rate of 83%-84% HRmax.
3. **82%-86% of MAS:** 1-3 repetitions of 15-16 minutes of effort and 7 minutes of rest. Aim for a target heart rate of 85%-87% HRmax.
4. **84%-86% of MAS:** 1-4 repetitions of 10-12 minutes of effort and 6 minutes of rest. Aim for a target heart rate of 88% HRmax.
5. **84%-88% of MAS:** 2-5 repetitions of 7-8 minutes of effort and 5 minutes of rest. Aim for a target heart rate of 89% HRmax.
6. **86%-90% of MAS:** 3-6 repetitions of 4-6 minutes of effort and 4-6 minutes of rest. Aim for a target heart rate of 90% HRmax.

Technique #21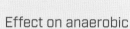

Perceived effort

■ ■ ■ ■ ☐

Effect on anaerobic alactic system

■ ☐ ☐ ☐ ☐

Effect on anaerobic lactic system

■ ■ ☐ ☐ ☐

Effect on aerobic system

■ ■ ■ ■ ☐

Experience required

■ ☐ ☐

✓ Accumulation method

☐ Intensification method

Trainer Tips

For optimal development, your cardiovascular training plan should incorporate 1 session per week of each of the following techniques:

1. Maximum aerobic speed (MAS)
2. Limited aerobic endurance
3. Long-term aerobic endurance

LONG-TERM AEROBIC ENDURANCE

HOW DOES IT WORK?

This technique simply consists of accomplishing long training sessions in order to learn how to regulate your speed, pace, and cadence for the competition or event. Activities over 20 minutes fall into this category.[26]

ADVANTAGES

→ It teaches you to regulate your pace in events of 5 kilometers and longer.
→ It allows you to acclimate to your body's reaction to the use of energy substrates in events lasting longer than an hour.
→ It can be done anywhere.

DISADVANTAGES

→ None.

PRESCRIPTION TABLE

Intensity (% of maximal speed)	Number of repetitions per set	Number of sets per exercise	Duration of a repetition	Target heart rate
61%-75%	1	1	More than 20 minutes	74%-81% HRmax

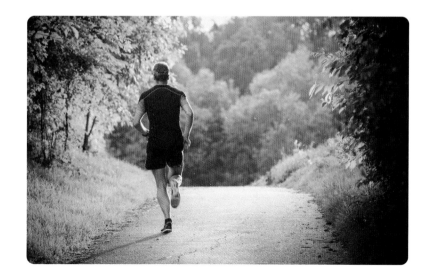

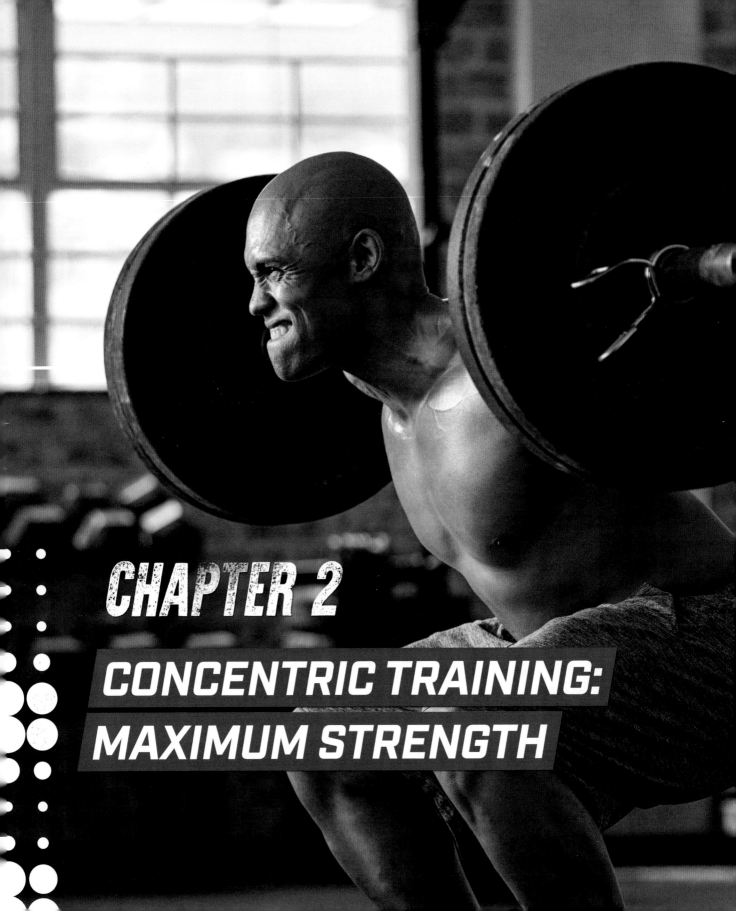

CHAPTER 2

CONCENTRIC TRAINING:
MAXIMUM STRENGTH

TRAINING PROGRAM

+ Intensity: **85%-100%**

+ Number of repetitions: **1-5, or 2-15 seconds of effort**

+ Speed of execution: **Maximal in concentric phase**

+ Rest between sets: **1-5 minutes**

+ Max reps per muscle group per workout: **50**

+ Max sets per muscle group: **16**

+ Max muscle groups per workout: **2**

+ Rest between workouts: **24-72 hours**

CONCENTRIC TRAINING: MAXIMUM STRENGTH

The techniques included in this section will help develop your muscular strength regardless of your current fitness level. Indeed, there are as many techniques for beginners as there are for more advanced individuals. However, I encourage you to progress sequentially through your training and not jump to the techniques with a level 3 rating before first completing the prerequisite level 1 and 2 techniques. As my colleague Christian Thibaudeau often says when he sees beginners using techniques that are too advanced for them, this is akin to killing a fly with a sledgehammer—that is, not necessary and possible to accomplish through much simpler methods! Advancing too quickly is not appropriate and only increases the risk of injury. Be mindful in your approach and use your best judgment.

Strength training is commonly used by powerlifters and strongmen to develop their ability to lift heavy loads, which is the basis of their respective sports. Many other athletes also use these methods to improve the strength component of power (power = strength × speed) or to help handle the heavy loads required by their sport (e.g., a defensive player in football). All of these athletes use the basic techniques presented here, such as the general standards 1RM-5RM (technique #22), maximum weight 1 and 2 (techniques #25 and #26), and 5 × 5 (technique #27). These techniques can also be made more difficult for more advanced athletes. For optimal planning of your strength training sessions, refer to the Prilepin chart (appendix #7).

Several years ago, I worked in a strength club led primarily by Jean-François Caron, a famous strongman holding several Canadian and North American titles and a participant in the World's Strongest Man competition. He holds Canadian records in deadlift, back squat, and bench press; won the title of "North America's Strongest Man" in 2012; and won the title of "Strongest Man in Canada" seven times (from 2011 to 2017), thus surpassing the record set by Hugo Girard. Through the classes offered by the strength club, I helped Jean-François incorporate new strength methods that, despite his extensive training experience, he had never used before. These methods have helped many advanced athletes break through stubborn plateaus and continue to progress. Now it's your turn to try them out!

Strength can be considered from three different perspectives: as absolute strength, as relative strength, or as relative strength as determined by the Wilks coefficient.

→ **Absolute strength.** Absolute strength is simple: This is the load that you are able to lift, full stop. If you lift 100 kg (220 lb) and your friend lifts 90 kg (198 lb), you have more absolute strength than him.

→ **Relative strength.** Relative strength is absolute strength divided by your body weight. Therefore, if you lift 100 kg (220 lb) in the bench press and weigh 90 kg (198 lb), your relative strength is 1.11 (100/90). If your friend weighs 80 kg (176 lb) and has lifted 90 kg (198 lb), he has a relative strength of 1.13 (90/80), so he has better relative strength than you.

→ **Wilks coefficient (appendix #6).** The Wilks coefficient goes beyond relative strength by allowing us to consider the maximum loads already lifted in the world by weight category. This avoids the biases that relative strength can present. For example, the world record for a clean and jerk in the 56 kg (bantamweight) category is 168.0 kg (370 lb), which is three times the athlete's body weight. If an athlete in the 130 to 140 kg (super heavyweight) category wishes to achieve better relative strength than this, then he should lift more than 390 kg—an impossible feat, because the current world record in this category is 263.5 kg. This is where the Wilks coefficient comes in.

Consider a male athlete who weighs 61.2 kg and who lifted 180 kg in the deadlift (relative strength of 2.9) and a male athlete who weighs 104.5 kg and who lifted 250 kg on the same exercise (relative strength of 2.4). The latter has the best absolute strength and the former has the best relative strength. But who is the strongest according to the Wilks coefficient? We can go to the table shown in appendix #6 to find the coefficient for each athlete. At the junction of lines 61 and 0.2 (for 61.2 kg) we get the number 0.8378, and at the junction of lines 104 and 0.5 (for 104.5 kg) we get the number 0.5986. As a result, our 61.2 kg athlete's Wilks score is 150.80 (180 kg × 0.8378) and our 104.5 kg athlete's score is 149.65 (250 kg × 0.5986). This score confirms that our 61.2 kg athlete actually has a higher relative strength than our 104.5 kg athlete.

The Wilks coefficient has been studied[23] and is considered valid for adjusting results in powerlifting. However, it does not take into account new world records over the years and only applies to powerlifting lifts, namely the bench press, squat, and deadlift. However, it remains a good means of comparing strength athletes to one another.

Technique #22

Perceived effort

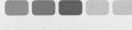

Effect on hypertrophy

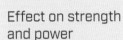

Effect on strength and power

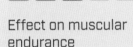

Effect on muscular endurance

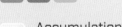

Experience required

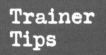

☐ Accumulation method

☑ Intensification method

Trainer Tips

Create your own rounds for each session (see the examples). This will introduce some variety into your workouts while developing your strength. Make sure to warm up before you start.

GENERAL STANDARDS 1RM-5RM

HOW DOES IT WORK?
This method—sometimes referred to as the bulk method—involves completing several sets of 1RM-5RM. You simply need to choose one exercise and complete it with a heavy weight. Your goal will be to do 1-5 repetitions maximum with an eccentric phase always under control (3-5 seconds).

ADVANTAGES
→ This technique is great as an introduction to heavier loads following hypertrophy training. The level of difficulty is low, which helps emphasize the technical control of movements with heavy loads.

DISADVANTAGES
→ A spotter is required during the bench press and squat exercises.

PRESCRIPTION TABLE

Load	Number of repetitions per set	Number of sets per exercise	Number of exercises per muscle group	Rest between sets
85%-100%	1-5	5-8	1-2	3-5 minutes

EXAMPLES OF POSSIBLE TRAINING SESSIONS INCLUDE THE FOLLOWING:
1. 2 × 5, 2 × 4, 2 × 3, 2 × 2 (8 sets)
2. 4 × 4, 4 × 3 (stage style over 8 sets)
3. 1 × 5, 1 × 4, 1 × 3, 1 × 2, 1 × 1 (5 sets)
4. 1 × 5, 1 × 1, 1 × 4, 1 × 1, 1 × 3, 1 × 1, 1 × 2, 1 × 1 (8 sets)
5. Your own creation: _____

Technique #23

Perceived effort

▪▪▪▫▫

Effect on hypertrophy

▪▪▪▫▫

Effect on strength and power

▪▪▪▫▫

Effect on muscular endurance

▪▪▫▫▫

Experience required

▪▫▫

☑ Accumulation method

☐ Intensification method

16-WEEK EVOLUTION

HOW DOES IT WORK?

This technique evolves over 16 weeks of training by gradually increasing the intensity while decreasing the number of reps. The sequences of repetitions and loads will be as follows:

→ **Weeks 1-3:** 12 repetitions at 70%
→ **Weeks 4-6:** 10 repetitions at 75%
→ **Weeks 7-9:** 8 repetitions at 80%
→ **Weeks 10-12:** 6 repetitions at 85%
→ **Weeks 13-15:** 4 repetitions at 90%
→ **Week 16:** 2 repetitions at 95%

ADVANTAGES

→ It improves maximum strength among beginners and intermediate athletes.
→ It can be incorporated into all types of training plans.

DISADVANTAGES

→ Performing the same exercises for 16 weeks risks becoming monotonous. Incorporate variety into your assistance exercises.

PRESCRIPTION TABLE

Load	Number of repetitions per set	Number of sets per exercise	Number of exercises per muscle group	Rest between sets
70%, 75%, 80%, 85%, 90%, 95%	12, 10, 8, 6, 4, 2	3-5	1-3	1-3 minutes

EXAMPLE SEQUENCE OF A FULL-BODY WORKOUT

Exercises	Weeks 1-3 S	1-3 R	4-6 S	4-6 R	7-9 S	7-9 R	10-12 S	10-12 R	13-15 S	13-15 R	16 S	16 R
Squat	4	12	4	10	4	8	4	6	5	4	5	2
Leg press	3	12	3	10	3	8	4	6	5	4	5	2
Bench press	4	12	4	10	4	8	4	6	5	4	5	2
Dip	3	12	3	10	3	8	4	6	5	4	5	2
Standing barbell military press	3	12	3	10	3	8	4	6	5	4	5	2
Barbell upright row	3	12	3	10	3	8	4	6	5	4	5	2
Seated row	4	12	4	10	4	8	4	6	5	4	5	2
Scott curl	3	12	3	10	3	8	4	6	5	4	5	2

S: sets; R: repetitions.

Technique #24

Perceived effort

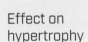

Effect on hypertrophy

Effect on strength and power

Effect on muscular endurance

Experience required

☐ Accumulation method

☑ Intensification method

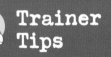

Trainer Tips

Because the workout sequences change every week and the loads change after 3 weeks, this technique requires enough experience in strength training to know your loads relatively well. In weeks 1 and 4, you may also prioritize training all three lifts in powerlifting.

STRENGTH IN MULTIPLE SPLITS

HOW DOES IT WORK?

This method is basically a 6-week workout plan that varies both the intensity and frequency of the muscle groups worked. In weeks 1-3 you will complete sets of 6-8 reps (80%); in weeks 4-6 you will perform sets of 2-3 reps (90%-95%). The distribution of your sessions will be as follows:

→ **Weeks 1 and 4.** You will complete a full-body split training plan (technique #57) with 3 workouts per week. You will choose 1 exercise per muscle group.

→ **Weeks 2 and 5.** You will complete a push–pull split training plan (technique #60) with 4 workouts per week. You will choose 2 exercises per muscle group.

→ **Weeks 3 and 6.** You will complete a squat–bench–deadlift split training plan (technique #48) with 3 workouts per week. You will choose 3 exercises per muscle group.

PRESCRIPTION TABLE

Load	Number of repetitions per set	Number of sets per exercise	Number of exercises per muscle group	Rest between sets
80%, 90%-95%	6-8, 2-3	3-4	1-3	2-3 minutes

EXAMPLE SEQUENCE FOR WEEKS 2 AND 5, PUSH–PULL TRAINING

	Exercises	Weeks			
		1-3		4-6	
		S	R	S	R
PUSH	Squat	4	6-8	4	2-3
	Hack squat	3	6-8	3	2-3
	Leg press	3	6-8	3	2-3
	Bench press	4	6-8	4	2-3
	Chest press	3	6-8	3	2-3
	Seated barbell military press	3	6-8	3	2-3
PULL	Deadlift	4	6-8	4	2-3
	Lying leg curl	3	6-8	3	2-3
	Lat pull-down	4	6-8	4	2-3
	Seated row	3	6-8	3	2-3
	Barbell standing curl	4	6-8	4	2-3
	Crunches (with machine)	3	6-8	3	2-3

S: sets; R: repetitions.

Technique #25

Perceived effort

Effect on
hypertrophy

Effect on strength
and power

Effect on muscular
endurance

Experience required

☐ Accumulation
method

☑ Intensification
method

Trainer Tips

It is best to use fractional plates for barbell and dumbbell exercises so you can add weight in 1 kg increments. Make sure you have a partner to spot each of your sets on bench press or squat!

MAXIMUM WEIGHT 1

HOW DOES IT WORK?

This method uses a narrow pyramid approach. Complete 5 sets in the following order:

3 × 90%

1 × 95%

1 × 97%

1 × 100%

1 × 100% + 1 kg

ADVANTAGES

→ This technique allows you to slightly increase your 1RM at each session.

DISADVANTAGES

→ You risk doing only the eccentric phase of the last set (a spotter is essential).

→ Adding as little load as 1 kg will require fractional plates.

PRESCRIPTION TABLE

Load	Number of repetitions per set	Number of sets per exercise	Number of exercises per muscle group	Rest between sets
90%-100% + 1 kg	1-3	5	1	3-5 minutes

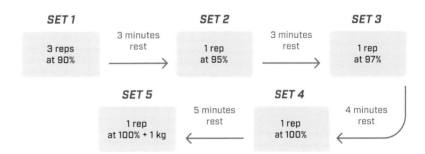

SET 1: 3 reps at 90% → 3 minutes rest → SET 2: 1 rep at 95% → 3 minutes rest → SET 3: 1 rep at 97% → 4 minutes rest → SET 4: 1 rep at 100% → 5 minutes rest → SET 5: 1 rep at 100% + 1 kg

Technique #26

Perceived effort

Effect on hypertrophy

Effect on strength and power

Effect on muscular endurance

Experience required

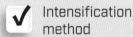

☐ Accumulation method

☑ Intensification method

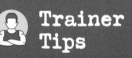

Trainer Tips

Depending on your muscle fiber type distribution (distribution of type I and type II fibers), your fourth and fifth sets may only be achievable at 90%-98% of your maximum because of the fatigue caused. This will generally occur in muscles made up mainly of fast-twitch fibers (e.g., the triceps).

MAXIMUM WEIGHT 2

HOW DOES IT WORK?

This technique involves performing 5 sets of your 1RM. With each new training session, you should try to improve your performance. For progression with small increments, you can use fractional plates. This is a technique that has been commonly used by Bulgarian weightlifters.

ADVANTAGES

→ This method is relatively simple.

DISADVANTAGES

→ This technique is recommended only for athletes and well-trained individuals due to its difficulty, stress on the tendons, and high-intensity load.
→ It requires great concentration at each repetition and can cause significant fatigue.

PRESCRIPTION TABLE

Load	Number of repetitions per set	Number of sets per exercise	Number of exercises per muscle group	Rest between sets
100%	1	5	1	3-5 minutes

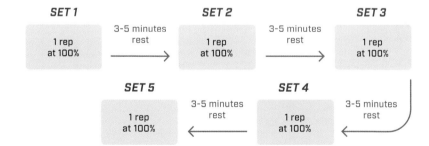

Technique #27

Perceived effort

■ ■ ■ ◻ ◻

Effect on hypertrophy

■ ■ ■ ◻ ◻

Effect on strength and power

■ ■ ◻ ◻ ◻

Effect on muscular endurance

■ ◻ ◻ ◻ ◻

Experience required

■ ◻ ◻

◻ Accumulation method

✓ Intensification method

Trainer Tips

Do not increase the load until you are able to complete your 5 sets of 5 repetitions. Once these are accomplished, the increase in load should be 2%-5%.

5 × 5

Ⓢ

HOW DOES IT WORK?

This method involves performing 5 sets of 5 repetitions beginning at 85% load. It is a derivative version of the general standards 1RM-5RM (technique #22) because it requires specific work within your 1RM-5RM.

ADVANTAGES

→ It allows you to work hard without being too close to your 1RM, therefore allowing beginners to become familiar with handling a higher intensity load without the risk of negatively affecting technique (often seen in 1RM).

DISADVANTAGES

→ It can become monotonous.
→ Advanced individuals will quickly stagnate with this technique.

PRESCRIPTION TABLE

Load	Number of repetitions per set	Number of sets per exercise	Number of exercises per muscle group	Rest between sets
85%	5	5	1-2	3 minutes

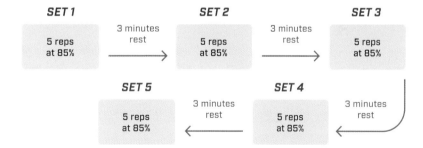

SET 1: 5 reps at 85% → 3 minutes rest → SET 2: 5 reps at 85% → 3 minutes rest → SET 3: 5 reps at 85% → 3 minutes rest → SET 4: 5 reps at 85% → 3 minutes rest → SET 5: 5 reps at 85%

Technique #28

Perceived effort

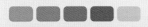

Effect on hypertrophy

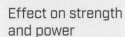

Effect on strength and power

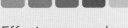

Effect on muscular endurance

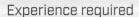

Experience required

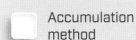

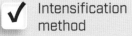

☐ Accumulation method

✓ Intensification method

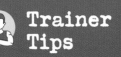

Trainer Tips

Because this technique is very demanding, be careful not to use it on one muscle group more than once a week. You can use this technique for up to 8 weeks.

5 × 5 HIGHER STRENGTH

HOW DOES IT WORK?

This technique is based on research carried out in Japan.[7] It demonstrated that individuals who performed very high reps on the last set of a maximal strength exercise had more gains in strength and muscle hypertrophy than those who only trained low reps. For this technique, therefore, you will need to perform 6 sets: the first 5 sets will be 5 reps at 85%, and the last set will be 25-30 reps at 45%-50%.

ADVANTAGES

→ It improves strength (+5%), endurance, and muscle hypertrophy.

→ It is easy to use with any exercise.

→ It helps to reach higher levels of growth hormone release, which provides additional gains in strength and hypertrophy.

DISADVANTAGES

→ It can be too demanding if performed more than once per week on a muscle group.

PRESCRIPTION TABLE

Load	Number of repetitions per set	Number of sets per exercise	Number of exercises per muscle group	Rest between sets
85%, 45%-50%	5, 25-30	6	2-3	1-3 minutes

EXAMPLE BENCH PRESS SEQUENCE

Exercises	Sets	Reps	Rest
Dumbbell bench press	5	5	3 min
	1	25-30	1 min
Barbell decline bench press	5	5	3 min
	1	25-30	1 min
Seated dumbbell shoulder press	5	5	2 min
	1	25-30	1 min
Dip	5	5	2 min
	1	25-30	1 min
Triceps push-down	5	5	2 min
	1	25-30	1 min

Technique #29

Perceived effort

■ ■ ■ □ □

Effect on hypertrophy

■ ■ ■ □ □

Effect on strength and power

■ ■ ■ □ □

Effect on muscular endurance

■ ■ ■ □ □

Experience required

■ ■ □

□ Accumulation method

☑ Intensification method

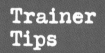

Trainer Tips

Vary the intensity of stages. For example, you could perform the following stages:
- 4RM-2RM (3 sets of 4 at 88% and 3 sets of 2 at 94%)
- 3RM-1RM (3 sets of 3 at 90% and 3 sets of 1 at 100%)
- 5RM-1RM (3 sets of 5 at 85% and 3 sets of 1 at 100%)
- 4RM-1RM (3 sets of 4 at 88% and 3 sets of 1 at 100%)
- 5RM-2RM (3 sets of 5 at 85% and 3 sets of 2 at 94%)

STAGE 5RM-3RM

HOW DOES IT WORK?

This technique consists of performing 3 consecutive sets at 5RM and 3 consecutive sets at 3RM.

ADVANTAGES

→ This method allows you to gradually incorporate higher intensity work so that you can learn to handle heavier loads. The number of repetitions can be varied (see the Trainer Tips).

DISADVANTAGES

→ It can become monotonous.
→ Advanced individuals will quickly stagnate with this technique.

PRESCRIPTION TABLE

Load	Number of repetitions per set	Number of sets per exercise	Number of exercises per muscle group	Rest between sets
85%, 90%	5, 3	6	1-2	3-4 minutes

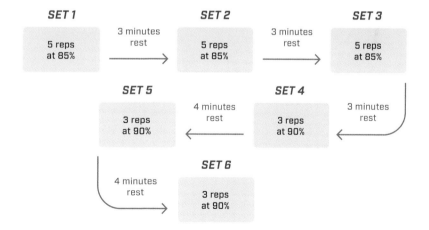

Technique #30

Perceived effort

■ ■ ■ ■ ■

Effect on
hypertrophy

■ ■ ■ ■ ■

Effect on strength
and power

■ ■ ■ ■ ■

Effect on muscular
endurance

■ ■ ■ ■ ■

Experience required

■ ■ ■

☐ Accumulation
method

☑ Intensification
method

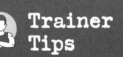
Trainer Tips

To take advantage of the elastic energy generated by the muscle, use solid structures such as blocks to control the rebound during a bench press. You can create your own blocks with 5 cm × 15 cm wood planks.

Ⓢ

PARTIAL REPS WITH MAX EFFORT

HOW DOES IT WORK?

This method consists of executing only part of the range of a movement in the region where you are strongest. This will allow you to use more weight in order to overload the movement. Research has shown significant gains in strength with this technique despite the lack of a full range of motion.[14,15]

ADVANTAGES

→ This method allows you to gradually incorporate higher intensity work so that you can learn to handle heavier loads without actually using it in a full range of motion.

DISADVANTAGES

→ Because it does not use a full range of motion, this should be combined with movements in a full range of motion to avoid creating understimulated portions of the movement.
→ This method should only be used once you have become proficient at the technique for a movement and a base level of strength has been attained through other methods in this book. It should not be used to simply lift heavier loads.

PRESCRIPTION TABLE

Load	Number of repetitions per set	Number of sets per exercise	Number of exercises per muscle group	Rest between sets
85%-110%	1-5	3-8	1-2	3-5 minutes

Technique #31

Perceived effort

▢▢▢▢▢

Effect on hypertrophy

▢▢▢▢▢

Effect on strength and power

▢▢▢▢▢

Effect on muscular endurance

▢▢▢▢▢

Experience required

▢▢▢

☐ Accumulation method

☑ Intensification method

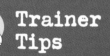

Trainer Tips

Each week, try increasing your initial loads for each muscle group by 1%. For example:
- Week 1: 95%, 90%, 85%, 80%, 75%
- Week 2: 96%, 91%, 86%, 81%, 76%
- Week 3: 97%, 92%, 87%, 82%, 77%

INTERSET DECREASING LOADS

HOW DOES IT WORK?

This method consists of a sequence in which you decrease the load while increasing the number of repetitions with each set. Be sure to warm up well before starting with your 1RM to avoid injury. Do at least 2-5 warm-up sets with gradually increasing loads.

ADVANTAGES

→ This technique allows you to recruit fast-twitch fibers using heavy loads.
→ It allows you to start training while fresh and rested for your heaviest sets, which will maximize the weight of the lifted loads.

DISADVANTAGES

→ This method can be very time consuming because of the extended warm-up period.

PRESCRIPTION TABLE

Load	Number of repetitions per set	Number of sets per exercise	Number of exercises per muscle group	Rest between sets
70%-100%	1-12	2-6	1-3	3-4 minutes

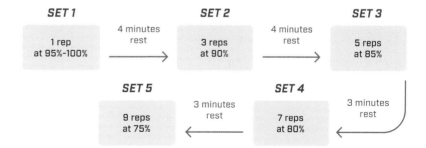

SET 1 — 1 rep at 95%-100% → 4 minutes rest → SET 2 — 3 reps at 90% → 4 minutes rest → SET 3 — 5 reps at 85% → 3 minutes rest → SET 4 — 7 reps at 80% → 3 minutes rest → SET 5 — 9 reps at 75%

Technique #32

Perceived effort

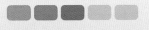

Effect on hypertrophy

Effect on strength and power

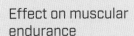

Effect on muscular endurance

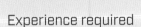

Experience required

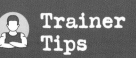

☐ Accumulation method

☑ Intensification method

GROUPING DROPSET

HOW DOES IT WORK?

Choose a load that allows you to perform a maximum of 4 reps (your 4RM), then rest for 10-15 seconds. Reduce the load by 10%-15% and try to complete as many reps as possible. Take another 10- to 15-second pause, remove 10%-15% of the load again, then complete as many reps as possible a second time.

ADVANTAGES

→ This technique is a prerequisite to grouping (technique #33). Start with this method and move on when you are comfortable.
→ It is very effective at fatiguing both fast- and slow-twitch muscle fibers.

DISADVANTAGES

→ You will need a spotter because you will work to muscle failure three times in a set.
→ It requires a change of loads.

PRESCRIPTION TABLE

Load	Number of repetitions per set	Number of sets per exercise	Number of exercises per muscle group	Rest between sets
58%-88%	4 + max + max	2-4	1-2	3-4 minutes

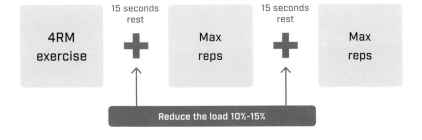

Technique #33

Perceived effort

■ ■ ■ □ □

Effect on
hypertrophy

■ ■ ■ □ □

Effect on strength
and power

■ ■ ■ ■ □

Effect on muscular
endurance

■ ■ □ □ □

Experience required

■ ■ □

☐ Accumulation
method

☑ Intensification
method

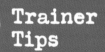

Trainer Tips

The first week, use a 5RM to do the sequence of 4 reps + 1-2 reps + 1-2 reps. This represents a more gradual approach. If you do more than 2 repetitions when grouping, this means you haven't used a load close enough to your 4RM; increase the loads in the next series.

GROUPING

HOW DOES IT WORK?

Choose a load that allows you to perform a maximum of 4 repetitions (your 4RM), then rest for 10-15 seconds. Then try to complete 1-2 reps. Rest another 10-15 seconds, then try to complete 1-2 reps a second time.

ADVANTAGES

→ This technique is based on the same principle as extended 7's (technique #100), but with an emphasis on strength work. It actually allows you to get a better volume of work at high intensity in your session.

DISADVANTAGES

→ You will need a spotter because you will work to muscle failure three times in a set.

PRESCRIPTION TABLE

Load	Number of repetitions per set	Number of sets per exercise	Number of exercises per muscle group	Rest between sets
88%	4 + 1-2 + 1-2	2-4	1-2	3-4 minutes

4RM exercise	+	15 seconds rest 1-2 reps	+	15 seconds rest 1-2 reps

Technique #34

Perceived effort

Effect on hypertrophy

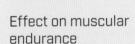

Effect on strength and power

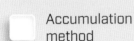

Effect on muscular endurance

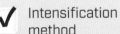

Experience required

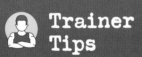

☐ Accumulation method

☑ Intensification method

Trainer Tips

When you successfully complete all 8 sets of 2 repetitions required at 85%, decrease the rest time by 5-10 seconds at the next session (e.g., 50 seconds between sets) or increase the load slightly.

1-MINUTE INTERVALS AT 85%

Ⓢ

HOW DOES IT WORK?
Do 2 repetitions at 85% of your 1RM with 1 minute of recovery between sets for a total of 8 consecutive sets.

85% is roughly equivalent to your 5RM. If, for example, you do 3 sets of 5RM (9 reps) spaced 3.5 minutes apart, it will take you about 8 minutes to finish. This technique allows you to take the same time to get to 16 reps—essentially equal work. However, this technique becomes more beneficial when you decrease the rest time. For example, if you take 45 seconds of rest between your sets, you'll accomplish your 16 reps in just over 6 minutes. This means an increase in the density of your workout and then more strength gains!

ADVANTAGES
→ It is easy to use with any exercise.
→ There is no need to change the load.

DISADVANTAGES
→ A spotter is required for the last sets during a bench press or squat.

PRESCRIPTION TABLE

Load	Number of repetitions per set	Number of sets per exercise	Number of exercises per muscle group	Rest between sets
85%	2	8	1	1 minute

Technique #35

Perceived effort

■ ■ ■ ▢ ▢

Effect on
hypertrophy

■ ■ ■ ▢ ▢

Effect on strength
and power

■ ■ ■ ▢ ▢

Effect on muscular
endurance

■ ■ ▢ ▢ ▢

Experience required

■ ■ ▢

▢ Accumulation
method

☑ Intensification
method

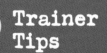

Trainer Tips

When you successfully complete all 10 sets of 1 repetition required at 90%, decrease the rest time by 5-10 seconds at the next session (e.g., 50 seconds between sets) or increase the load slightly.

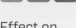

1-MINUTE INTERVALS AT 90%

Ⓢ

HOW DOES IT WORK?

Do 1 repetition at 90% of your 1RM with 1 minute of recovery between sets for a total of 10 consecutive sets.

90% is roughly equivalent to your 3RM. If, for example, you do 3 sets of 3RM (9 reps) spaced 4 minutes apart, it will take you about 9 minutes to finish. This technique allows you to take the same time to get to 10 reps—essentially equal work. However, this technique becomes more beneficial when you decrease the rest time. For example, if you take 30 seconds of rest between your sets, you'll accomplish your 10 reps in just 6 minutes. This means an increase in the density of your workout and more strength gains!

ADVANTAGES

→ It is easy to use with any exercise.
→ There is no need to change the load.

DISADVANTAGES

→ A spotter is required for the last sets during a bench press or squat.

PRESCRIPTION TABLE

Load	Number of repetitions per set	Number of sets per exercise	Number of exercises per muscle group	Rest between sets
90%	1	10	1	1 minute

Technique #36

Perceived effort

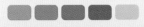

Effect on hypertrophy

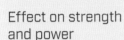

Effect on strength and power

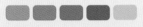

Effect on muscular endurance

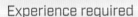

Experience required

☐ Accumulation method

☑ Intensification method

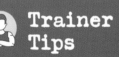

Trainer Tips

This technique is useful not only for the gains in strength it provides but also for the gains in hypertrophy caused by cumulative time under tension. It can therefore be used in a hypertrophy program.

SUPER-PLETNEV

HOW DOES IT WORK?

This technique consists of performing 4 consecutive exercises with different intensification methods and no rest between exercises. **The first** will be 4 eccentric repetitions performed at 100%-110% of your maximum load while a partner assists during the concentric phase. **The second** will consist of 6 explosive repetitions at 30% of your 1RM. **The third** will be an isometric repetition that will last 20-40 seconds, and **the fourth** will be a strength exercise performed at 3RM-5RM. Ideally, use basic exercises like push-ups, squats, deadlifts, and bent-over rows for all 4 consecutive exercises, but for the eccentric repetitions (first exercise), use an exercise that allows you to do the concentric phase with two arms or legs and the eccentric phase with one arm or leg.

ADVANTAGES

→ This technique helps to fatigue a wide range of muscle fibers because it uses all modes of contraction. It therefore has a great impact on strength gains and hypertrophy.

DISADVANTAGES

→ It is very demanding and should only be performed by advanced individuals.
→ A partner is required to perform the concentric phase of the first exercise.

PRESCRIPTION TABLE

Load	Number of repetitions or seconds per set	Number of sets per exercise	Number of exercises per muscle group	Rest between sets
30%-110%	4 reps + 6 reps + 20-40 seconds + 3-5 reps	2-4	1-2	3-5 minutes

ECCENTRIC EXERCISE

Eccentric leg press:
4 reps

or

Fly to press:
5 reps

→

EXPLOSIVE EXERCISE

Jump squat:
6 reps

or

Clap push-up:
6 reps

↓

STRENGTH EXERCISE

Lunge:
3 reps per leg

or

Dumbbell chest press:
5 reps

←

ISOMETRIC EXERCISE

Isometric barbell front
squat at 90 degrees:
20 seconds

or

Isometric push-up:
30 seconds

Technique #37

Perceived effort

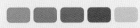

Effect on
hypertrophy

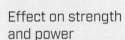

Effect on strength
and power

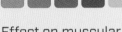

Effect on muscular
endurance

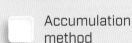

Experience required

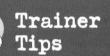

☐ Accumulation
method

☑ Intensification
method

Trainer Tips

Vary the working angles to which manual isometric tension will be applied. You can, for example, vary the isometric position with each repetition:

- Repetitions 1 and 4: 1/4 movement
- Repetitions 2 and 5: 1/2 movement
- Repetitions 3 and 6: 3/4 movement

HEAVY LIFTING AND MANUAL ISOMETRICS

HOW DOES IT WORK?

A partner applies a manual overload during the concentric phase of the movement, preventing you from continuing the movement. This pressure is applied for only 2-3 seconds before it is removed and you can complete your repetition. This may be done to only some of the repetitions or all repetitions of a set.

For this technique, your partner should control her strength so that the bar stays in an isometric position for 2-3 seconds. Pushing too hard would lower the bar, involving a supramaximal eccentric phase, which is not the goal and which would increase the risk of injury. In addition, the direction of the pressure emitted should mirror the exercise. For example, in a pull-up your partner will need to exert a downward body pull, whereas in a lat pull-down she will need to exert upward pressure on the bar.

ADVANTAGES

→ This technique has the advantages of overcoming isometric training and improves its weak points. For example, if the most difficult phase of the bench press for you is the elbow lockout, you might ask your partner to apply pressure to the bar when 3/4 of the movement has been completed.

DISADVANTAGES

→ It requires a partner to complete.
→ It is difficult to perform on certain exercises in which you are stronger than your partner (e.g., squat, deadlift).
→ It is impossible to execute on explosive movements (e.g., snatch, clean).

PRESCRIPTION TABLE

Load	Number of repetitions per set	Number of sets per exercise	Number of exercises per muscle group	Rest between sets
70%-83%	2-6 (1-6 overloads)	2-5	1-2	2-3 minutes

Technique #38

Perceived effort

Effect on hypertrophy

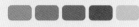

Effect on strength and power

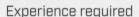

Effect on muscular endurance

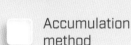

Experience required

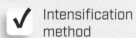

☐ Accumulation method

☑ Intensification method

Trainer Tips

Wait until you are experienced in strength training before using this method; otherwise you will be excessively fatigued by the beginning of the training session and be unable to take full advantage of the post-tetanic effect following the activation phase.

KULESZA METHOD

HOW DOES IT WORK?

Start with 2 progressive warm-up sets of 3 repetitions at 70% and 80%, 1 minute apart. Then continue with 3 progressive sets toward your 1RM, consisting of 3 reps at 90%, 2 reps at 95%, and 1 rep at 100%, spaced with a rest of 3-5 minutes between sets. Finally, perform 3-5 sets of 2-3 repetitions at 85%-90%, spaced with a rest of 3-5 minutes between sets.

ADVANTAGES

→ This variant uses a specific muscular response called post-tetanic facilitation. Researchers have shown that there was an increase in contractile force and speed after a period of rest following maximum exertion.[6,8] This could allow the loads to be increased by 1%-2% on subsequent series.

DISADVANTAGES

→ It requires a long phase of preparation before the training session. However, the activation phase still results in strength gains.

PRESCRIPTION TABLE

Load	Number of repetitions per set	Number of sets per exercise	Number of exercises per muscle group	Rest between sets
70%-100%	1-3	8-10	1	3-5 minutes

WARM-UP PHASE

3 reps at 70% + 3 reps at 80% + 1 minute rest between sets

ACTIVATION PHASE

3 reps at 90% + 2 reps at 95% + 1 rep at 100% + 3-5 minutes rest between sets

TRAINING SESSION

3-5 sets of 2-3 reps at 85%-90% + 3-5 minutes rest between sets

Technique #39

Perceived effort

Effect on hypertrophy

Effect on strength and power

Effect on muscular endurance

Experience required

☐ Accumulation method

✓ Intensification method

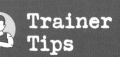

Trainer Tips

Wait until you are experienced in strength training before using this method; otherwise you will be excessively fatigued by the beginning of the training session and be unable to take full advantage of the post-tetanic effect following the activation phase.

BULGARIAN METHOD

HOW DOES IT WORK?

This technique uses the same principle as overload in big waves (technique #111), but at very high intensity. Perform progressive warm-up sets (e.g., 2 reps each at 60% and 70% and 1 rep each at 80% and 90%), then start your first set with a single rep at 100%. After 3-5 minutes rest, do 2-3 repetitions at 85%-89%, then 1 repetition at 90%, then repeat 1 repetition at 100%. Each set should be followed by 3-5 minutes of rest. Alternate this sequence, trying to slightly increase the load used to perform 2-3 repetitions. Ideally, do no more than 2-3 waves. It might look like this: 100% + 85% + 90% + 100% + 86% + 91% + 100%.

ADVANTAGES

→ This variant uses a specific muscular response called post-tetanic facilitation. Researchers have demonstrated an increase in contractile force and speed after a period of rest following maximum exertion.[6,8]

→ This could allow the loads to be increased by 1%-2% on subsequent series.

DISADVANTAGES

→ As in all maximum strength techniques, it requires a spotter on the squat and bench press.

PRESCRIPTION TABLE

Load	Number of repetitions per set	Number of sets per exercise	Number of exercises per muscle group	Rest between sets
85%-100%	1-3	6-9	1	3-5 minutes

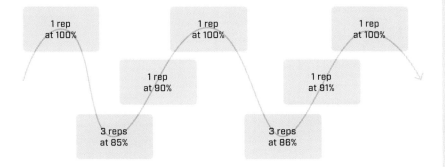

Technique #40

Perceived effort

■ ■ ■ □ □

Effect on hypertrophy

■ ■ ■ □ □

Effect on strength and power

■ ■ ■ □ □

Effect on muscular endurance

■ ■ □ □ □

Experience required

■ ■ □

☐ Accumulation method

✓ Intensification method

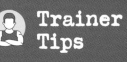

Trainer Tips

This is one of the wave overloading techniques that I enjoy the most. It is simple and efficient. You can also vary the repetitions (e.g., 7RM-2RM waves or 8RM-3RM waves) as long as you stay under 3RM during your even series in order to maintain the post-tetanic effect.

OVERLOAD IN SMALL WAVES

HOW DOES IT WORK?

This method consists of repeating 2-3 waves made up of 2 sets performed at 6RM (83%) and 1RM (100%). Try to increase the load of your sets of 6RM by at least 1% with each new wave. To do this, you can use fractional plates.

ADVANTAGES

→ This technique uses post-tetanic facilitation by increasing the intensity of work at 6RM as the waves progress.

→ It allows you to reassess your 1RM.

→ It is easy to apply and can be used in the first year of training because it includes fewer sets than overload in big waves (technique #111).

DISADVANTAGES

→ As in all maximum strength techniques, it requires a spotter on the squat and bench press.

PRESCRIPTION TABLE

Load	Number of repetitions per set	Number of sets per exercise	Number of exercises per muscle group	Rest between sets
83%-100%	1-6	4-6	1	3-5 minutes

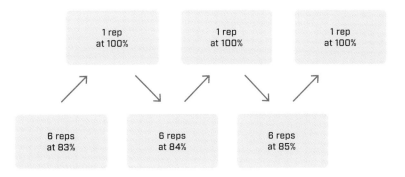

Technique #41

Perceived effort
▪▪▪▫▫

Effect on hypertrophy
▪▪▪▪▫

Effect on strength and power
▪▪▪▪▪

Effect on muscular endurance
▪▪▫▫▫

Experience required
▪▪▫

✓ Accumulation method

✓ Intensification method

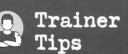

Trainer Tips

This technique causes constant adaptation of the muscles by varying the loads week after week. The first few weeks you may not be able to complete your 25 (5 × 5) and 100 (10 × 10) reps at the prescribed loads, which is normal. Continue the method for 8 weeks or until you can get all your reps.

5 × 10

HOW DOES IT WORK?

This method is actually a 6-8 week training plan that involves alternating a 5 × 5 (technique #27) and a 10 × 10, or German volume phase 1 (technique #132), on the same exercise. This is a technique that works very well with a 3-day split such as the squat–bench–deadlift split (technique #48).

→ **Weeks 1, 3, 5, and 7:** Choose two exercises for the same muscle group and complete 5 sets of 5 reps (5 × 5) at 85% followed by additional exercises. You will take 2-3 minutes of recovery between sets.

→ **Weeks 2, 4, 6, and 8:** Choose one of the exercises you used for 5 × 5 and complete 10 sets of 10 reps (10 × 10) at 65%-70%. You will take 2 minutes of recovery between sets and add 1 or 2 assistance exercises.

ADVANTAGES

→ It allows excellent gains in strength and muscle hypertrophy.

DISADVANTAGES

→ Due to the high volume, this method should not be used by novices.

PRESCRIPTION TABLE

Load	Number of repetitions per set	Number of sets per exercise	Number of exercises per muscle group	Rest between sets
85%, 65%-70%	5, 10	5, 10	2, 1	2-3 minutes

EXAMPLE DEADLIFT SEQUENCE

Exercises	Weeks 1, 3, 5, and 7			Weeks 2, 4, 6, and 8		
	Sets	Reps	Rest	Sets	Reps	Rest
Deadlift	5	5	3 min	10	10	2 min
Romanian deadlift	5	5	3 min	3	8-10	2 min
Lying leg curl	3	4-6	3 min	3	8-10	2 min
Lat pull-down	3	4-6	3 min	3	8-10	2 min
Barbell standing curl	3	4-6	2 min	3	8-10	2 min
Crunches with machine	3	4-6	2 min	3	8-10	2 min

Technique #42

Perceived effort

■ ■ ■ ☐ ☐

Effect on hypertrophy

■ ■ ■ ☐ ☐

Effect on strength and power

■ ■ ■ ■ ☐

Effect on muscular endurance

■ ■ ☐ ☐ ☐

Experience required

■ ■ ☐

☐ Accumulation method

✓ Intensification method

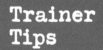

Trainer Tips

Before trying this technique, start with variable resistance training (technique #159), which is in fact the same technique as this one, but with less intensity.

MAX EFFORT WITH VARIABLE RESISTANCE

HOW DOES IT WORK?

This technique is the same as the general standards 1RM-5RM (technique #22), but with the addition of chains or superbands.

ADVANTAGES

→ This method allows you to take advantage of the mechanical ability of the muscle. When muscles are in a lengthened position, there is greater passive tension (tendons) and less active tension (muscles). You are therefore weaker in these positions. Conversely, the more the muscle is shortened, the more the active tension increases and the stronger you are (to a certain degree). The overload created by chains or superbands therefore increases the total tension placed on the muscles and increases the strength gains.

DISADVANTAGES

→ This technique is not possible in all training facilities due to the required equipment and ground anchors (for deadlift with superbands, for example).

PRESCRIPTION TABLE

Load	Number of repetitions per set	Number of sets per exercise	Number of exercises per muscle group	Rest between sets
85%-100%	1-5	5-8	1-2	3-5 minutes

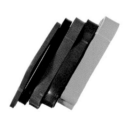

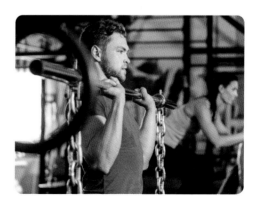

Technique #43

Perceived effort

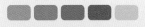

Effect on hypertrophy

Effect on strength and power

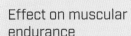

Effect on muscular endurance

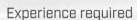

Experience required

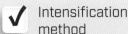

✓ Accumulation method

✓ Intensification method

Trainer Tips

This technique was used by Bob Hoffman, founder of the York Barbell Company and creator of *Muscular Development* magazine, for his weightlifting athletes in the 1960s. In addition, Mike Mentzer, a professional bodybuilder, extolled the virtues of isometric training for gains in strength and muscle hypertrophy.

ISOMETRIC STRENGTH

HOW DOES IT WORK?

This technique consists of performing 2 sets where you will hold a load of 90% at 4-8 cm before the end of the movement for 10-20 seconds, spaced with 2 minutes of rest. Once these 2 sets have been completed, you will then complete, on the same exercise, 3 sets of 6 repetitions at 80% load. The Smith machine is very useful for this type of training technique.

ADVANTAGES

→ It increases muscle density and improves maximum strength in the last phase of a movement.

DISADVANTAGES

→ It requires a workout partner on certain exercises to count the time under tension.

PRESCRIPTION TABLE

Load	Number of seconds or repetitions per set	Number of sets per exercise	Number of exercises per muscle group	Rest between sets
80%-90%	10-20 seconds + 6 reps	5	1-3	2 minutes

EXAMPLE OF AN ISOMETRIC STRENGTH TRAINING SESSION FOR BENCH PRESS

Exercises	Sets	Time under tension/Reps	Rest
Bench press with Smith machine	2	10-20 s	2 min
	3	6 reps	2 min
Dumbbell incline bench press	2	10-20 s	2 min
	3	6 reps	2 min
Seated military press with Smith machine	2	10-20 s	2 min
	3	6 reps	2 min
Barbell closed-grip bench press	2	10-20 s	2 min
	3	6 reps	2 min
Triceps push-down	2	10-20 s	2 min
	3	6 reps	2 min

Technique #44

Perceived effort

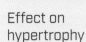

Effect on hypertrophy

Effect on strength and power

Effect on muscular endurance

Experience required

 Accumulation method

✓ Intensification method

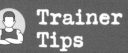 **Trainer Tips**

This technique is preferably used on basic exercises, such as the bench press, squat, and deadlift. You will need to use a power rack in order to properly adjust the height of the safety bars to guide your range of motion.

THE INCH PROGRAM

HOW DOES IT WORK?

This method involves performing partial repetitions with a 110% load, gradually increasing the distance to be covered each week by 4-5 cm. This method should be combined with full repetitions to ensure you are working through the full range of motion. Typically you will start with 2 sets of partial reps (110%) followed by 3 sets of full reps (75%-90%).

ADVANTAGES

→ This technique allows you to gradually increase your strength by adding more range of motion to your reps each week. On average, you will be able to increase your strength on a movement 10% over the course of 8 weeks.

DISADVANTAGES

→ It should be supplemented by full-amplitude exercises.
→ A spotter is necessary when handling loads above your 1RM.
→ It requires a power rack with moveable safety bars.

PRESCRIPTION TABLE

Load on partial repetition	Number of repetitions per set	Number of sets per exercise	Number of exercises per muscle group	Rest between sets
110%	1-3	2	1	2-3 minutes

EXAMPLE OF PROGRESSION OVER THE COURSE OF 8 WEEKS

Week	Placement of safety bars (power rack)
1	8 cm from the start of the movement
2	12 cm from the start of the movement
3	16 cm from the start of the movement
4	20 cm from the start of the movement
5	24 cm from the start of the movement
6	28 cm from the start of the movement
7	32 cm from the start of the movement
8	Complete repetition

Technique #45

Perceived effort

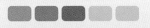

Effect on hypertrophy

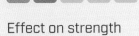

Effect on strength and power

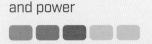

Effect on muscular endurance

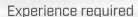

Experience required

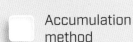

☐ Accumulation method

✓ Intensification method

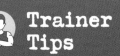

WENDLER METHOD

HOW DOES IT WORK?

This technique is based on the book by Jim Wendler,[34] a powerlifter who once did a 450 kg squat in competition. The plan is designed for 4 days a week (each day targets either standing press, deadlift, squat, or bench press) for 4 weeks:

→ **Week 1:** 3 sets of 5 repetitions at 75%, 80%, and 85%

→ **Week 2:** 3 sets of 3 repetitions at 80%, 85%, and 90%

→ **Week 3:** 1 set of 5 repetitions, 1 set of 3 repetitions, and 1 set of 1 repetition at 75%, 85%, and 95%, respectively

→ **Week 4:** 3 sets of 5 repetitions at 40%, 50%, and 60%

ADVANTAGES

→ It helps improve muscle strength on powerlifting lifts.

DISADVANTAGES

→ It allows a very low volume at maximal strength. According to the Prilepin chart (appendix #7), with a weight between 80%-90% of 1RM, the goal is 10-20 repetitions, with 15 being optimal. This technique achieves only a maximum of 9 repetitions (5 + 3 + 1).

→ Only 1 set per exercise will go to failure.

PRESCRIPTION TABLE

Load	Number of repetitions per set	Number of sets per exercise	Number of exercises per muscle group	Rest between sets
40%-95%	5, 3, 5 + 3 + 1, 5	1-3	1	2-3 minutes

EXAMPLE OF 4 WEEKS OF THE WENDLER METHOD

Training week	Day 1	Day 2	Day 3	Day 4
	Warm-up			
	Standing press	Deadlift	Squat	Bench press
Week 1	5 × 75%, 5 × 80%, maximum reps at 85% (5 or more)			
Week 2	3 × 80%, 3 × 85%, maximum reps at 90% (3 or more)			
Week 3	5 × 75%, 3 × 85%, maximum reps at 95% (1 or more)			
Week 4	5 × 40%, 5 × 50%, 5 × 60% (deload week)			
	Continue with assistance exercises			

Technique #46

Perceived effort

■ ■ ■ □ □

Effect on hypertrophy

■ ■ ■ □ □

Effect on strength and power

■ ■ ■ ■ □

Effect on muscular endurance

■ ■ □ □ □

Experience required

■ ■ □

☐ Accumulation method

☑ Intensification method

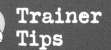

Trainer Tips

After 10 weeks of maximum strength, switch to lower intensity, higher volume training. This will spare your tendons and your nervous system, which will have been strongly stimulated during the application of this technique.

5-3-2 SPLIT

HOW DOES IT WORK?

This method involves performing 10 weeks of maximum strength training. The weeks will be divided into a 5-3-2 split:

1. The first 5 weeks, you will complete 5 sets of 5 repetitions.
2. The next 3 weeks, you will complete 3 sets of 3 repetitions.
3. The next 2 weeks, you will complete 2 sets of 2 repetitions.

ADVANTAGES

→ It allows you to work progressively toward your 1RM and to develop your maximum strength.
→ It is ideal for training the main lifts, such as the squat, deadlift, and bench press.

DISADVANTAGES

→ A spotter is required to monitor lifts where you may get stuck (e.g., bench press, squat).
→ It is advisable to have at least a year of training experience before undertaking this technique.

PRESCRIPTION TABLE

Load	Number of repetitions per set	Number of sets per exercise	Number of exercises per muscle group	Rest between sets
85%, 90%, 95%	5, 3, 2	5, 3, 2	2-3	3-5 minutes

EXAMPLE TRAINING PLAN FOR PUSH DAYS

Exercises	Weeks 1-5		Weeks 6-8		Weeks 9-10	
	Sets	Reps	Sets	Reps	Sets	Reps
Squat	5	5	3	3	2	2
Leg press	5	5	3	3	2	2
Leg extension	5	5	3	3	2	2
Bench press	5	5	3	3	2	2
Dumbbell bench press	5	5	3	3	2	2
Dip	5	5	3	3	2	2
Seated barbell shoulder press	5	5	3	3	2	2

Technique #47

Perceived effort

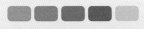

Effect on
hypertrophy

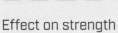

Effect on strength
and power

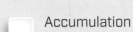

Effect on muscular
endurance

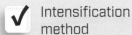

Experience required

☐ Accumulation
method

☑ Intensification
method

Trainer Tips

On dynamic effort days, Louie Simmons suggests doing sets of 3 reps for the bench press, 2 reps for the squat, and 1 rep for the deadlift. The box squat is another essential exercise that you must integrate. For more information, see one of his books.

WESTSIDE METHOD

HOW DOES IT WORK?

This method was popularized by Louie Simmons[30] in the late 1980s and early 1990s. It consists of performing strength and power work on powerlifting lifts (squat, bench press, and deadlift) spread over 2 days (maximal effort [90%-100%] and dynamic effort [40%-60%]) spaced 72 hours apart. For example, your weekly schedule might look like this:

→ **Monday:** Maximal effort on squat or deadlift
→ **Wednesday:** Maximal effort on bench press
→ **Friday:** Dynamic effort on squat or deadlift
→ **Sunday:** Dynamic effort on bench press

A Westside session consists of an average of 4 exercises: the main lift; an assistance exercise to the main lift (e.g., triceps for the bench press in 4-5 sets of 5 repetitions); and 2 assistance exercises (e.g., latissimus, shoulders, abdominals). On maximum effort days, the use of chains or weight releasers is recommended, while on dynamic effort days, chains or superbands are recommended in order to promote acceleration at the end of the movement. Also, because the deadlift is more demanding on the nervous system than the squat or bench press, perform the optimal number of repetitions according to the Prilepin chart (appendix #7).

PRESCRIPTION TABLE

Load	Number of repetitions per set	Number of sets per exercise	Number of exercises per muscle group	Rest between sets
90%-100%, 40%-60%	1-3, 3-6	3-10, 8-12	1	2-5 minutes, 45-60 seconds

DAY 1: MAXIMAL

Squat or deadlift + assistance exercises for hamstrings and lower back

DAY 2: MAXIMAL

Bench press + assistance exercises for pectorals and triceps

DAY 3: DYNAMIC

Squat or deadlift + assistance exercises for quadriceps and abdominals

DAY 4: DYNAMIC

Bench press + assistance exercises for shoulders and triceps

Technique #48

Perceived effort

▦ ▦ ▦ ▢ ▢

Effect on hypertrophy

▦ ▦ ▦ ▢ ▢

Effect on strength and power

▦ ▦ ▦ ▢ ▢

Effect on muscular endurance

▦ ▦ ▢ ▢ ▢

Experience required

▦ ▢ ▢

☐ Accumulation method

☑ Intensification method

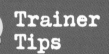

Trainer Tips

Incorporate about 4-5 exercises (2 on your main lift and 3 assistance exercises) per day on which you will complete 3 or 4 sets. For example, for day 1, you could do a squat exercise, box squat exercise, leg extension exercise, calf exercise, and sit-ups. For day 2, you could do two bench press exercises, a shoulder exercise, a triceps exercise, and an abdominal exercise.

SQUAT–BENCH–DEADLIFT SPLIT

HOW DOES IT WORK?

This method focuses primarily on powerlifting lifts: the squat, bench press, and deadlift. As a result, you will split your training over 3 days (48 hours apart) and work on one lift per day. Some people prefer this plan because it ensures they have an equal allocation of practice time for each lift. You can use this method as long as you want, with a slight variation in the repetition scheme every 4 weeks.

ADVANTAGES

→ It is ideal for beginners who want to familiarize themselves with the lifts in powerlifting.
→ It only requires 3 days of training a week.

DISADVANTAGES

→ It does not allow you to do a high volume of work on each muscle group.
→ Each lift (squat, bench press, deadlift) is only trained once a week.

PRESCRIPTION TABLE

Load	Number of repetitions per set	Number of sets per exercise	Number of main lift exercises per muscle group	Rest between sets
70%-90%	3-12	3-4	2	1-3 minutes

DAY 1	DAY 2	DAY 3
Squat training	Bench press training	Deadlift training

Technique #49

Perceived effort

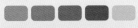

Effect on hypertrophy

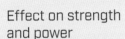

Effect on strength and power

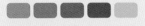

Effect on muscular endurance

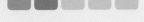

Experience required

☐ Accumulation method

✓ Intensification method

Trainer Tips

In order to limit exhaustion, do a cluster technique for a maximum of 4 weeks, then do a more traditional training technique for the next 4 weeks before repeating another cluster technique.

Ⓢ

EXTENDED 5'S CLUSTER

HOW DOES IT WORK?

You begin with 5 repetitions at 5RM (85%), then rest 7-12 seconds. Then do only 1 repetition and rest for another 7-12 seconds. Repeat the same pattern of 1 rep and 7-12 seconds rest until you reach 10 repetitions. At the end of the set, rest for 3-5 minutes. Repeat this set 3-5 times.

ADVANTAGES

→ This technique allows you to perform more total work at high intensity, leading to gains in strength and muscle hypertrophy.

DISADVANTAGES

→ Cluster training is very demanding on the muscles and nervous system. Too much work will limit progress or even cause regression. This technique should not be used on more than one muscle group at a time to avoid central nervous system (CNS) exhaustion.

PRESCRIPTION TABLE

Load	Number of repetitions per set	Number of sets per exercise	Number of exercises per muscle group	Rest between sets
85%	10	3-5	1	3-5 minutes

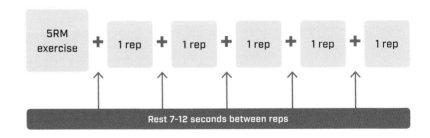

Technique #50

Perceived effort

Effect on hypertrophy

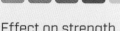

Effect on strength and power

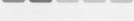

Effect on muscular endurance

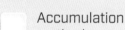

Experience required

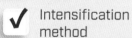

☐ Accumulation method

✓ Intensification method

Trainer Tips

In order to limit exhaustion, do a cluster technique for a maximum of 4 weeks, then do a more traditional training technique for the next 4 weeks before repeating another cluster technique.

CLASSIC CLUSTER

HOW DOES IT WORK?

Perform only 1 repetition at a time at 87%-92%, with a 7-12 second rest between each repetition, for a total of 5 reps.

ADVANTAGES

→ This technique will allow you to get a better total workout at high intensity because instead of doing 3 reps per set at 87%-92%, you will accomplish 5 reps per set at 87%-92% (i.e., 5 reps at ~3RM intensity instead of 3 reps at ~3RM intensity).

DISADVANTAGES

→ Cluster training is very demanding on the muscles and nervous system. Too much work will limit progress or even cause regression. This technique should not be used on more than one muscle group at a time to avoid central nervous system (CNS) exhaustion.

PRESCRIPTION TABLE

Load	Number of repetitions per set	Number of sets per exercise	Number of exercises per muscle group	Rest between sets
87%-92%	5	3-5	1	3-5 minutes

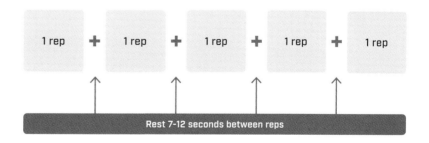

Technique #51

Perceived effort

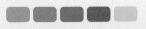

Effect on hypertrophy

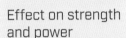

Effect on strength and power

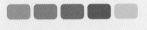

Effect on muscular endurance

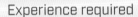

Experience required

- [ ] Accumulation method
- [✓] Intensification method

 Trainer Tips

In order to limit exhaustion, do a cluster technique for a maximum of 4 weeks, then do a more traditional training technique for the next 4 weeks before repeating another cluster technique.

ANTAGONIST CLUSTER

(S)

HOW DOES IT WORK?

This technique is similar to the classic cluster (technique #50), except that it includes 2 exercises that are performed in an alternating fashion. You will perform 5 total reps for each exercise at 87%-92%, alternating 1 rep at a time without rest between exercises until all 10 repetitions are accomplished. Antagonist means "the opposite," so you should combine chest with upper back, lats with shoulders, quadriceps with hamstrings, biceps with triceps, or glutes and lower back with abdominals.

ADVANTAGES

→ This technique will allow you to get a better total workout at high intensity because instead of doing 3 reps per set at 87%-92%, you will accomplish 5 reps per set at 87%-92% (i.e., 5 reps at ~3RM intensity instead of 3 reps at ~3RM intensity).

→ It saves time by allowing you to perform two exercises simultaneously.

DISADVANTAGES

→ This technique should not be used on more than one exercise per muscle group at a time to avoid central nervous system (CNS) exhaustion.

PRESCRIPTION TABLE

Load	Number of repetitions per set	Number of sets per exercise	Number of exercises per muscle group	Rest between sets
87%-92%	10 (5 each exercise)	3-5	1	3-5 minutes

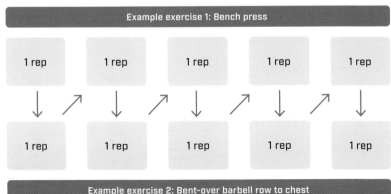

Example exercise 1: Bench press

Example exercise 2: Bent-over barbell row to chest

Technique #52

Perceived effort

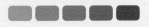

Effect on hypertrophy

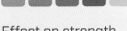

Effect on strength and power

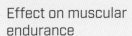

Effect on muscular endurance

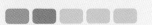

Experience required

☐ Accumulation method

☑ Intensification method

Trainer Tips

In order to limit exhaustion, do a cluster technique for a maximum of 4 weeks, then do a more traditional training technique for the next 4 weeks before repeating another cluster technique.

MENTZER CLUSTER

HOW DOES IT WORK?

You will perform 3 reps at 95%-100% of your maximum, performing 1 rep at a time with 7-12 seconds of rest between each repetition, then decrease the load by 10% in order to perform a final repetition separated by the same rest time (7-12 seconds).

ADVANTAGES

→ This technique allows you to do several repetitions at very high intensity, procuring great gains in strength.

DISADVANTAGES

→ The classic cluster (technique #50) is a prerequisite before performing this technique.

→ This technique should not be used on more than one muscle group at a time to avoid central nervous system (CNS) exhaustion.

→ A training partner may be needed to change the load between repetitions.

PRESCRIPTION TABLE

Load	Number of repetitions per set	Number of sets per exercise	Number of exercises per muscle group	Rest between sets
95%-100% + 85%-90%	4	3-5	1	3-5 minutes

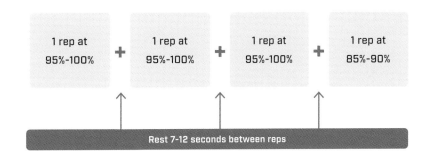

Technique #53

Perceived effort

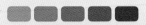

Effect on hypertrophy

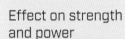

Effect on strength and power

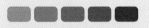

Effect on muscular endurance

Experience required

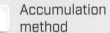

☐ Accumulation method

☑ Intensification method

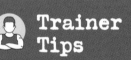

Trainer Tips

Appendix #8 includes a dropset cluster chart to help you in the progression of your loads according to your 1RM in the bench press and in the squat.

DROPSET CLUSTER

HOW DOES IT WORK?

This technique comes from the internal pyramid method (technique #114), but is performed at higher intensity. It consists of doing 4-6 repetitions with a rest time of 7-12 seconds between each repetition. The load will decrease by 5% for each repetition. For example, a dropset cluster of 4 repetitions might be done at 95%, 90%, 85%, and 80%. You can use up to 6 reps per set (add 1 rep at 75% and 1 rep at 70%).

ADVANTAGES

→ This technique allows for higher volume at higher intensity than 4 reps per set at 88%. This cluster is recommended as a prerequisite to using the Mentzer cluster (technique #52).

DISADVANTAGES

→ It requires a very precise change in loads (5%), which requires a preliminary calculation of the loads to be used (see appendix #8 for the predicted absolute maximum based on number of repetitions for the bench press and the squat).

PRESCRIPTION TABLE

Load	Number of repetitions per set	Number of sets per exercise	Number of exercises per muscle group	Rest between sets
70%-95%	2-6	2-4	1	3-5 minutes

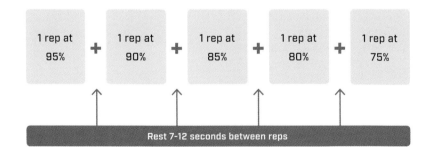

Technique #54

Perceived effort

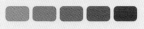

Effect on hypertrophy

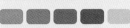

Effect on strength and power

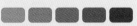

Effect on muscular endurance

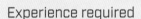

Experience required

☐ Accumulation method

✓ Intensification method

 Trainer Tips

In order to limit exhaustion, do a cluster technique for a maximum of 4 weeks, then do a more traditional training technique for the next 4 weeks before repeating another cluster technique.

ACCENTUATED ECCENTRIC CLUSTER

HOW DOES IT WORK?

This technique is the same as the classic cluster (technique #50), except for each repetition, a partner will exert additional resistance during the eccentric portion of the movement, which you must control for 5 seconds. If you can't keep up the 5-second pace, your partner is pushing too hard. As with the classic cluster, you will rest for 7-12 seconds between each repetition.

ADVANTAGES

→ This technique allows you to perform higher volume at high intensity because instead of doing 3 reps per set at 87%-92%, you will accomplish 5 reps per set at 87%-92% (i.e., 5 reps at ~3RM intensity instead of 3 reps at ~3RM intensity).

→ The eccentric overload can also provide more strength gains.

DISADVANTAGES

→ This technique should not be used on more than one muscle group at a time to avoid central nervous system (CNS) exhaustion.

→ It requires a training partner to provide the resistance.

PRESCRIPTION TABLE

Load	Number of repetitions per set	Number of sets per exercise	Number of exercises per muscle group	Rest between sets
87%-92%	5	2-4	1	3-5 minutes

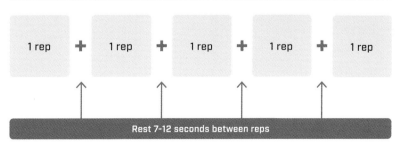

A partner must add resistance in the eccentric phase of each repetition

1 rep + 1 rep + 1 rep + 1 rep + 1 rep

Rest 7-12 seconds between reps

Technique #55

Perceived effort

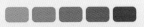

Effect on hypertrophy

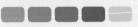

Effect on strength and power

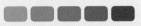

Effect on muscular endurance

Experience required

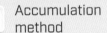

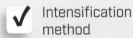 Accumulation method

✓ Intensification method

Trainer Tips

In order to limit exhaustion, do a cluster technique for a maximum of 4 weeks, then do a more traditional training technique for the next 4 weeks before repeating another cluster technique.

FUNCTIONAL ISOMETRIC CLUSTER

Ⓢ

HOW DOES IT WORK?

You will perform 6 isometric repetitions held for 5-10 seconds each with 7-12 second pauses between each repetition. Ideally, choose 3 positions in the movement and perform 2 repetitions per position (e.g., at the start, middle, and end of the movement).

ADVANTAGES

→ This technique uses isometric contractions, which increase strength by 10%-15%;[2] therefore, larger loads can be used.

DISADVANTAGES

→ Given the intensity of the contractions, you will need a partner to help you return to the starting position between repetitions.

→ You must use more than one position for each movement to be sure your strength gains are transferred through the full range of motion.

PRESCRIPTION TABLE

Load	Number of repetitions per set	Number of sets per exercise	Number of exercises per muscle group	Rest between sets
70%-100%	6	2-4	1	3-5 minutes

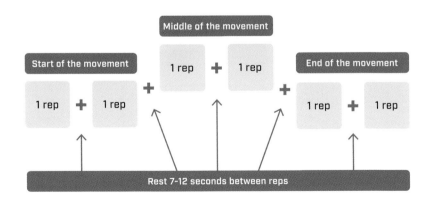

Technique #56

Perceived effort

■■■□□

Effect on hypertrophy

■■■■□

Effect on strength and power

■■□□□

Effect on muscular endurance

■□□□□

Experience required

■■□

☐ Accumulation method

☑ Intensification method

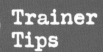

Trainer Tips

In order to limit exhaustion, do a cluster technique for a maximum of 4 weeks, then do a more traditional training technique for the next 4 weeks before repeating another cluster technique.

MAXIMUM CONTRACTION CLUSTER

HOW DOES IT WORK?

This method is a combination of the accentuated eccentric cluster (technique #54) and functional isometric cluster (technique #55). You will perform 5 reps (1 rep at a time) at 80%-90% load with a partner putting pressure on the bar during the eccentric phase for 5 seconds. Then push or pull the barbell halfway through the concentric portion and hold for 5-10 seconds, during which your partner will again exert additional pressure. Finally, complete the last concentric portion by yourself or with help. A 7-12 second rest is required between each repetition.

ADVANTAGES

→ This technique allows high-quality work at high intensity, because the imposed load varies within a repetition according to the force exerted.

DISADVANTAGES

→ This technique requires a partner in order to exert the additional eccentric and isometric pressures.

PRESCRIPTION TABLE

Load	Number of repetitions per set	Number of sets per exercise	Number of exercises per muscle group	Rest between sets
80%-90%	5	2-4	1	3-5 minutes

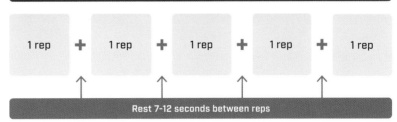

Eccentric phase: Pressure from a partner (5 seconds)
Concentric phase: Pause halfway through and isometric hold 5-10 seconds with pressure from a partner, then complete alone or with help

1 rep + 1 rep + 1 rep + 1 rep + 1 rep

Rest 7-12 seconds between reps

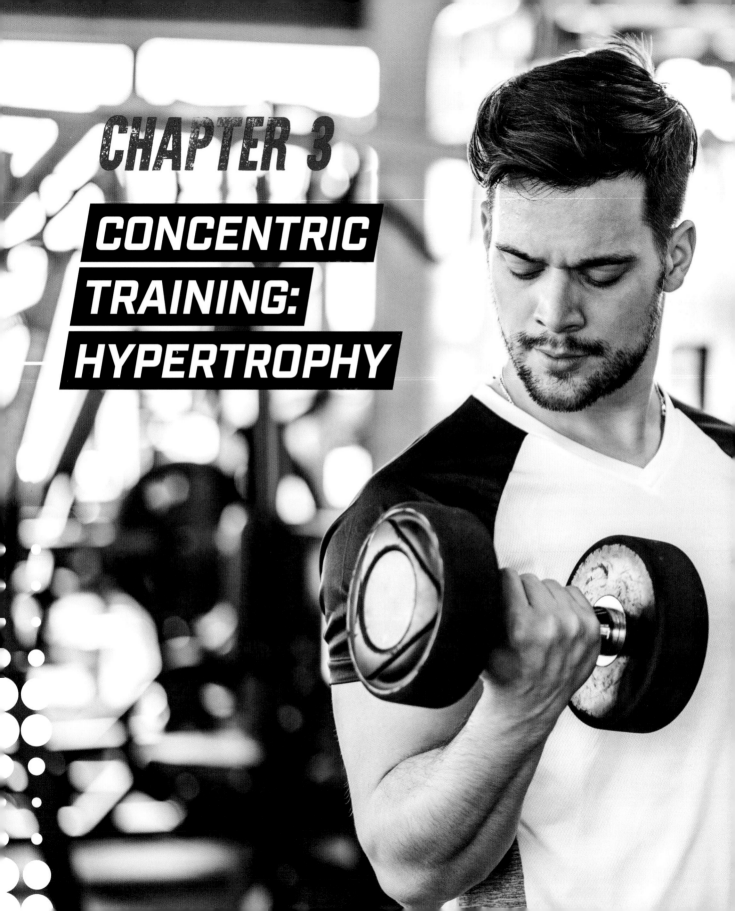

CHAPTER 3

CONCENTRIC TRAINING: HYPERTROPHY

TRAINING PROGRAM

+ Intensity: **50%-85%** (in some cases less, after a first failure with this intensity)

+ Number of repetitions: **6-12, or 15-50 seconds of effort** (we also use endurance parameters in this chapter to promote hypertrophy)

+ Speed of execution: **Maximal in concentric phase**

+ Rest between sets: **30 seconds to 3 minutes**

+ Max reps per muscle group per workout: **200**

+ Max sets per muscle group: **16**

+ Max muscle groups per workout: **2** (12-16 sets each); **6** (4-5 sets each)

+ Rest between workouts: **24-48 hours**

#3

CONCENTRIC TRAINING: HYPERTROPHY

Concentric training techniques are the techniques seen most often in gyms today. This section provides an introduction to the wide range of those available to you as you design your programs. For trainers, I strongly recommend that you begin to incorporate these methods into your own workouts before prescribing them to your clients. This will not only help deepen your understanding of the techniques but also give you the experience needed to best educate your clients on their use and the logic behind them. Think of the gym as a laboratory in which you have to experiment with the techniques you want to apply before advising your clients.

Each Repetition Must Be Perfect

One important point about the application of the techniques in this chapter (and all the other techniques in this book that do not specifically mention speed of execution) is the use of control during the eccentric phase of a movement and acceleration during the concentric phase. Try it and see the results for yourself: Take a session in which you do your workout without worrying about these details, then repeat this same session a week later. The second time, focus on controlling the eccentric portion for 2-3 seconds and accelerating the weight as quickly as possible in the concentric phase. Note the difference in the level of difficulty and any soreness felt in the following days. Without having introduced any other training techniques, you will already see a difference in the effectiveness of your workouts.

In training, the goal is not to just complete your 6, 8, or 15 reps, but rather to complete your reps in such a way that each one takes you closer to your goal. If you want to develop your power, then each repetition must be done in a way that maximizes your strength or speed. If you want to build muscle mass, then each rep should create a certain amount of fatigue requiring further muscular adaptations (hypertrophy or hyperplasia). Most people who are unaware of these elements perform only 1 or 2 reps per set that take them closer to their goal (usually the last 2 reps, which are the most difficult). In fact, a perfect repetition must consist of three main elements: control in the eccentric phase, a slight controlled rebound in the transition phase, and maximum acceleration in the concentric phase.

→ **Control in the eccentric phase.** The eccentric phase promotes greater adaptation in muscle hypertrophy than the concentric phase. In fact, eccentric muscle action is a necessary stimulus for muscle growth. It produces better neural adaptation, greater strength, a higher level of stress per motor unit, better recruitment of fast-twitch fibers, and more muscle microtears. To perform it well, this phase should be performed over 2-3 seconds, contracting the target muscles (e.g., if you are doing a back exercise, you should not feel the strain primarily in your biceps) without any muscle relaxation during the movement. Keep in mind that when you exercise, you are not lifting weights, you are contracting your muscles against resistance. This small detail will make all the difference.

→ **Rebound in the transition phase.** During the eccentric–concentric transition, it is best to activate what is called the myotatic stretch reflex (prestretch). It is a nervous system reflex that causes increased recruitment of fast-twitch (type II) fibers generated by neuromuscular spindles, which are specialized fibers in the muscle that protect it from stretching too quickly. This recruitment therefore allows greater fatigue of type II fibers and will lead to better muscle gains. In addition, prestretching adds the forces of the elastic components of the tendons during the concentric phase, providing an advantage for your concentric strength. To perform this prestretch properly, you must perform the last quarter of the eccentric phase in a short and quick fashion while making sure to contract the target muscles.

→ **Maximum acceleration in the concentric phase.** Newton's second law states that force is equal to mass (in kilograms) multiplied by acceleration (in square meters per second). Therefore, to increase the force generated by the muscle fibers, we can either increase the lifted mass or increase its acceleration. The higher the force required, the greater the number of muscle fibers involved, thus creating greater fatigue. One of the best ways to generate maximum recruitment for each of the reps is to take on a moderate to heavy load and perform the concentric phase as quickly as possible. Note that it is the intention to speed up the bar that counts, not the speed of the bar. This will recruit more total fibers through a set than when this criterion is not taken into account. This method is called compensatory acceleration training, or CAT (the load is accelerated in order to compensate for the use of a lighter load).

In summary, each repetition done using the training techniques in this section should be accomplished this way: Perform the eccentric phase with control over 2-3 seconds, make a fast and controlled transition, then speed up the concentric phase as much as possible. If this isn't the way you train already, apply this basic principle first and it will be a great start.

Perceived effort

▭▭▭▭▭

Effect on hypertrophy

▭▭▭▭▭

Effect on strength and power

▭▭▭▭▭

Effect on muscular endurance

▭▭▭▭▭

Experience required

▭▭▭

✓ Accumulation method

☐ Intensification method

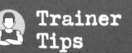

Trainer Tips

This training distribution is ideal for beginners because their muscle capacity is not high enough to withstand too much training volume. Thus, performing 1 or 2 exercises per muscle group 3 times per week will be optimal. After 6-8 weeks of training, they can then switch to a push-pull split (technique #60).

FULL-BODY SPLIT

HOW DOES IT WORK?

This method involves working the whole body in each of your workouts with 1 or 2 exercises per muscle group.

ADVANTAGES

→ This technique allows you to increase muscle adaptations without requiring too much training volume.

→ It includes exercises that utilize large muscle groups, which promotes fat loss.

→ Because it works every body part, this technique increases metabolism.

DISADVANTAGES

→ Advanced athletes will quickly stagnate with this technique due to the lack of volume per muscle group. This type of split will be more effective if it is used for muscular strength needs (e.g., strength in multiple splits, technique #24).

PRESCRIPTION TABLE

Load	Number of repetitions per set	Number of sets per exercise	Number of exercises per muscle group	Rest between sets
60%-83%	6-20	2-4	1-2	1-2 minutes

EXAMPLE OF A FULL-BODY SPLIT FOR BEGINNERS

Exercises	Sets	Reps	Rest
Bench press	3	8-10	90 seconds
One-arm dumbbell row	3	8-10	90 seconds
Leg press	3	8-10	90 seconds
Seated row to chest	3	8-10	90 seconds
Seated shoulder press with machine	3	8-10	90 seconds
Triceps push-down	3	8-10	90 seconds
Standing barbell curl	3	8-10	90 seconds
Weighted crunch	3	8-10	90 seconds

Technique #58

Perceived effort

■ ■ ▢ ▢ ▢

Effect on hypertrophy

■ ■ ▢ ▢ ▢

Effect on strength and power

■ ■ ▢ ▢ ▢

Effect on muscular endurance

■ ■ ▢ ▢ ▢

Experience required

■ ▢ ▢

☑ Accumulation method

☐ Intensification method

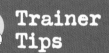

Trainer Tips

Just because this workout plan is over 2 days doesn't mean you only need to work out 2 days a week. In fact, it is very effective when alternated over 4 days of training (e.g., day 1, day 2, day 1, day 2).

2-DAY SPLIT

HOW DOES IT WORK?

This technique involves dividing your full-body workouts into 2 days, similar to the push–pull split (technique #60) and the lower- and upper-body split (technique #59). The only difference is that upper-body (arm) exercises are included with the leg exercises. The distribution of muscle groups will be as follows:

→ **Day 1:** Chest, back, shoulders, trapezius, and abdominals
→ **Day 2:** Quadriceps, hamstrings, calves, biceps, and triceps

ADVANTAGES

→ It allows frequent training of all muscle groups with a little more volume than the full-body split (technique #57).

DISADVANTAGES

→ None.

PRESCRIPTION TABLE

Load	Number of repetitions per set	Number of sets per exercise	Number of exercises per muscle group	Rest between sets
66%-83%	6-15	2-4	1-2	1-2 minutes

EXAMPLE OF A 2-DAY SPLIT

	Exercises	Sets	Reps
DAY 1	Bench press	3	6-8
	Cable fly	3	8-10
	Lat pull-down	3	6-8
	Seated row	3	8-10
	Upright dumbbell row	4	6-8
	Dumbbell shrug	3	6-8
	Weighted crunch	4	10-12

	Exercises	Sets	Reps
DAY 2	Leg press	3	6-8
	Alternating leg extension	3	10-12
	Lying leg curl	4	6-8
	Standing calf with machine	4	12-15
	Standing barbell curl	4	6-8
	Lying dumbbell triceps extension	3	6-8
	Triceps push-down	3	6-8

Technique #59

Perceived effort

▪▪▪▫▫

Effect on
hypertrophy

▪▪▪▫▫

Effect on strength
and power

▪▪▪▫▫

Effect on muscular
endurance

▪▪▫▫▫

Experience required

▪▪▫

☑ Accumulation
method

☐ Intensification
method

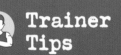

Trainer Tips

When you want to build muscle strength, focus on the squat on day 1 (with additional quadriceps exercises) and on the deadlift on day 3 (with additional hamstring exercises).

LOWER- AND UPPER-BODY SPLIT

HOW DOES IT WORK?

This method divides workouts into lower-body and upper-body exercises. It is effective for developing muscle mass as well as muscle strength because it allows these muscle groups to be worked twice a week. Perform exercises labeled with the same letter as supersets with no rest between them, then rest for 2 minutes between supersets (i.e., perform A1 and A2, 2-minute rest; perform B1 and B2, 2-minute rest; then perform C1, C2, and C3, 2-minute rest).

ADVANTAGES

→ This method is easy to plan and execute.

→ It is ideal for beginners or for those who want to learn about strength training.

→ Many powerlifters use an advanced version of this style of training plan, such as the Westside method (technique #47).

DISADVANTAGES

→ It doesn't allow you to do a large amount of training with each muscle group.

PRESCRIPTION TABLE

Load	Number of repetitions per set	Number of sets per exercise	Number of exercises per muscle group	Rest between sets
70%-85%	6-12	2-4	1-3	1-3 minutes

EXAMPLE SEQUENCE OF LOWER-BODY EXERCISES (DAYS 1 AND 3)

Exercises	Sets	Reps
A1 Back squat superset	4	6-8
A2 Lying leg curl	4	6-8
B1 Walking dumbbell lunge superset	4	8-10
B2 Seated leg curl	4	8-10
C1 Barbell hip thrust superset	3	10-12
C2 Leg extension superset	3	10-12
C3 Back extension	3	10-12

EXAMPLE SEQUENCE OF UPPER-BODY EXERCISES (DAYS 2 AND 4)

Exercises	Sets	Reps
A1 Barbell bench press superset	4	6-8
A2 Bent-over barbell row	4	6-8
B1 Lat pull-down superset	4	8-10
B2 Upright barbell row	4	8-10
C1 Dumbbell curl with a supination	3	10-12
C2 Dip	3	10-12
C3 Reverse crunch	3	10-12

Technique #60

Perceived effort

⬛⬛⬛⬜⬜

Effect on hypertrophy

⬛⬛⬛⬜⬜

Effect on strength and power

⬛⬛⬛⬜⬜

Effect on muscular endurance

⬛⬛⬜⬜⬜

Experience required

⬛⬜⬜

☑ Accumulation method

☐ Intensification method

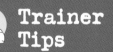

Trainer Tips

Complete the first push day with the leg exercises and, on the second push day, start with the bench press exercises. Do the same pattern for the pull day (refer to the example program).

PUSH–PULL SPLIT

HOW DOES IT WORK?

This method divides workouts into exercises that include a push (moving a weight away from the body) and those that include a pull (bringing a weight closer to the body). Examples include the following:

1. **Pushing exercises:** Bench press (with bar, machine, or dumbbells), seated press (with barbell, machine, or dumbbells), dips, leg machine press, squat, standing calf curl
2. **Pulling exercises:** Deadlift, leg curl (lying, sitting, or standing), seated row or bent-over row (with bar, pulley, or dumbbells), curl (with bar, dumbbells, or machine), pull-up, chin-up

ADVANTAGES

→ It allows you to work a single muscle group several times a week.
→ It is ideal for beginners in training.

DISADVANTAGES

→ It doesn't allow you to do a large amount of training with a single muscle group in one session.

PRESCRIPTION TABLE

Load	Number of repetitions per set	Number of sets per exercise	Number of exercises per muscle group	Rest between sets
70%-83%	6-12	2-4	1-3	1-3 minutes

EXAMPLE OF A PUSH–PULL SPLIT

	Exercises	Sets	Reps
DAY 1 (push)	Front squat	4	6-8
	Leg press	4	6-8
	Bench press with Smith machine	4	8-10
	Dip	4	8-10
	Barbell military press	3	8-10
	Diamond push-up	3	8-10
	Seated calf with machine	3	10-12

	Exercises	Sets	Reps
DAY 2 (pull)	Barbell Romanian deadlift	4	6-8
	Lying leg curl	4	6-8
	Pull-up	4	8-10
	Seated row	4	8-10
	Bent-over barbell row to chest	3	8-10
	Standing barbell curl (EZ bar)	3	10-12
	Dumbbell hammer curl	3	10-12

	Exercises	Sets	Reps
DAY 3 (push)	Bench press with Smith machine	4	6-8
	Dip	4	6-8
	Barbell military press	4	8-10
	Diamond push-up	4	8-10
	Front squat	3	8-10
	Leg press	3	8-10
	Seated calf with machine	3	10-12

	Exercises	Sets	Reps
DAY 4 (pull)	Pull-up	4	6-8
	Seated row	4	6-8
	Bent-over barbell row to chest	4	8-10
	Barbell Romanian deadlift	4	8-10
	Lying leg curl	3	8-10
	Standing barbell curl (EZ bar)	3	10-12
	Dumbbell hammer curl	3	10-12

Perceived effort

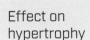

Effect on
hypertrophy

Effect on strength
and power

Effect on muscular
endurance

Experience required

✓ Accumulation
method

☐ Intensification
method

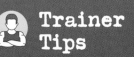

Trainer Tips

In this workout split, preferably choose 3 exercises for large muscle groups (pecs, quads, back, upper back, hamstrings) and 2 exercises for smaller muscle groups (triceps, biceps, trapezius, calves, abdominals, forearms).

3-DAY SPLIT

HOW DOES IT WORK?

This technique involves dividing your workouts into 3 days. One specific example is the squat–bench–deadlift split (technique #48); the difference is that the exercises in this technique are divided according to their function and not according to specific lifts. The distribution of muscle groups will be done as follows:

1. **Day 1 (pushing, upper body):** Chest, shoulders, trapezius, and triceps
2. **Day 2 (lower body):** Quadriceps, hamstrings, glutes, and calves
3. **Day 3 (pulling, upper body):** Back, upper back, biceps, forearms, and abdominals

ADVANTAGES

→ It allows a greater volume of exercises than the full-body split (technique #57) and the 2-day split styles (techniques #58, #59, and #60).

DISADVANTAGES

→ None.

PRESCRIPTION TABLE

Load	Number of repetitions per set	Number of sets per exercise	Number of exercises per muscle group	Rest between sets
66%-83%	6-15	2-4	1-3	1-2 minutes

EXAMPLE OF A 3-DAY SPLIT

Exercises			Sets	Reps
Day 1	Day 2	Day 3		
Barbell bench press	Squat	Pull-up	3	8-10
Incline dumbbell bench press	Leg press	Seated row	3	8-10
Dumbbell fly	Walking dumbbell lunge	Incline dumbbell row	3	8-10
Seated shoulder press with machine	Barbell Romanian deadlift	Seated row to chest	3	8-10
Upright dumbbell row	Lying leg curl	Bent-over dumbbell rear delt fly	3	8-10
Dumbbell lateral raise	Hip abduction with machine	Barbell Scott curl	3	8-10
Barbell shrug	Cable glute kick-back	Dumbbell hammer curl	3	8-10
Overhead dumbbell triceps extension	Standing calf with machine	Barbell wrist flexion	3	8-10
Triceps push-down	Seated calf with machine	High-pulley crunch with rope	3	8-10

Technique #62

Perceived effort

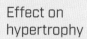

Effect on
hypertrophy

Effect on strength
and power

Effect on muscular
endurance

Experience required

✓ Accumulation
method

☐ Intensification
method

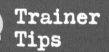

Trainer Tips

In this workout split, preferably choose 3 exercises for large muscle groups (pecs, quads, back, upper back, hamstrings) and 2 exercises for smaller muscle groups (triceps, biceps, trapezius, calves, abdominals, forearms).

PUSH–PULL–ISOLATION TRAINING

HOW DOES IT WORK?

This technique is derived from the push–pull split (technique #60), which is used mainly to develop muscle strength but rarely includes isolation exercises. The aim of this technique is therefore to promote more muscle hypertrophy by introducing movements that complement the basic exercises. As with a push–pull split, you will train each muscle group twice a week. On the isolation exercise, you can sometimes use endurance parameters (up to 20 reps).

ADVANTAGES

→ It stimulates muscle groups twice a week, which leads to very good gains in muscle hypertrophy.
→ It helps build strength because the first two training sessions of the week are done at a higher intensity.

DISADVANTAGES

→ None.

PRESCRIPTION TABLE

Load	Number of repetitions per set	Number of sets per exercise	Number of exercises per muscle group	Rest between sets
74%-85%, 60%-74%	6-10, 10-20	2-4	1-3	1-2 minutes

EXAMPLE OF PUSH–PULL–ISOLATION TRAINING EXERCISES
FOR 4 TRAINING SESSIONS

DAY 1: PUSH

Chest (incline barbell bench press), quadriceps (back squat), shoulders (barbell military press), triceps (close-grip bench press), calves (standing calves), abdominals (crunches with machine)

DAY 2: PULL

Back (lat pull-down), upper back (seated row to chest), biceps (chin-up), forearms (barbell reverse curl), hamstrings (barbell Romanian deadlift), trapezius (dumbbell shrug)

DAY 3: ISOLATION 1

Chest (cable fly), quadriceps (leg extension), shoulders (lateral raise), triceps (rope push-down), calves (standing calves), abdominals (crunches with machine)

DAY 4: ISOLATION 2

Back (straight-arm pull-down), upper back (rear delt fly), biceps (barbell Scott curl), forearms (dumbbell wrist extension), hamstrings (lying leg curl), trapezius (dumbbell shrug)

Technique #63

Perceived effort

▮▮▮▯▯

Effect on
hypertrophy

▮▮▮▮▯

Effect on strength
and power

▮▮▮▯▯

Effect on muscular
endurance

▮▮▯▯▯

Experience required

▮▮▯

✓ Accumulation
method

☐ Intensification
method

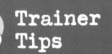

Trainer Tips

This is a training plan that allows an optimal ratio between the number of training days and the number of rest days. A great way to plan it out for the week is to work out on Monday, Tuesday, Thursday, and Saturday.

4-DAY SPLIT

HOW DOES IT WORK?

This technique involves dividing your workouts into 4 days. Several choices are then possible in the distribution of the days. You can combine complementary muscle groups (e.g., chest and triceps; back and biceps; quadriceps and hamstrings; shoulders and trapezius), antagonistic exercises (e.g., chest and upper back; quadriceps and hamstrings; back and shoulders; triceps and biceps) or combine a large muscle group with a small muscle group (chest and biceps; back and shoulders; quadriceps and triceps; upper back and hamstrings).

ADVANTAGES

→ It allows you to work muscle groups with greater volume than a full-body split (technique #57), 2-day split styles (techniques #58, #59, and #60), or a 3-day split (technique #61).
→ It is ideal for advanced athletes in bodybuilding.

DISADVANTAGES

→ None.

PRESCRIPTION TABLE

Load	Number of repetitions per set	Number of sets per exercise	Number of exercises per muscle group	Rest between sets
66%-85%	6-15	2-4	1-3	1-2 minutes

EXAMPLE OF A 4-DAY TRAINING SPLIT WITH ANTAGONIST COMBINATIONS

Exercises				Sets	Reps
Day 1 Chest and upper back	Day 2 Quads and hamstrings	Day 3 Back and shoulders	Day 4 Triceps and biceps		
Incline barbell bench press	Squat	Pull-up	Barbell close-grip bench press	4	6-8
Dumbbell bench press	Leg press	One-arm dumbbell row	Lying dumbbell triceps extension	3	8-10
Chest press	Step-up	Seated row	Dip	3	8-10
Pec deck	Leg extension	Straight-arm lat pull-down	Triceps rope push-down	3	12-15
Seated row to chest	Barbell Romanian deadlift	Standing barbell military press	Barbell curl (supinated grip)	4	6-8
One-arm dumbbell row to chest	Seated leg curl	Seated dumbbell military press	Dumbbell hammer curl	3	8-10
Inverted row with Smith machine	Lying leg curl	Upright barbell row	Curl with machine (supinated grip)	3	8-10
Rear delt dumbbell fly	Nordic leg curl	Lateral raise	Pronated barbell curl	3	12-15

Technique #64

Perceived effort

▪▪▫▫▫

Effect on
hypertrophy

▪▪▪▫▫

Effect on strength
and power

▪▪▪▫▫

Effect on muscular
endurance

▪▪▫▫▫

Experience required

▪▫▫

☑ Accumulation
method

☐ Intensification
method

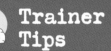

Trainer Tips

The majority of training plans neglect unilateral training. This technique will prevent an imbalance in strength and muscle mass between the two sides of your body, thus ensuring better symmetry while capitalizing on the slight advantage of strength that comes from training one limb at a time.

UNILATERAL SPLIT

HOW DOES IT WORK?

This technique involves using exercises that target only one side of the body at a time, integrating your preferred techniques (e.g., agonist superset, technique #71). Your training will be spread over 4 days:

→ **Day 1:** Upper body, right side
→ **Day 2:** Upper body, left side
→ **Day 3:** Lower body, right side
→ **Day 4:** Lower body, left side

ADVANTAGES

→ This technique potentiates the effects of higher forces produced by working one side at a time.
→ The resting side still receives nerve stimulation from the increased blood supply caused by working out on the other side, promoting muscle growth.

DISADVANTAGES

→ None.

PRESCRIPTION TABLE

Load	Number of repetitions per set	Number of sets per exercise	Number of exercises per muscle group	Rest between sets
70%-83%	6-12	2-4	2-5	1-2 minutes

EXAMPLE OF UNILATERAL SPLIT EXERCISES FOR 4 TRAINING SESSIONS

DAY 1: UPPER BODY, RIGHT SIDE

Chest (chest press, right arm), shoulders (upright dumbbell row, right arm), trapezius (dumbbell shrug with low pulley, right arm), triceps (triceps kick-back with pulley, right arm), back (one-arm dumbbell row, right arm), biceps (hammer curl with low pulley, right arm)

DAY 2: UPPER BODY, LEFT SIDE

Chest (chest press, left arm), shoulders (upright dumbbell row, left arm), trapezius (dumbbell shrug with low pulley, left arm), triceps (triceps kick-back with pulley, left arm), back (one-arm dumbbell row, left arm), biceps (hammer curl with low pulley, left arm)

DAY 3: LOWER BODY, RIGHT SIDE

Quadriceps (leg extension, right leg), hamstrings (lying leg curl, right leg), glutes (one-leg hip thrust, right leg), calves (standing calf with dumbbell, right calf)

DAY 4: LOWER BODY, LEFT SIDE

Quadriceps (leg extension, left leg), hamstrings (lying leg curl, left leg), glutes (one-leg hip thrust, left leg), calves (standing calf with dumbbell, left calf)

Technique #65

Perceived effort

■ ■ ■ □ □

Effect on hypertrophy

■ ■ ■ ■ □

Effect on strength and power

■ ■ ■ □ □

Effect on muscular endurance

■ ■ ■ □ □

Experience required

■ □ □

✓ Accumulation method

☐ Intensification method

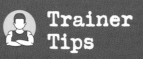 **Trainer Tips**

This is one of the training plans that has given me the most gains in muscle mass and strength. Because you will be exercising more frequently, however, avoid exceeding 90 minutes per workout.

5-DAY SPLIT

HOW DOES IT WORK?

This technique involves dividing your workouts into 5 days. You can use the 4-day split (technique #63) and add a fifth day to work neglected muscle groups (e.g., abdominals, calves, glutes, forearms, trapezius) or to repeat work on your weakest muscle groups (e.g., work the chest and shoulders a second time on day 5).

ADVANTAGES

→ It allows you to use a very high training volume per muscle group (up to 16 total sets per muscle group) if you choose to work only 1 muscle group per day.

→ It allows you to work the whole body without neglecting certain muscle groups.

DISADVANTAGES

→ It can be time consuming.

PRESCRIPTION TABLE

Load	Number of repetitions per set	Number of sets per exercise	Number of exercises per muscle group	Rest between sets
66%-83%	6-15	2-4	3-5	1-2 minutes

EXAMPLE OF A RECOMMENDED 5-DAY SPLIT

Day 1	Day 2	Day 3	Day 4	Day 5
Chest	Quadriceps	Back	Glutes	Upper back
Biceps	Abdominals	Shoulders	Triceps	Hamstrings

EXAMPLE OF AN OPTIMAL 5-DAY SPLIT

Day 1	Day 2	Day 3	Day 4	Day 5
Chest	Quadriceps	Back	Glutes	Upper back
Biceps	Abdominals	Shoulders	Triceps	Hamstrings
Forearms	Calves	Trapezius	Hip adductors	Lower back

Technique #66

Perceived effort

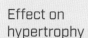

Effect on
hypertrophy

Effect on strength
and power

Effect on muscular
endurance

Experience required

✓ Accumulation
method

☐ Intensification
method

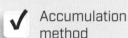
Trainer Tips

This is a technique I love that gives good results quickly. One way to do this type of technique is to divide the training into 3 days—a push day, a pull day, and a lower-body day—that intersect over 4 consecutive training sessions (see the example).

BACK-TO-BACK TRAINING

HOW DOES IT WORK?

For this technique, you will train the same muscle group on 2 consecutive days. The first workout should be done with heavy loads (6-12 reps) and the second workout with lighter loads (15-20 reps). During the first workout, add accumulation techniques such as dropsets, double dropsets, or rest–pause sets. Perform 12-16 sets per muscle group and go to failure on each set. For the second workout, complete 6-8 sets per muscle group and don't go to failure on any set.

ADVANTAGES

→ It helps increase blood flow (rich in amino acids, glucose, testosterone, and growth hormone) to damaged muscles the day after the session, thereby promoting muscle recovery.

DISADVANTAGES

→ You must have the opportunity to train on 2 consecutive days, with the potential for 4 consecutive days.

PRESCRIPTION TABLE

Load	Number of repetitions per set	Number of sets per exercise	Number of exercises per muscle group	Rest between sets
70%-83%, 60%-70%	6-12, 15-20	3-4, 2-3	3-4, 2-3	2-3 minutes

EXAMPLE OF 4 TRAINING SESSIONS

MONDAY
Chest, shoulders, triceps (6-12 reps)
+
abdominals (15-20 reps)

TUESDAY
Back, upper back, biceps (6-12 reps)
+
chest, shoulders, triceps (15-20 reps)

WEDNESDAY
Lower body (6-12 reps)
+
back, upper back, biceps (15-20 reps)

THURSDAY
Abdominals (6-12 reps)
+
lower body (15-20 reps)

Perceived effort

⬛⬛⬛⬜⬜

Effect on hypertrophy

⬛⬛⬛⬛⬜

Effect on strength and power

⬛⬛⬜⬜⬜

Effect on muscular endurance

⬛⬛⬜⬜⬜

Experience required

⬛⬛⬜

✓ Accumulation method

☐ Intensification method

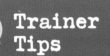

Trainer Tips

Because you will be doing the same workout twice in the same day, I suggest that you reverse the order of the exercises in the second workout. Thus, you will start with isolation exercises and end with basic exercises. This helps prevent monotony.

TWICE-A-DAY TRAINING

HOW DOES IT WORK?

This method is similar to back-to-back training (technique #66), except that the rest time between the sessions is shorter (6-8 hours compared to 24 hours). You will therefore need to train either in the morning and the afternoon, or in the morning and evening, or in the afternoon and evening. The first workout should be done with heavy loads (6-10 reps) and the second workout with lighter loads of the same exercises (15-20 reps).

ADVANTAGES

→ It helps increase blood flow (rich in amino acids, glucose, testosterone, and growth hormone) to damaged muscles shortly after the start of muscle recovery, thereby promoting better muscle growth.

DISADVANTAGES

→ You must have the opportunity to train twice in the same day.
→ Because of the physical difficulty and short recovery period, you must be experienced with strength training before using this technique.

PRESCRIPTION TABLE

Load	Number of repetitions per set	Number of sets per exercise	Number of exercises per muscle group	Rest between sets
60%-83%	6-10, 15-20	3-4, 2-3	3-4, 2-3	2-3 minutes

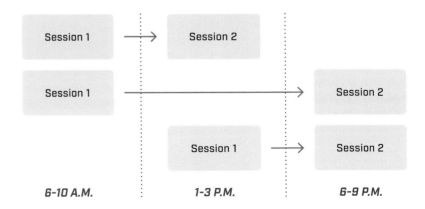

Technique #68

Perceived effort

Effect on hypertrophy

Effect on strength and power

Effect on muscular endurance

Experience required

✓ Accumulation method

☐ Intensification method

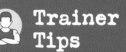

Trainer Tips

Submaximal sets are a great technique for beginners or those coming back to the gym after a long break. When you come back, your muscles will have lost their adaptations, so beginning with lighter and submaximal weights is a good strategy to prevent injuries.

SUBMAXIMAL SET

S

HOW DOES IT WORK?

Complete a set using any load and stop before muscle failure. For example, if you do only 6-8 reps using your 10RM, you have completed a submaximal set. Doing 10 reps with your 10RM, however, would be a failure set (technique #69). This technique uses a low load to work your cardiovascular system through strength training. The Tabata method (technique #221) and German volume training (techniques #132-#135) are good examples of a submaximal set.

ADVANTAGES

→ For beginners, submaximal training can lead to gains in strength and muscle mass.

→ It can be useful during the rehabilitation of an injured muscle.

DISADVANTAGES

→ Given the low level of muscular and nervous fatigue caused by this technique, the development of various physical qualities will be limited.

PRESCRIPTION TABLE

Load	Number of repetitions per set	Number of sets per exercise	Number of exercises per muscle group	Rest between sets
Your choice	6-20	2-4	2-3	15-60 seconds

Technique #69

Perceived effort

▮▮▯▯▯

Effect on
hypertrophy

▮▮▮▯▯

Effect on strength
and power

▮▮▮▯▯

Effect on muscular
endurance

▮▮▯▯▯

Experience required

▮▯▯

✓ Accumulation
method

☐ Intensification
method

🏋 Trainer Tips

Only start a rep you can complete without partner assistance. Missing reps is very demanding on your central nervous system (CNS) and will decrease the quality of subsequent sets.

FAILURE SET

HOW DOES IT WORK?
This technique simply requires that you perform reps until failure (in RM or reps maximum). In general, for each exercise, beginners will complete 2-4 sets of 12-15 reps, intermediate individuals will do 3-5 sets of 8-12 reps, and more advanced athletes will do 4-6 sets of 6-8 reps.

Because this technique involves muscle failure at the end of the set, always ask for supervision on lifts where you risk getting stuck (e.g., bench press or squat). This will improve your confidence when performing the final reps of your set.

ADVANTAGES
→ It makes it possible to achieve muscle failure by creating localized fatigue in the fibers used during exercise (unlike a submaximal set, technique #68).
→ It is simple and easy to use.
→ It allows the development of strength and power in individuals advanced in strength training.[4]

DISADVANTAGES
→ It can become monotonous.
→ The body adapts quickly, so while this technique works well for beginners, advanced lifters will need to add other techniques rapidly to progress their strength and muscle mass.
→ It requires the assistance of a spotter during certain exercises.

PRESCRIPTION TABLE

Load	Number of repetitions per set	Number of sets per exercise	Number of exercises per muscle group	Rest between sets
66%-70% (beginner), 70%-78% (intermediate), or 78%-83% (advanced)	12-15 (beginner), 8-12 (intermediate), or 6-8 (advanced)	2-4 (beginner), 3-5 (intermediate), or 4-6 (advanced)	2-3	1-3 minutes

Technique #70

Perceived effort

▪▪▫▫▫

Effect on
hypertrophy

▪▪▫▫▫

Effect on strength
and power

▪▪▫▫▫

Effect on muscular
endurance

▪▪▫▫▫

Experience required

▪▫▫

✓ Accumulation
method

☐ Intensification
method

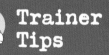

Trainer Tips

Do not stop at the required number of reps. If you are able to do 7 reps using last week's 6RM load, do it. Once you are able to do 2 more reps than is required, increase the load.

 (S)

HYPERTROPHY 12RM-10RM-8RM-6RM

HOW DOES IT WORK?

This method is one of the oldest and most commonly used by trainers with beginners. Perform 4 total sets, one each at 12RM, 10RM, 8RM, and 6RM while increasing the load.

ADVANTAGES

→ It makes it possible to achieve muscle failure by creating localized fatigue in the fibers used during exercise (unlike a submaximal set, technique #68).
→ It is ideal for beginners because it exposes them to both light and heavy loads.
→ It is simple and easy to use.

DISADVANTAGES

→ It can become monotonous.
→ The body adapts quickly, so while this technique works well for beginners, advanced lifters will need to add other techniques rapidly to progress their strength and muscle mass.
→ It requires the assistance of a spotter during certain exercises.

PRESCRIPTION TABLE

Load	Number of repetitions per set	Number of sets per exercise	Number of exercises per muscle group	Rest between sets
70%-83%	12, 10, 8, 6	4	1-4	1-3 minutes

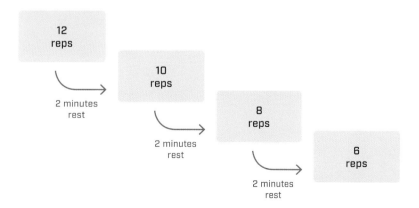

Technique #71

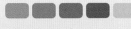

Perceived effort

■ ■ ■ ■ □

Effect on
hypertrophy

■ ■ ■ ■ □

Effect on strength
and power

■ ■ ■ □ □

Effect on muscular
endurance

■ ■ ■ □ □

Experience required

■ ■ □

 ✓ Accumulation
method

☐ Intensification
method

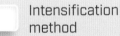 ## Trainer Tips

To increase the variety in your supersets, include explosive (potentiation), unstable (activation), or high-speed movements with elastic bands (timed sets, technique #79).

 (S)

AGONIST SUPERSET

HOW DOES IT WORK?
Also known simply as a superset, this technique involves performing, without rest, 2 exercises that use the same muscle group. You must do repetitions until failure in both exercises. Prefatigue, postfatigue, and dropset methods are all examples of this technique. The loads and repetitions will ideally be the same for both exercises.

ADVANTAGES
→ This technique results in greater muscle fatigue by including two consecutive sets that use the same muscle group.

DISADVANTAGES
→ Although it is a basic technique that is useful for beginners, it is usually quickly replaced by pre- and postfatigue techniques, which are much more effective in rebalancing the weaker parts of a particular muscle group.

PRESCRIPTION TABLE

Load	Number of repetitions per set	Number of sets per exercise	Number of exercises per muscle group	Rest between sets
70%-83%	6-12	2-4	1-3 supersets	2-3 minutes

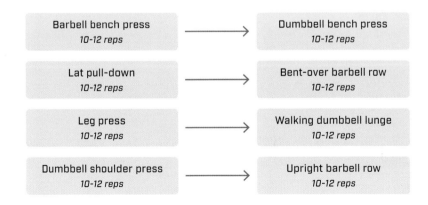

Barbell bench press 10-12 reps	→	Dumbbell bench press 10-12 reps
Lat pull-down 10-12 reps	→	Bent-over barbell row 10-12 reps
Leg press 10-12 reps	→	Walking dumbbell lunge 10-12 reps
Dumbbell shoulder press 10-12 reps	→	Upright barbell row 10-12 reps

Technique #72

Perceived effort

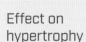

Effect on
hypertrophy

Effect on strength
and power

Effect on muscular
endurance

Experience required

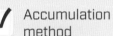

✓ Accumulation
method

☐ Intensification
method

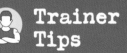

Trainer Tips

Most people think that the pecs and lats are antagonists, but this is wrong: The pectoralis major and latissimus dorsi are both internal rotators of the shoulder. So make sure to work your pecs with your upper back (middle trapezius, rhomboids) and your shoulders with your lats!

ANTAGONIST SUPERSET

HOW DOES IT WORK?

This method involves performing, without rest, 2 exercises for opposing muscle groups (e.g., biceps and triceps, upper back and pectorals, back and shoulders, hip adductors and hip abductors, quadriceps and hamstrings, wrist flexors and wrist extensors).

The loads can vary from 70%-83% for each exercise. If you choose to complete 12 reps, you will use 70% load, whereas an 83% load will limit you to 6 reps. You may select the number of reps to perform. However, if you are a beginner, you will only do 2 or 3 sets of a single superset, whereas an intermediate or advanced individual may do 3 or 4 sets of 3 different supersets. The rest time between sets will also vary depending on the load used (e.g., 1-2 minutes for 70%; 2-3 minutes for 80%).

ADVANTAGES

→ This technique cuts back on the time spent in the gym by reducing total rest time.
→ It ensures the muscular balance of a joint by providing equal work for the opposing muscles.
→ It's simple and very easy to incorporate into your workouts.

DISADVANTAGES

→ Compared to the agonist superset (technique #71), it does not create very pronounced muscle fatigue for each muscle group.

PRESCRIPTION TABLE

Load	Number of repetitions per set	Number of sets per exercise	Number of exercises per muscle group	Rest between sets
70%-83%	6-12	2-4	1-4 supersets	1-3 minutes

Technique #73

Perceived effort

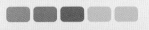

Effect on hypertrophy

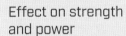

Effect on strength and power

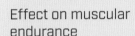

Effect on muscular endurance

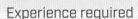

Experience required

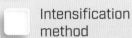

 ✓ Accumulation method

☐ Intensification method

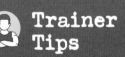

Trainer Tips

I often use this kind of superset with my clients to work their abs and lower back more effectively (e.g., bench press followed by weighted crunches) because they tend to neglect the core at the end of the workout.

COMPLEMENTARY SUPERSET

HOW DOES IT WORK?

This method consists of performing, without rest, two exercises that use neighboring muscle groups (e.g., quadriceps and hip adductors, pectorals and rotator cuff, biceps and shoulders). The loads and repetitions will be heavier for the first exercise and lighter for the second exercise. Both will be done until failure.

ADVANTAGES

→ This technique cuts back on the time spent in the gym by reducing total rest time.
→ It is often used to work understimulated areas or those that are not often targeted.
→ It is simple and very easy to incorporate into your workouts.

DISADVANTAGES

→ Compared to the agonist superset (technique #71), it does not create very pronounced muscle fatigue for each muscle group.

PRESCRIPTION TABLE

Load	Number of repetitions per set	Number of sets per exercise	Number of exercises per muscle group	Rest between sets
70%-83%	6-12	2-4	1-4 supersets	1-2 minutes

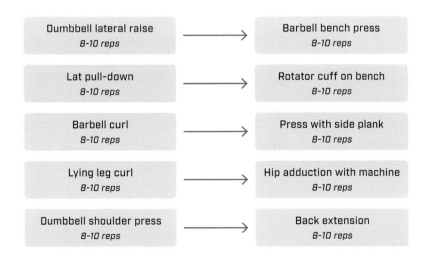

Technique #74

Perceived effort

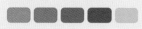

Effect on hypertrophy

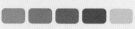

Effect on strength and power

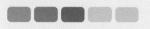

Effect on muscular endurance

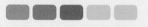

Experience required

✓ Accumulation method

☐ Intensification method

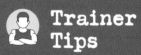

DROPSET

HOW DOES IT WORK?

This method is a type of agonist superset (technique #71). Instead of performing two different exercises, however, you perform an exercise for max reps, then decrease the load in order to perform a second set of the same exercise until failure.

ADVANTAGES

→ This technique results in greater muscle fatigue by including two consecutive sets that use the same muscle group.

→ It is a basic technique that is useful for beginners.

→ It helps train a motor pattern without rest.

DISADVANTAGES

→ Because this technique does not let you isolate deficient muscle groups within a single multijoint movement, you will need to include isolation exercises in your workout.

→ It works best with exercises that use machines or free weights to facilitate changing the load.

PRESCRIPTION TABLE

Load	Number of repetitions per set	Number of sets per exercise	Number of exercises per muscle group	Rest between sets
70%-80% + 40%-60%	6-12	2-5	1-4 dropsets	1-2 minutes

Leg press with 130 kg
6-8 reps

20%-30% load reduction
→

Leg press with 100 kg
6-8 reps

Technique #75

Perceived effort

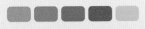

Effect on
hypertrophy

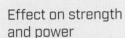

Effect on strength
and power

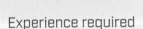

Effect on muscular
endurance

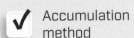

Experience required

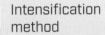

✓ Accumulation
method

☐ Intensification
method

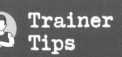

Trainer Tips

Some bodybuilders prefer to perform 3 dropsets per workout over 2 exercises per muscle group (a multijoint exercise and an isolation exercise). Other bodybuilders perform a double dropset only in the last set of each exercise (descending sets 1, technique #128).

DOUBLE DROPSET

HOW DOES IT WORK?

This method is an extended version of the dropset (technique #74), or an agonist triset. It consists of performing an exercise for max reps, then reducing the load by 20%-30% for the second sequence on the same exercise, then reducing the load again by 20%-30% for the third sequence until failure.

ADVANTAGES

→ This technique results in greater muscle fatigue by including two consecutive sets that use the same muscle group.
→ It is a basic technique that is useful for beginners.
→ It helps train a motor pattern without rest.

DISADVANTAGES

→ Because this technique does not let you isolate deficient muscle groups within a single multijoint movement, you will need to include isolation exercises in your workout.
→ It works best with exercises that use machines or free weights to facilitate changing the load.

PRESCRIPTION TABLE

Load	Number of repetitions per set	Number of sets per exercise	Number of exercises per muscle group	Rest between sets
70%-80% + 40%-60% + 10%-40%	6-12	2-5	1-4 double dropsets	2-3 minutes

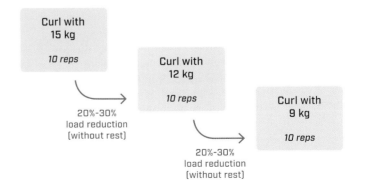

Technique #76

Perceived effort

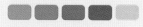

Effect on hypertrophy

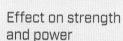

Effect on strength and power

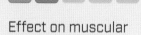

Effect on muscular endurance

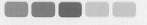

Experience required

✓ Accumulation method

☐ Intensification method

HOLISTIC SET

Ⓢ

HOW DOES IT WORK?

A holistic set is a series of sets whose reps combine to form a cohesive whole. (It is also sometimes known as a *triple drop* or *breakdown*.) Start with a set at 6RM, immediately followed by a decrease in load, then a 12RM, then a second decrease in load, then a 24RM (without rest). This is 1 set.

ADVANTAGES

→ This technique is similar to a triset, but it fatigues all muscle fibers, from fast-twitch fibers in the beginning of the set to slow-twitch fibers at the end.

DISADVANTAGES

→ It works best with exercises that use machines or free weights to facilitate changing the load. For all movements with a barbell or dumbbells, you need to change the weight twice (for example, you will need three pairs of dumbbells).

PRESCRIPTION TABLE

Load	Number of repetitions per set	Number of sets per exercise	Number of exercises per muscle group	Rest between sets
80%-85% + 40%-50% + 20%-30%	6 + 12 + 24	2-4	1-3	2-3 minutes

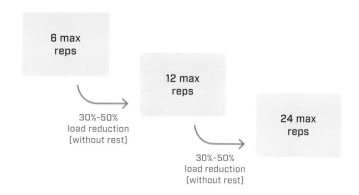

Technique #77

Perceived effort

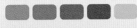

Effect on hypertrophy

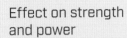

Effect on strength and power

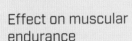

Effect on muscular endurance

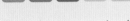

Experience required

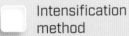 Accumulation method

Intensification method

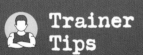 **Trainer Tips**

Some individuals have difficulty recruiting their pecs during a bench press. This method will improve erroneous motor patterns by preceding, for example, a bench press with a cable fly.

PREFATIGUE

HOW DOES IT WORK?

This method is considered a superset. Complete 2 consecutive exercises for the same muscle without rest between sets, with the multijoint movement after the isolation movement. The goal is to maximize the recruitment of weak muscles. For example, if you have difficulty recruiting your pectorals during a bench press (your shoulders and triceps do the work for them), perform a cable fly before doing your bench press. Because your pectorals will be already exhausted from the cable fly, but your shoulders and triceps will not, you will feel more work on your pectorals when doing the bench press.

Isolation exercise + multijoint exercise

ADVANTAGES

→ This technique is useful for targeting less-developed muscle groups (e.g., if your triceps are the weak link in your bench press, use this technique to target this area).

DISADVANTAGES

→ This technique is less effective than the postfatigue method (technique #78) for general hypertrophy because of the lighter load used in the basic exercises.

PRESCRIPTION TABLE

Load	Number of repetitions per set	Number of sets per exercise	Number of exercises per muscle group	Rest between sets
60%-80%	6-15	2-5	1-3 supersets	1-3 minutes

ISOLATION EXERCISE

Standing barbell curl
8-10 reps

Lateral raise
8-10 reps

Leg extension
8-10 reps

Lying leg curl
8-10 reps

Triceps push-down
8-10 reps

MULTIJOINT EXERCISE

Lat pull-down
8-10 reps

Dumbbell shoulder press
8-10 reps

Leg press
8-10 reps

Barbell Romanian deadlift
8-10 reps

Barbell bench press
8-10 reps

Technique #78

Perceived effort

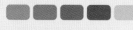

Effect on hypertrophy

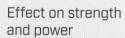

Effect on strength and power

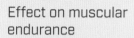

Effect on muscular endurance

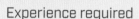

Experience required

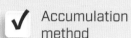

✓ Accumulation method

☐ Intensification method

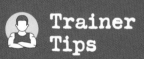

Trainer Tips

Use this method for your weaker muscle groups. Once your weaknesses have been corrected, then you can have fun using it with your strongest muscle groups!

POSTFATIGUE

Ⓢ

HOW DOES IT WORK?

This method is considered a superset. Complete 2 consecutive exercises for the same muscle without rest between sets, this time performing the isolation movement after the multijoint movement. Because the weakest muscles are the first to fatigue in a multijoint exercise (weakest link principle), the major muscles do not always receive optimal stimulation. For example, during a bench press, the triceps and deltoids are likely to fatigue before the pectorals, causing efforts to cease without having optimized pectoral development. This technique continues to stimulate these muscles.

Multijoint exercise + isolation exercise

ADVANTAGES

→ It works the understimulated muscles in order to maximize their development.

DISADVANTAGES

→ The isolation exercise only develops one muscle at a time.

PRESCRIPTION TABLE

Load	Number of repetitions per set	Number of sets per exercise	Number of exercises per muscle group	Rest between sets
60%-80%	6-15	2-5	1-3 supersets	1-3 minutes

MULTIJOINT EXERCISE		ISOLATION EXERCISE
Barbell bench press *8-10 reps*	→	Dumbbell fly *8-10 reps*
Back squat *8-10 reps*	→	Leg extension *8-10 reps*
Bent-over barbell row *8-10 reps*	→	Straight-arm pull-down *8-10 reps*
Upright barbell row *8-10 reps*	→	Lateral raise with cable *8-10 reps*

Technique #79

Perceived effort

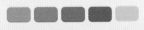

Effect on hypertrophy

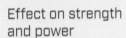

Effect on strength and power

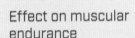

Effect on muscular endurance

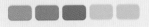

Experience required

✓ Accumulation method

☐ Intensification method

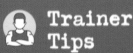

Trainer Tips

Series shorter than 20 seconds should be excluded because they mainly use the anaerobic alactic system, as should those longer than 60 seconds if you want repetitions of a certain quality. Keep in mind that fast-twitch fibers are not very resistant to fatigue.

TIMED SETS

HOW DOES IT WORK?

This technique is rarely used in gyms because many people underestimate the effectiveness of elastic bands, reserving them for beginners or travelers. On the contrary, they are very useful! Using an elastic band with handles or a superband, do as many reps as possible as fast as possible in a set period of time, usually 20-60 seconds.

ADVANTAGES

→ Although you can use free weights with this technique, bands with handles are more effective because they help decelerate the load given the fast speed of the movements, something that is not possible when using free weights.

→ This technique is often used to increase energy expenditure and promote fat loss. The secret lies in its impact on the accumulation of metabolic acidosis (H+ ions), which stimulates the release of growth hormone.

DISADVANTAGES

→ It does not allow the use of heavy loads, so the impact on hypertrophy will be lower than that of other techniques.

→ It is very difficult to use with lower-body exercises.

PRESCRIPTION TABLE

Load	Number of seconds per set	Number of sets per exercise	Number of exercises per muscle group	Rest between sets
Elastic band only	20-60 seconds	2-4	1-2	30-60 seconds

To perform a push or pull metabolic exercise, secure the elastic band to an apparatus pole, squat cage, or other stationary surface to create an anchor point. For arm or shoulder exercises, place your feet on the middle of the elastic to create the anchor point. Perform metabolic work for the prescribed time without changing the technique of movement.

Perceived effort

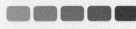

Effect on hypertrophy

Effect on strength and power

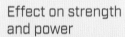

Effect on muscular endurance

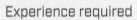

Experience required

✓ Accumulation method

☐ Intensification method

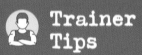

Trainer Tips

An elastic band or superband are ideal accessories for performing metabolic exercises. Anchor them to a stable surface and adjust your position (farther or closer) to increase or decrease the difficulty of the effort.

METABOLIC PREFATIGUE

HOW DOES IT WORK?

This method is considered a superset. Complete 2 consecutive exercises for the same muscle without rest between sets, performing the metabolic movement (rapid movement of any kind of exercise for 20-40 seconds) before the multijoint movement (6-15 repetitions). On the metabolic exercise, stop the movement when you are not able to maintain a fast speed.

Metabolic exercise + multijoint exercise

ADVANTAGES

→ It promotes quality work on the metabolic exercise (better position, less compensation), compared to metabolic postfatigue (technique #81).

→ It is easy to perform using an elastic band (ideal for training at home).

DISADVANTAGES

→ It does not allow the use of heavy loads on the multijoint exercise.

PRESCRIPTION TABLE

Load	Number of seconds or repetitions per set	Number of sets per exercise	Number of exercises per muscle group	Rest between sets
Elastic band + 60%-80%	20-40 seconds + 6-15 reps	2-4	1-3 supersets	1-3 minutes

METABOLIC EXERCISE		MULTIJOINT EXERCISE
Rapid lateral raise with band *30 seconds*	→	Dumbbell shoulder press *8-10 reps*
Rapid high-position alternate punching with band: *30 seconds*	→	Cable fly *8-10 reps*
Rapid low-position pulling with band: *30 seconds*	→	Close-grip lat pull-down *8-10 reps*
Rapid standing curl with band *30 seconds*	→	Barbell Scott curl *8-10 reps*
Rapid triceps extension with band: *30 seconds*	→	Overhead dumbbell triceps extension: *8-10 reps*

Technique #81

Perceived effort

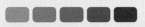

Effect on hypertrophy

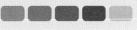

Effect on strength and power

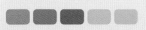

Effect on muscular endurance

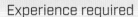

Experience required

✓ Accumulation method

☐ Intensification method

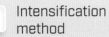

Trainer Tips

Start with this technique before trying the giant sets that include metabolic exercises (techniques #91-#96). In training, it's all about progression.

METABOLIC POSTFATIGUE

(S)

HOW DOES IT WORK?

This method is considered a superset. Complete 2 consecutive exercises for the same muscle without rest between sets, this time performing the metabolic movement (rapid movement of any kind of exercise for 20-40 seconds) after the multijoint movement (6-15 repetitions). On the metabolic exercise, stop the movement when you are not able to maintain a fast speed.

Multijoint exercise + metabolic exercise

ADVANTAGES

→ It promotes the complete fatigue of the fast-twitch fibers due to the metabolic movement in the second exercise, allowing the slow-twitch fibers to work.

→ It is ideal for a fat loss goal.

→ It is easy to perform at home using an elastic band.

DISADVANTAGES

→ There is a risk of compensating in the metabolic movement because of the accumulated fatigue. Make sure you maintain great technique.

PRESCRIPTION TABLE

Load	Number of repetitions or seconds per set	Number of sets per exercise	Number of exercises per muscle group	Rest between sets
60%-80% + elastic band	6-15 reps + 20-40 seconds	2-4	1-3 supersets	1-3 minutes

MULTIJOINT EXERCISE		METABOLIC EXERCISE
Barbell bench press *8-10 reps*	→	Rapid high-position alternate punching with band: *30 seconds*
Lateral raise with machine *8-10 reps*	→	Rapid alternate vertical pull with band: *30 seconds*
Shoulder press *8-10 reps*	→	Rapid alternate front foot raise with band: *30 seconds*
Pull-up *8-10 reps*	→	Rapid high-position alternate pulling with band: *30 seconds*

Technique #82

Perceived effort

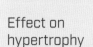

Effect on hypertrophy

Effect on strength and power

Effect on muscular endurance

Experience required

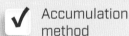

✓ Accumulation method

☐ Intensification method

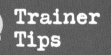

Trainer Tips

For activating (unstable) movements, you can also use a superband (i.e., elastic band) that has been passed through a plate (e.g., 2.5, 5, or 10 kg) so that it is suspended on the end of a bar. The rebound will then create the desired instability.

PREACTIVATION

HOW DOES IT WORK?

This method is considered a superset. Complete, without rest, an activation exercise (e.g., using a Swiss ball, BOSU ball, or balance disc) followed by a traditional exercise. In this technique, you will use a low load for the unstable movement (e.g., body weight or 30%-40% of your maximum strength) and a higher load for the traditional movement (70%-83%). You may select the number of reps to perform.

Activation exercise + traditional exercise

ADVANTAGES

→ It helps to develop a high degree of stability.
→ Fatigue of fast-twitch fibers during unstable movement stimulates their hypertrophy.
→ This technique can be useful if you have trouble properly stimulating a particular muscle group.

DISADVANTAGES

→ The instability increases the recruitment of muscles secondary to movement, which can tire prematurely. This can limit the development of the target muscle if the secondary muscles are too weak.
→ Performing the activation exercise first will decrease the load used for the traditional exercise; therefore, the gains in hypertrophy will be lower.

PRESCRIPTION TABLE

Load	Number of repetitions per set	Number of sets per exercise	Number of exercises per muscle group	Rest between sets
30%-40% + 70%-83%	6-12 + 6-12	2-4	1-3 supersets	2-3 minutes

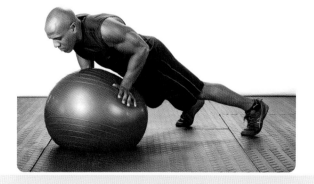

Technique #83

Perceived effort

■ ■ ■ □ □

Effect on hypertrophy

■ ■ ■ ■ □

Effect on strength and power

■ ■ ■ □ □

Effect on muscular endurance

■ ■ ■ □ □

Experience required

■ □ □

☑ Accumulation method

☐ Intensification method

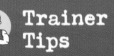

Trainer Tips

When using superbands with loads to add instability (e.g., at the ends of an Olympic bar), concentrate on performing the concentric phase explosively. This will increase the shaking movements at the end of the concentric phase and will require more effort from fast-twitch fibers.

POSTACTIVATION

 (S)

HOW DOES IT WORK?

This method is considered a superset. Complete, without rest, a traditional exercise followed by an activation (unstable) exercise (e.g., using a Swiss ball, BOSU ball, or balance disc).

Traditional exercise + activation exercise

ADVANTAGES

→ It helps to develop a high degree of stability.
→ Fatigue of fast-twitch fibers during unstable movement stimulates their hypertrophy.
→ This technique can be useful if you have trouble properly stimulating a particular muscle group.

DISADVANTAGES

→ The instability increases the recruitment of muscles secondary to movement, which can tire prematurely. This can limit the development of the target muscle if the secondary muscles are too weak.

PRESCRIPTION TABLE

Load	Number of repetitions per set	Number of sets per exercise	Number of exercises per muscle group	Rest between sets
70%-83% + 30%-40%	6-12 + 6-12	2-4	1-3 supersets	2-3 minutes

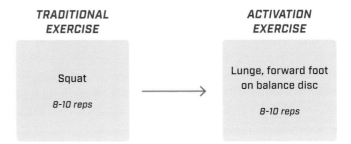

TRADITIONAL EXERCISE

Squat

8-10 reps

ACTIVATION EXERCISE

Lunge, forward foot on balance disc

8-10 reps

Technique #84

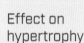

Perceived effort

⬛⬛⬛⬜⬜

Effect on
hypertrophy

⬛⬛⬛⬛⬜

Effect on strength
and power

⬛⬛⬛⬛⬜

Effect on muscular
endurance

⬛⬛⬛⬜⬜

Experience required

⬛⬛⬜

✓ Accumulation
method

☐ Intensification
method

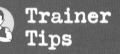

Trainer Tips

Try not to overexert yourself during the potentiation exercise in order to optimize performance during the traditional exercise. Be explosive and don't aim for max failure in the first exercise. Rather, aim for quality in each of your repetitions.

PREPOTENTIATION

HOW DOES IT WORK?

This method is considered a superset. Complete, without rest, a potentiation exercise followed by a traditional exercise. A potentiation exercise is simply an exercise done with power without a deceleration phase at the end of the concentric phase (e.g., long jump, box jump, or clap push-up). For example, a regular bench press is not a potentiation exercise, but if you perform it on the Smith machine and throw the bar with high speed at the end of the movement, it's a potentiation exercise.

Potentiation exercise + traditional exercise

ADVANTAGES

→ The introduction of a potentiation exercise requires more effort from fast-twitch fibers in order to generate enough power.

→ The resulting fatigue of fast-twitch fibers promotes larger gains in hypertrophy and power.

DISADVANTAGES

→ It is not suitable for beginners because it is necessary to develop some muscle strength before undertaking power exercises.

→ Performing the potentiation exercise first will decrease the load used for the traditional exercise; therefore, the gains in hypertrophy will be lower.

PRESCRIPTION TABLE

Load	Number of repetitions per set	Number of sets per exercise	Number of exercises per muscle group	Rest between sets
30%-50% + 70%-83%	6-8 + 6-12	2-4	1-3 supersets	2-3 minutes

POTENTIATION EXERCISE [30%-50%]		TRADITIONAL EXERCISE [70%-83%]
Clap push-up 6-8 reps	→	Dumbbell bench press 8-10 reps
Clap pull-up 6-8 reps	→	Bent-over dumbbell row 8-10 reps
Inverted row, alternating close- to wide-grip: 6-8 reps	→	Bent-over barbell row to chest 8-10 reps
Skater jump 6-8 reps	→	Front squat 8-10 reps

Technique #85

Perceived effort

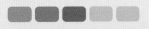

Effect on hypertrophy

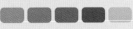

Effect on strength and power

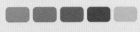

Effect on muscular endurance

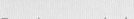

Experience required

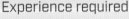

 ✓ Accumulation method

☐ Intensification method

Trainer Tips

If you find yourself losing speed during the power exercise, take 10-20 seconds of rest between exercises in order to maximize your effort during the second exercise.

 Ⓢ

POSTPOTENTIATION

HOW DOES IT WORK?

This method is considered a superset. Complete, without rest, a traditional exercise followed by a potentiation exercise (described in technique #84).

Traditional exercise + potentiation exercise

ADVANTAGES

→ It increases the recruitment of fast-twitch fibers during the traditional exercise.
→ It increases the stimulation of fast-twitch fibers by emphasizing power during the second exercise.
→ The resulting fatigue of fast-twitch fibers promotes larger gains in hypertrophy and power.

DISADVANTAGES

→ It is not suitable for beginners because it is necessary to develop some muscle strength before undertaking power exercises.

PRESCRIPTION TABLE

Load	Number of repetitions per set	Number of sets per exercise	Number of exercises per muscle group	Rest between sets
70%-83% + 30%-50%	6-12 + 6-8	2-4	1-3 supersets	2-3 minutes

TRADITIONAL EXERCISE (70%-83%)		POTENTIATION EXERCISE (30%-50%)
Hack squat 8-10 reps	→	Long jump 6-8 reps
Dumbbell bench press 8-10 reps	→	Superman push-up 6-8 reps
Leg extension 8-10 reps	→	Box jump 6-8 reps
Seated row 8-10 reps	→	Two-height pull-up 6-8 reps

Technique #86

Perceived effort

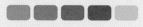

Effect on hypertrophy

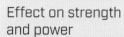

Effect on strength and power

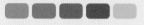

Effect on muscular endurance

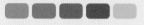

Experience required

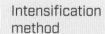

 ✓ Accumulation method

☐ Intensification method

Trainer Tips

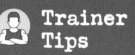

For trisets that target a single muscle group (and for better hypertrophy), refer to the following techniques: uniangular triset (technique #89), mechanical dropset (technique #88), and pre-post-fatigue (technique #87).

TRISET

HOW DOES IT WORK?

Perform 3 exercises one after the other with little to no rest between exercises. You can work 3 different muscles, a single muscle from three different angles, or a single muscle in the same position using different machines. The uniangular triset (technique #89) and mechanical dropset (technique #88) are variations of this method. Other variants can be created by combining different types of exercises (traditional, activation, potentiation, and metabolic).

ADVANTAGES

→ Performing 3 exercises for the same muscle group has great potential for gains in hypertrophy.

→ The high level of energy expended by combining exercises that recruit separate muscle groups can be very effective for fat loss.

DISADVANTAGES

→ This technique has a high cardiovascular demand; if this is a limiting factor, add 15-30 seconds of rest between exercises.

PRESCRIPTION TABLE

Load	Number of repetitions per set	Number of sets per exercise	Number of exercises per muscle group	Rest between sets
70%-83%	6-12 + 6-12 + 6-12	2-4	1-3 trisets	2-3 minutes

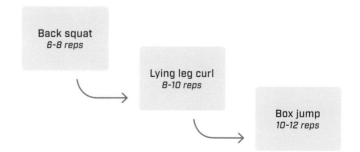

Back squat
6-8 reps

Lying leg curl
8-10 reps

Box jump
10-12 reps

Technique #87

Perceived effort

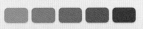

Effect on hypertrophy

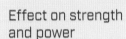

Effect on strength and power

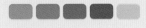

Effect on muscular endurance

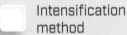

Experience required

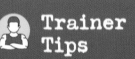

 ✓ Accumulation method

☐ Intensification method

Trainer Tips

More advanced individuals may choose a multijoint movement and then decide to perform two pre-post-fatigue techniques for the same agonist muscle groups while maintaining a similar basis of movement. For example, for the bench press, you might choose to isolate either the pecs, triceps, or shoulders.

PRE-POST-FATIGUE

HOW DOES IT WORK?

This method is considered a triset. Complete 3 consecutive exercises for the same muscle or for agonist muscles with no rest between exercises. Execute the movements in the following order: isolation movement, then multijoint movement, and finally another isolation movement. The isolation exercises can be applied in two ways: by targeting the same muscle group twice or by targeting two different muscle groups.

Isolation exercise + multijoint exercise + isolation exercise

ADVANTAGES

→ It isolates more than one muscle group in order to promote their development.

→ This is one of the most difficult but effective hypertrophy methods.

DISADVANTAGES

→ This technique has a high cardiovascular demand; if this is a limiting factor, add 15-30 seconds of rest between exercises.

PRESCRIPTION TABLE

Load	Number of repetitions per set	Number of sets per exercise	Number of exercises per muscle group	Rest between sets
70%-83%	6-12 + 6-12 + 6-12	2-4	1-2 trisets	2-3 minutes

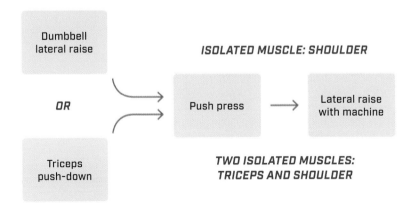

ISOLATED MUSCLE: SHOULDER

TWO ISOLATED MUSCLES: TRICEPS AND SHOULDER

Technique #88

Perceived effort

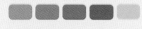

Effect on hypertrophy

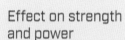

Effect on strength and power

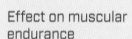

Effect on muscular endurance

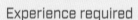

Experience required

✓ Accumulation method

☐ Intensification method

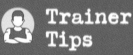

Trainer Tips

Choose 3 exercises. Consider which exercise is your strongest and place it at the end, and begin with your weakest exercise. For example, if seated military press is your weakest exercise, followed by incline bench press, then flat bench press, perform them in this order.

MECHANICAL DROPSET

HOW DOES IT WORK?

This technique uses 3 movements that target the same muscle group according to their particular biomechanical advantage. They are performed from the weakest to the strongest and use the same load. Perform 6-12 reps of the first exercise, then as many reps as possible of the following 2 exercises.

ADVANTAGES

→ It has a great potential for hypertrophy by varying the working angle.

→ It is very easy to use.

DISADVANTAGES

→ It requires at least 6 months of experience because several muscle patterns must have already been developed.

→ This technique has a high cardiovascular demand; if this is a limiting factor, add 15-30 seconds of rest between exercises.

PRESCRIPTION TABLE

Load	Number of repetitions per set	Number of sets per exercise	Number of exercises per muscle group	Rest between sets
70%-83%	6-12 + max + max	2-4	3-6	2-3 minutes

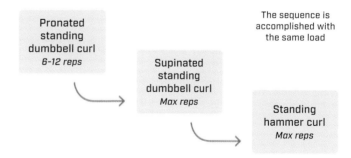

The sequence is accomplished with the same load

Pronated standing dumbbell curl
6-12 reps

Supinated standing dumbbell curl
Max reps

Standing hammer curl
Max reps

Technique #89

Perceived effort

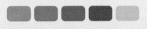

Effect on hypertrophy

Effect on strength and power

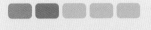

Effect on muscular endurance

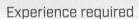

Experience required

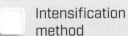

✓ Accumulation method

☐ Intensification method

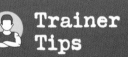

Trainer Tips

For each exercise, you can use a lighter load with which you reach failure only once (e.g., at the end of the triset) or a heavier load with which you reach failure three times (e.g., 5RM dumbbell bench press, 5RM barbell bench press, 5RM push-ups).

UNIANGULAR TRISET

HOW DOES IT WORK?

The uniangular triset involves using 3 slightly different exercises to target the same muscle group. There are two ways to use this method:

1. by varying factors such as starting position, equipment, grip width, or range of motion; or

2. by choosing different exercises that work the same muscle without changing the angle of work. The mechanical dropset (technique #88) and the 21 (technique #90) are examples of uniangular triset options.

ADVANTAGES

→ This technique maximizes the development of a motor pattern by using the same angle of work for all 3 exercises.

→ It can be applied to any exercise.

DISADVANTAGES

→ It may require several pieces of equipment.

PRESCRIPTION TABLE

Load	Number of repetitions per set	Number of sets per exercise	Number of exercises per muscle group	Rest between sets
70%-83%	5-12 + 5-12 + 5-12	2-4	1-2 trisets	2-3 minutes

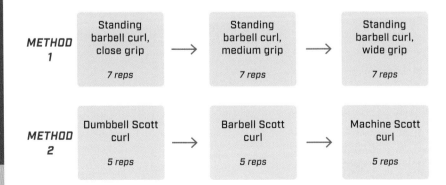

Technique #90

Perceived effort

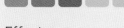

Effect on hypertrophy

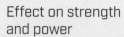

Effect on strength and power

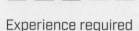

Effect on muscular endurance

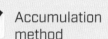

Experience required

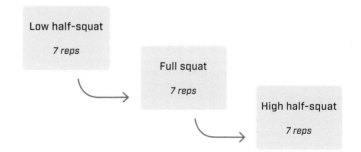

✓ Accumulation method

☐ Intensification method

Trainer Tips

The use of cables or machines to accomplish this training technique is a great way to maintain continuous tension in the muscle. Weights and free bars, through gravity, usually decrease the tension at the beginning or at the end of movement.

THE 21

Ⓢ

HOW DOES IT WORK?

This method is considered a triset and is the most well-known form of uniangular triset (technique #89). You will complete, without rest, a traditional exercise divided into three distinct ranges of motion, performing 7 repetitions at each range.

ADVANTAGES

→ It can be applied to any exercise.

→ It is suitable for beginners because the load used is light.

→ In multijoint exercises, it allows localization of the effort on a muscle group, particularly in the first phase (e.g., pectorals in bench press or glutes in squat).

DISADVANTAGES

→ None.

PRESCRIPTION TABLE

Load	Number of repetitions per set	Number of sets per exercise	Number of exercises per muscle group	Rest between sets
60%-65%	7 + 7 + 7	2-4	1-3 trisets	1-2 minutes

Low half-squat
7 reps

Full squat
7 reps

High half-squat
7 reps

Technique #91

Perceived effort

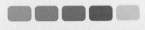

Effect on hypertrophy

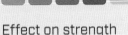

Effect on strength and power

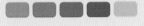

Effect on muscular endurance

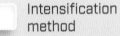

Experience required

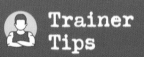

✓ Accumulation method

☐ Intensification method

Trainer Tips

Because you will perform the metabolic exercise to muscular fatigue, always keep in mind that your technique must be perfect. If you perform a push, pull, or raise motion, keep your torso straight without any rotation and your chest out.

GIANT ORGANIC SET 1

HOW DOES IT WORK?

This method is considered a triset. Perform, without rest, an activation exercise, followed by a traditional exercise, then a metabolic exercise for the same muscle group.

Activation exercise + traditional exercise + metabolic exercise

ADVANTAGES

→ It can be used for hypertrophy and fat loss.
→ It can be very effective at stimulating underworked muscle groups.

DISADVANTAGES

→ This technique is very physically demanding. Start by doing superset techniques that introduce activation and metabolic exercises until you are comfortable performing them.

PRESCRIPTION TABLE

Load	Number of repetitions or seconds per set	Number of sets per exercise	Number of exercises per muscle group	Rest between sets
60%-83% + 60%-83% + 20%-30%	6-12 reps + 6-15 reps + 20-40 seconds	2-4	1-3 trisets	2-3 minutes

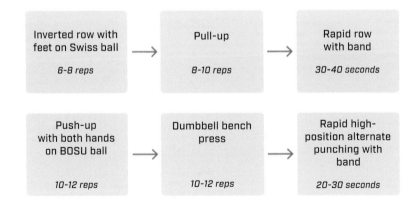

| Inverted row with feet on Swiss ball | | Pull-up | | Rapid row with band |
| 6-8 reps | → | 8-10 reps | → | 30-40 seconds |

| Push-up with both hands on BOSU ball | | Dumbbell bench press | | Rapid high-position alternate punching with band |
| 10-12 reps | → | 10-12 reps | → | 20-30 seconds |

Technique #92

Perceived effort

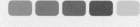

Effect on hypertrophy

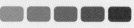

Effect on strength and power

Effect on muscular endurance

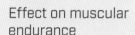

Experience required

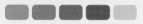

☑ Accumulation method

☐ Intensification method

Trainer Tips

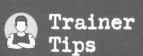

All giant organic set techniques are a great tool to increase your muscular capacity. You will increase your hypertrophy and your endurance. Just give them a try!

GIANT ORGANIC SET 2

HOW DOES IT WORK?

This method is considered a triset. Perform, without rest, a traditional exercise, followed by an activation exercise, then a metabolic exercise for the same muscle group.

Traditional exercise + activation exercise + metabolic exercise

ADVANTAGES

→ It can be used for hypertrophy and fat loss.

→ Of all the giant organic sets, this one will give you the best results in terms of body composition.

→ Performing the traditional exercise first allows you to use heavier loads and achieve higher intensity than the giant organic set 1 (technique #91) or 3 (technique #93).

DISADVANTAGES

→ This technique is very physically demanding. Start by doing superset techniques that introduce activation and metabolic exercises until you are comfortable performing them.

PRESCRIPTION TABLE

Load	Number of repetitions or seconds per set	Number of sets per exercise	Number of exercises per muscle group	Rest between sets
60%-83% + 60%-83% + 20%-30%	6-15 reps + 6-12 reps + 20-40 seconds	2-4	1-3 trisets	2-3 minutes

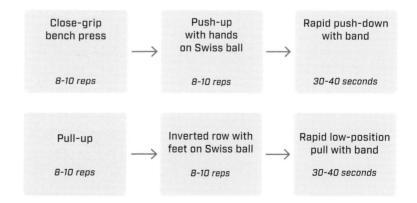

Technique #93

Perceived effort

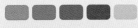

Effect on hypertrophy

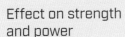

Effect on strength and power

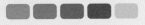

Effect on muscular endurance

Experience required

✓ Accumulation method

☐ Intensification method

GIANT ORGANIC SET 3 Ⓢ

HOW DOES IT WORK?

This method is considered a triset. Perform, without rest, a potentiation exercise, followed by a traditional exercise, then a metabolic exercise for the same muscle group.

Potentiation exercise + traditional exercise + metabolic exercise

ADVANTAGES

→ It can be used for hypertrophy and fat loss.
→ It is useful for athletes because it simulates the movements used in various sports (explosive acceleration, traditional defensive movements, and metabolic movements to improve anaerobic capacity).

DISADVANTAGES

→ This technique is very physically demanding. Start by doing superset techniques that introduce potentiation and metabolic exercises until you are comfortable performing them.

PRESCRIPTION TABLE

Load	Number of repetitions or seconds per set	Number of sets per exercise	Number of exercises per muscle group	Rest between sets
30%-50% + 65%-80% + 20%-30%	4-10 reps + 6-15 reps + 20-40 seconds	2-4	1-3 trisets	2-3 minutes

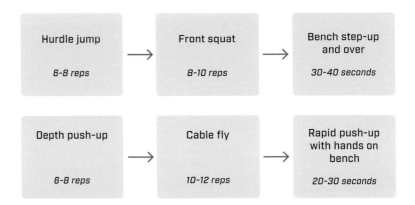

Technique #94

Perceived effort

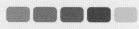

Effect on hypertrophy

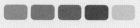

Effect on strength and power

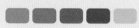

Effect on muscular endurance

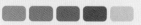

Experience required

✓ Accumulation method

☐ Intensification method

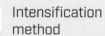
GIANT ORGANIC SET 4

HOW DOES IT WORK?

This method is considered a triset. Perform, without rest, a traditional exercise, followed by a potentiation exercise, then a metabolic exercise for the same muscle group.

Traditional exercise + potentiation exercise + metabolic exercise

ADVANTAGES

→ It can be used for hypertrophy and fat loss.

→ It is useful for athletes because it simulates the movements used in various sports (traditional defensive movements, explosive acceleration, and metabolic movements to improve anaerobic capacity).

DISADVANTAGES

→ This technique is very physically demanding. Start by doing superset techniques that introduce potentiation and metabolic exercises until you are comfortable performing them.

PRESCRIPTION TABLE

Load	Number of repetitions or seconds per set	Number of sets per exercise	Number of exercises per muscle group	Rest between sets
65%–80% + 30%–50% + 20%–30%	6-15 reps + 4-10 reps + 20-40 seconds	2-4	1-3 trisets	2-5 minutes

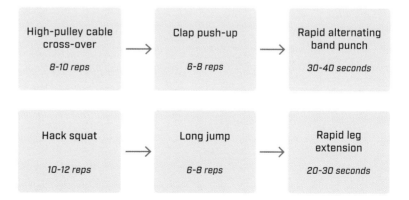

Technique #95

Perceived effort

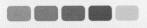

Effect on
hypertrophy

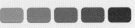

Effect on strength
and power

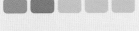

Effect on muscular
endurance

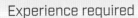

Experience required

- ✓ Accumulation
  method
- ☐ Intensification
  method

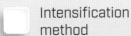

Trainer Tips

This technique is one of my favorite trisets for building muscle mass. It creates great muscular fatigue and causes rapid gains. This technique should not be underestimated!

GIANT ORGANIC SET 5

HOW DOES IT WORK?

This method is considered a triset. Perform, without rest, a traditional multijoint exercise, followed by a traditional isolation exercise, then a metabolic exercise for the same muscle group.

Multijoint exercise + isolation exercise + metabolic exercise

ADVANTAGES

→ It can be used for hypertrophy and fat loss.
→ Of all the giant organic sets, this one is the best for muscle growth because heavier loads can be used when combining traditional exercises.

DISADVANTAGES

→ This technique is very physically demanding. Start by doing superset techniques that introduce metabolic exercises until you are comfortable performing them.

PRESCRIPTION TABLE

Load	Number of repetitions or seconds per set	Number of sets per exercise	Number of exercises per muscle group	Rest between sets
65%-80% + 65%-80% + 20%-30%	6-15 reps + 6-15 reps + 20-40 seconds	2-4	1-3 trisets	2-3 minutes

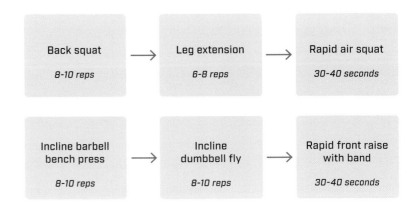

Technique #96

Perceived effort

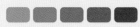

Effect on
hypertrophy

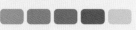

Effect on strength
and power

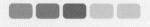

Effect on muscular
endurance

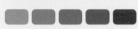

Experience required

✓ Accumulation
method

☐ Intensification
method

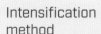

FULL GIANT ORGANIC SET

HOW DOES IT WORK?

This method is part of the circuit training category. Perform, without rest, a potentiation exercise, followed by a traditional exercise, then an activation exercise, and finally a metabolic exercise.

Potentiation exercise + traditional exercise + activation exercise + metabolic exercise

ADVANTAGES

→ Of all the giant organic sets, this one is the best for fat loss and for improving muscular anaerobic capacity.

DISADVANTAGES

→ This technique is very physically demanding. Start by doing superset techniques that introduce potentiation, activation, and metabolic exercises until you are comfortable performing them.

→ It should be performed only by individuals with at least 1-2 years of strength training experience.

PRESCRIPTION TABLE

Load	Number of repetition or seconds per set	Number of sets per exercise	Number of exercises per muscle group	Rest between sets
30%-50% + 65%-83% + 65%-83% + 20%-30%	4-10 reps + 6-15 reps + 6-15 reps + 20-40 seconds	2-4	1-3 circuits	2-3 minutes

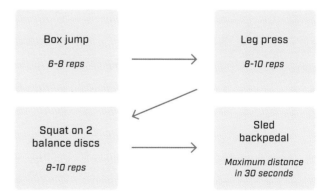

Box jump — 6-8 reps → Leg press — 8-10 reps

Squat on 2 balance discs — 8-10 reps → Sled backpedal — Maximum distance in 30 seconds

Technique #97

Perceived effort

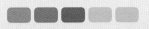

Effect on hypertrophy

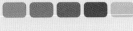

Effect on strength and power

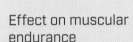

Effect on muscular endurance

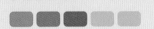

Experience required

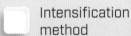

 ✓ Accumulation method

☐ Intensification method

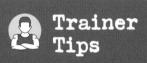

Trainer Tips

A good benchmark for this technique is to maintain the isometric hold for 10-15 seconds. If you exceed this time, it means your load is too light.

 Ⓢ

MAXIMAL FATIGUE

HOW DOES IT WORK?

Perform a regular set until muscle failure, then, after the last rep, maintain the load isometrically in a fully or semi-contracted position for as long as possible. For example, at the end of a dumbbell bench press, you will hold the weights with your elbows at 90 degrees (semi-contracted position). At the end of a bent-over barbell row, you will hold the bar in contact with your abdominals (fully contracted position).

ADVANTAGES

→ It increases the time under tension compared to a conventional set.
→ It uses isometric contraction, during which the muscle exerts more force, thus creating greater fatigue.

DISADVANTAGES

→ A spotter is required for exercises such as the bench press and back or front squats.

PRESCRIPTION TABLE

Load	Number of repetitions or seconds per set	Number of sets per exercise	Number of exercises per muscle group	Rest between sets
65%-83%	6-15 + max time isometric hold	2-5	2-3	1-2 minutes

Dumbbell lateral raise		Hold shoulders at 90 degrees at the end of the set for as long as possible

Technique #98

Perceived effort

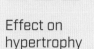

Effect on hypertrophy

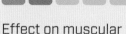

Effect on strength and power

Effect on muscular endurance

Experience required

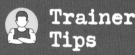

☑ Accumulation method

☐ Intensification method

POSTFATIGUE ISOMETRIC

HOW DOES IT WORK?

This technique, which uses isometric contractions after prefatiguing the muscle, is a maximal fatigue technique distributed throughout the entire range of motion. After reaching concentric fatigue for a set, perform 3 isometric pauses of 6 seconds each at three different points in the range of motion. This method is more demanding than maximal fatigue (technique #97) because it works multiple angles.

ADVANTAGES

→ It uses isometric work to extend the duration and intensity of a conventional set in which concentric fatigue has already been reached.

→ It is easy to use with exercises that utilize machines.

DISADVANTAGES

→ It requires a spotter or safety guards for barbell exercises (bench press, back squat, etc.).

PRESCRIPTION TABLE

Load	Number of repetitions or seconds per set	Number of sets per exercise	Number of exercises per muscle group	Rest between sets
70%-83%	6-12 reps + 6 seconds on each of 3 different positions	2-4	1-4	2-3 minutes

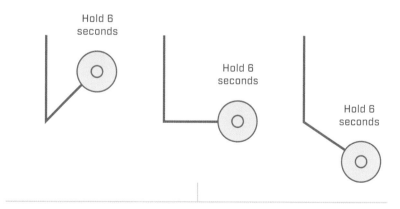

Last eccentric repetition of standing barbell curl

Technique #99

Perceived effort

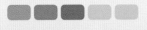

Effect on hypertrophy

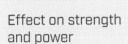

Effect on strength and power

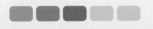

Effect on muscular endurance

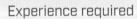

Experience required

✓ Accumulation method

☐ Intensification method

Trainer Tips

During your extra reps, aim for a maximum of half the number of reps already completed. If you can do more, then your starting load is too light.

REST-PAUSE

Ⓢ

HOW DOES IT WORK?

Do 6-12 max reps, then rest for 10-15 seconds before doing as many reps as possible with the same load (for large muscles) or a lighter load (for smaller muscles). This technique is also known as an extended set.

ADVANTAGES

→ Simply adding this technique to an exercise lets you do more work using a given load, increasing the volume of the workout. An easy way to maximize your workout!

DISADVANTAGES

→ None.

PRESCRIPTION TABLE

Load	Number of repetitions per set	Number of sets per exercise	Number of exercises per muscle group	Rest between sets
70%-83%	6-12 + 1-6	2-4	1-4	2-3 minutes

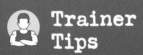

Seated row with V bar		Seated row with V bar
8-10 reps	**+**	+ 3 reps
	Rest 10-15 seconds	

Technique #100

Perceived effort

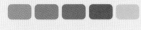

Effect on hypertrophy

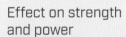

Effect on strength and power

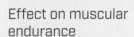

Effect on muscular endurance

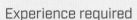

Experience required

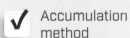

✓ Accumulation method

☐ Intensification method

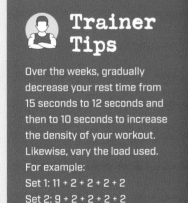

Trainer Tips

Over the weeks, gradually decrease your rest time from 15 seconds to 12 seconds and then to 10 seconds to increase the density of your workout. Likewise, vary the load used.
For example:
Set 1: 11 + 2 + 2 + 2 + 2
Set 2: 9 + 2 + 2 + 2 + 2
Set 3: 7 + 2 + 2 + 2 + 2

EXTENDED 7'S

HOW DOES IT WORK?

Using a load equal to your 7RM, complete multiple sets of 13-15 reps. Each set should consist of a first block of 7 reps, followed by clusters of 2, separated by 10-15 seconds of rest until you achieve the desired number of reps.

ADVANTAGES

→ This technique is very effective for hypertrophy because it uses high-intensity loads.
→ Repeating small blocks of reps punctuated by rest periods leads to a massive influx of blood in the muscle. This increase in internal pressure, coupled with nutrient-rich blood (especially if protein is ingested before the workout) and the fatigue of fast-twitch fibers, results in greater muscular hypertrophy.

DISADVANTAGES

→ This is a very demanding method that should be used sparingly.

PRESCRIPTION TABLE

Load	Number of repetitions per set	Number of sets per exercise	Number of exercises per muscle group	Rest between sets
80%	7 + 2 + 2 + 2 [+ 2]	2-4	1-4	2-3 minutes

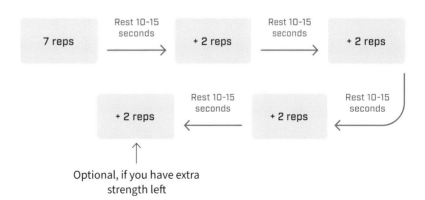

Optional, if you have extra strength left

Technique #101

Perceived effort

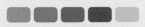

Effect on hypertrophy

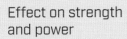

Effect on strength and power

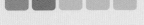

Effect on muscular endurance

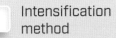

Experience required

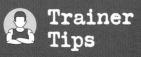

✓ Accumulation method

☐ Intensification method

🧑 Trainer Tips

If you are able to accomplish more than 1 rep in the last sequence, increase the load by 2.5-5 kg the next workout. If you can only complete 1 repetition, then the selected weight is adequate.

ALTERNATING REST-PAUSE

HOW DOES IT WORK?

This method is a variation of the rest-pause (technique #99) using unilateral exercises. When you work on one side, the other will be at rest. Using a load that allows you to complete 6-8 reps, you will perform the following sequence by alternating each of your arms or legs: 3, 3, 3, 2, 2, 1. By the end, you will have completed 14 repetitions per side with a load that only allows you to do 6-8 repetitions.

ADVANTAGES

→ It increases the density of your workout.
→ It is easy to use with any exercise.
→ It provides muscle pump quickly.
→ It is ideal when you do not have a lot of time to train.

DISADVANTAGES

→ It can be monotonous when done over several weeks in a row.

PRESCRIPTION TABLE

Load	Number of repetitions per set	Number of sets per exercise	Number of exercises per muscle group	Rest between sets
79%-83%	3 + 3 + 3 + 2 + 2 + 1	2-4	1-5	1-2 minutes

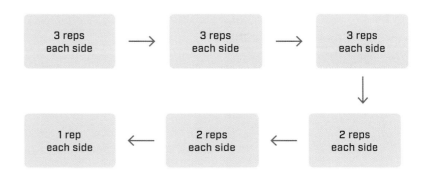

Technique #102

Perceived effort

Effect on hypertrophy

Effect on strength and power

Effect on muscular endurance

Experience required

✓ Accumulation method

☐ Intensification method

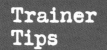

Trainer Tips

I like to use this basic technique to emphasize the importance of time spent under strain. Those of my clients who like to do 10 reps in less than 10 seconds find it a bit hard to grasp!

SUPER SLOW REPS 5-5

HOW DOES IT WORK?
Using a load equal to your 12RM (70%), do 6 reps with a slow tempo of 5 seconds in the eccentric phase and 5 seconds in the concentric phase.

ADVANTAGES
→ The momentum generated by doing reps too quickly prevents the neuromuscular system from receiving enough stimulation for optimal strength gains. This technique increases time under tension by slowing the movement.
→ Slow, high-intensity training is ideal for increasing the concentrations of glycogen, phosphagens, and several anaerobic metabolism enzymes.

DISADVANTAGES
→ It requires great concentration in order to count the time under tension in each phase of the movement.

PRESCRIPTION TABLE

Load	Number of repetitions per set	Number of sets per exercise	Number of exercises per muscle group	Rest between sets
70%	6	2-5	2-3	1-2 minutes

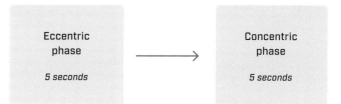

Eccentric phase

5 seconds

→

Concentric phase

5 seconds

Technique #103

Perceived effort

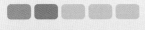

Effect on
hypertrophy

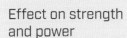

Effect on strength
and power

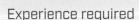

Effect on muscular
endurance

Experience required

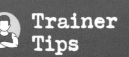

✓ Accumulation
method

☐ Intensification
method

SUPER SLOW REPS 10-4

HOW DOES IT WORK?

Using a load equal to your 12RM (70%), do 4-5 reps with a slow tempo of 10 seconds in the eccentric phase and 4 seconds in the concentric phase.

ADVANTAGES

→ The momentum generated by doing reps too quickly prevents the neuromuscular system from receiving enough stimulation for optimal strength gains. This technique increases time under tension by slowing the movement.

→ Slow, high-intensity training is ideal for increasing the concentrations of glycogen, phosphagens, and several anaerobic metabolism enzymes.

→ Because the eccentric phase causes more muscular damage than the concentric, this technique can have better hypertrophy results than super slow reps 5-5 (technique #102).

DISADVANTAGES

→ It requires great concentration in order to count the time under tension in each phase of the movement.

PRESCRIPTION TABLE

Load	Number of repetitions per set	Number of sets per exercise	Number of exercises per muscle group	Rest between sets
70%	4-5	2-5	2-3	1-2 minutes

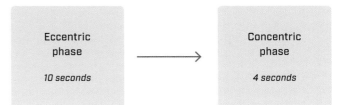

Technique #104

Perceived effort

■ ■ ■ ■ ■

Effect on
hypertrophy

■ ■ ■ ■ ■

Effect on strength
and power

■ ■ ■ ■ ■

Effect on muscular
endurance

■ ■ ■ ■ ■

Experience required

■ ■ ■

✓ Accumulation
method

☐ Intensification
method

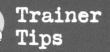
Trainer Tips

Always control your load at a constant speed. If your speed in the eccentric phase increases during negative reps, it may be time to end the set. If you continue, you risk injury.

NEGATIVE REPS

HOW DOES IT WORK?

At the end of a set performed to failure, do 1-3 additional reps, this time performing only the eccentric phase. Each eccentric phase should last 4-6 seconds. You will need the help of a partner to complete the concentric phase of the additional reps.

ADVANTAGES

→ Unlike most techniques, doing negative reps lets you reach both concentric and eccentric muscle failure.

→ Eccentric contractions are more damaging to the muscle than concentric contractions. Negative reps allow for eccentric failure, thus increasing muscle breakdown, which is great for hypertrophy.

→ Negative training leads to higher levels of growth hormone release.[24]

DISADVANTAGES

→ It requires a partner to perform the concentric phase of the additional repetitions.

PRESCRIPTION TABLE

Load	Number of repetitions per set	Number of sets per exercise	Number of exercises per muscle group	Rest between sets
70%-83%	6-12 + 1-3 additional negative reps	2-5	1-3	1-3 minutes

Standing
barbell curl

8-10 reps

Standing
barbell curl

+ 1-3 reps in 4-6 seconds each (eccentric phase only)

With partner assistance
(concentric phase)

Technique #105

Perceived effort

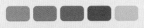

Effect on hypertrophy

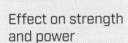

Effect on strength and power

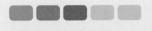

Effect on muscular endurance

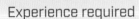

Experience required

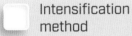

 ✓ Accumulation method

☐ Intensification method

Trainer Tips

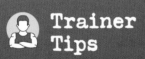

Use your imagination to safely add resistance. For example:
Pull-up: Pulling down on the feet
Bench press: Pushing down on the bar

SUPER NEGATIVE REPS

HOW DOES IT WORK?

At the end of a set performed to failure, do 2-3 additional reps, this time performing only the eccentric phase. Each eccentric phase should last 4-6 seconds, during which your partner will apply additional resistance. Your partner will need to assist you during the concentric phase of the additional reps.

ADVANTAGES

→ This technique is used to completely exhaust eccentric strength after reaching the threshold of concentric fatigue.
→ It increases microtears in the muscle by overloading and emphasizing the eccentric phase, which can lead to gains in hypertrophy.
→ Negative training leads to higher levels of growth hormone release.[24]

DISADVANTAGES

→ You will need a partner to add eccentric resistance during the additional reps.

PRESCRIPTION TABLE

Load	Number of repetitions per set	Number of sets per exercise	Number of exercises per muscle group	Rest between sets
70%-83%	6-12 + 2-3 additional reps	2-5	1-3	2-3 minutes

Barbell bench press

8-10 reps

Barbell bench press with additional resistance

+ 2-3 reps in 4-6 seconds each (eccentric phase only)

With partner assistance (concentric phase)

Technique #106

Perceived effort

■■□□□

Effect on
hypertrophy

■■■□□

Effect on strength
and power

■■□□□

Effect on muscular
endurance

■■■□□

Experience required

■□□

☑ Accumulation
method

☐ Intensification
method

Trainer Tips

If you find these prescriptive elements easy, do the same number of reps, but increase the amount of time spent in the eccentric phase up to 14 seconds per repetition.

SUPER SLOW ECCENTRIC REPS

HOW DOES IT WORK?

This technique is similar to the eccentric–concentric contrast (technique #138), but without a pause at the end of the movement. Control the eccentric phase for 4-14 seconds, depending on the load, then lift explosively during the concentric phase.

ADVANTAGES

→ This technique lets you focus on the eccentric part of a movement. It is also very effective at recruiting fast-twitch fibers, allowing for gains in hypertrophy using loads greater than 70% of your 1RM.

→ Lighter loads help develop endurance and hypertrophy of slow-twitch fibers (type I).

DISADVANTAGES

→ None.

PRESCRIPTION TABLE

Load	Number of repetitions per set	Number of sets per exercise	Number of exercises per muscle group	Rest between sets
60%-85%	1-5	3-6	1-3	1-2 minutes

The following is the recommended prescription based on your 1RM (%):

→ **60%:** 14 seconds in eccentric for 3-5 reps
→ **65%:** 12 seconds in eccentric for 3-5 reps
→ **70%:** 10 seconds in eccentric for 3-5 reps
→ **75%:** 8 seconds in eccentric for 3-5 reps
→ **80%:** 6 seconds in eccentric for 2-4 reps
→ **85%:** 4 seconds in eccentric for 2-4 reps

Technique #107

Perceived effort

▪▪▪▪▫

Effect on hypertrophy

▪▪▪▪▫

Effect on strength and power

▪▫▫▫▫

Effect on muscular endurance

▪▪▪▫▫

Experience required

▪▪▫

 ✓ Accumulation method

☐ Intensification method

Trainer Tips

For an advanced version, ask your partner to place light pressure with their hands on the bar or the free weights during the eccentric phase, then remove their hands during the concentric phase. That way, you can do fewer repetitions with higher intensity (e.g., if you do 6 repetitions instead of 9, you will begin with an eccentric of 6 seconds).

REGRESSIVE ECCENTRIC REPS

Ⓢ

HOW DOES IT WORK?

Perform your repetitions with a shorter and shorter eccentric phase. You start with a first repetition lasting 10 seconds (1 second in concentric and 9 seconds in eccentric), followed by a second repetition lasting 9 seconds (1 second in concentric and 8 seconds in eccentric), and continue the pattern until the last repetition, which will be accomplished in 1 second each in the eccentric and concentric phases. A set will last 54 seconds.

ADVANTAGES

→ It increases the time under tension in the eccentric phase.
→ The low velocity used during the eccentric phase can improve movement technique.

DISADVANTAGES

→ None.

PRESCRIPTION TABLE

Load	Number of repetitions per set	Number of sets per exercise	Number of exercises per muscle group	Rest between sets
50%-65%	9	2-4	1-3	1-2 minutes

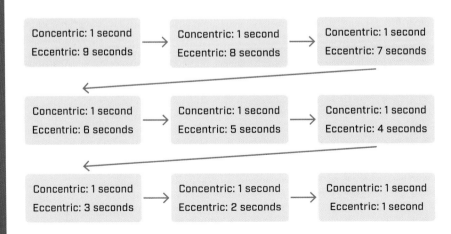

Technique #108

Perceived effort

■■□□□

Effect on
hypertrophy

■■■□□

Effect on strength
and power

■■□□□

Effect on muscular
endurance

■■□□□

Experience required

■■■

✓ Accumulation
method

☐ Intensification
method

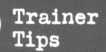

Trainer Tips

Use the half-rep to target a specific muscle or weakness. For example, if you wanted to focus on your pecs during a bench press, you would perform a low double contraction. However, if you wanted to work your triceps more, you would opt for a high double contraction.

DOUBLE CONTRACTION

HOW DOES IT WORK?

This technique involves performing a full movement followed by a partial rep (1/4 or 1/2) of the same movement. You can do this partial rep using the lower part (low double contraction) or the upper part (high double contraction) of the movement.

ADVANTAGES

→ This method lets you focus on weaker muscle groups in a single set.

→ It increases the total time under tension, leading to better muscle gains.

→ It can be accomplished with relatively heavy loads.

DISADVANTAGES

→ None.

PRESCRIPTION TABLE

Load	Number of repetitions per set	Number of sets per exercise	Number of exercises per muscle group	Rest between sets
70%-83%	6-12	2-5	1-2	2-3 minutes

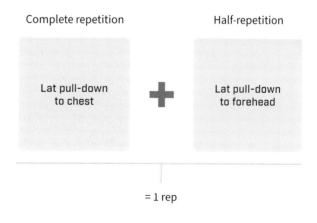

Complete repetition   Half-repetition

Lat pull-down to chest   +   Lat pull-down to forehead

= 1 rep

Perceived effort

Effect on
hypertrophy

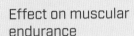

Effect on strength
and power

Effect on muscular
endurance

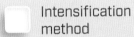

Experience required

 ✓ Accumulation
method

☐ Intensification
method

HYPERTROPHY CIRCUIT

HOW DOES IT WORK?

This technique combines different exercises that target the same muscle group at each set change. No exercise may be performed in 2 consecutive sets. For example, you can do 12 sets with 12 different exercises (1 set/exercise) or you can choose 4 exercises and alternate them for 12 total sets (3 sets/exercise). Apply a new technique from this book on each set.

ADVANTAGES

→ This method is less monotonous than a traditional workout because you are moving from one exercise to another with each set.
→ It allows you to use several training techniques for the same exercise.

DISADVANTAGES

→ You should have at least 1 or 2 years of training experience in order to have an adequate selection of exercises and knowledge of your loads.

PRESCRIPTION TABLE

Load	Number of repetitions per set	Number of sets per exercise	Number of exercises per muscle group	Rest between sets
70%-83%	6-12	1-3	4-12	2-3 minutes

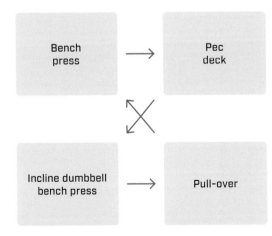

Rest between exercises: 2 minutes

Set 1:
Double contraction
(technique #108)
Set 2:
Maximal fatigue
(technique #97)
Set 3:
Holistic set
(technique #76)

Technique #110

Perceived effort

■ ■ ■ □ □

Effect on hypertrophy

■ ■ ■ □ □

Effect on strength and power

■ □ □ □ □

Effect on muscular endurance

■ ■ ■ □ □

Experience required

■ □ □

☑ Accumulation method

☐ Intensification method

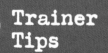

Trainer Tips

It is essential to use the correct load, which is the equivalent of a 12RM-13RM. Use the first set (without counting it) to determine your true 12RM-13RM. Once determined, note the load in your program so that you do not need to repeat this step in the second week of training.

4 × 10 PER MINUTE

HOW DOES IT WORK?

Using a load equal to your 12RM-13RM, perform 10 reps per set, with only 1 minute of rest between sets.

ADVANTAGES

→ This technique is great if you are short on time—in only 6 minutes, you will have completed your first exercise!

→ It is mainly used for hypertrophy because it increases the density (amount of work per time unit) of your workout.

DISADVANTAGES

→ The reps are submaximal in the first sets, but quickly become closer to maximal in the last sets given that there is little rest time.

PRESCRIPTION TABLE

Load	Number of repetitions per set	Number of sets per exercise	Number of exercises per muscle group	Rest between sets
70%	10	4	1-4	1 minute

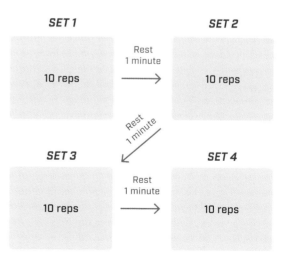

Technique #111

Perceived effort

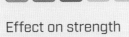

Effect on
hypertrophy

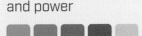

Effect on strength
and power

Effect on muscular
endurance

Experience required

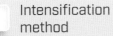

✓ Accumulation
method

☐ Intensification
method

OVERLOAD IN BIG WAVES

HOW DOES IT WORK?

Complete 2-3 waves, each wave consisting of 2-3 sets of 3-12 reps each. Decrease your reps by 2 throughout the wave, and try to increase the load by 1% for each new wave. For example:

Example 1 (6 sets): 10 + 8 + 6 + 10 + 8 + 6 (2 waves)

Example 2 (6 sets): 12 + 10 + 8 + 12 + 10 + 8 (2 waves)

Example 3 (9 sets): 11 + 9 + 7 + 11 + 9 + 7 + 11 + 9 + 7 (3 waves)

ADVANTAGES

→ It uses post-tetanic potentiation by adding a bit more weight to the 4th and 7th sets.

→ This potentiation maintains the activation of fast-twitch fibers throughout the lift.

DISADVANTAGES

→ The higher number of sets make this technique very time consuming.

PRESCRIPTION TABLE

Load	Number of repetitions per set	Number of sets per exercise	Number of exercises per muscle group	Rest between sets
70%-85%	3-12	6 or 9	1	2-3 minutes

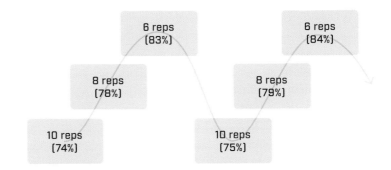

Technique #112

Perceived effort

▦ ▦ ▦ ▢ ▢

Effect on hypertrophy

▦ ▦ ▦ ▢ ▢

Effect on strength and power

▦ ▦ ▢ ▢ ▢

Effect on muscular endurance

▦ ▦ ▦ ▢ ▢

Experience required

▦ ▢ ▢

- ✓ Accumulation method
- ☐ Intensification method

👤 Trainer Tips

You can vary the repetitions for each stage. For example, you could use the following steps to increase strength with a combination of sets in hypertrophy (>6 reps) and sets in strength gains (<6 reps):

1. Stage 8RM-4RM
   [3 × 8RM + 2 × 4RM]
2. Stage 7RM-3RM
   [3 × 7RM + 2 × 3RM]
3. Stage 6RM-2RM
   [3 × 6RM + 2 × 2RM]
4. Stage 5RM-1RM
   [3 × 5RM + 2 × 1RM]

STAGE 10RM-6RM

HOW DOES IT WORK?

Complete 3 consecutive sets at 10RM and 2 consecutive sets at 6RM. Each set is separated by 2-3 minutes of rest and you can vary the number of reps in each stage. This technique must be done before stage 6RM-10RM (technique #113).

ADVANTAGES

→ It lets you add progressive strength work after completing sets at lower intensity.
→ Performing 5 sets of the same exercise may improve movement technique.

DISADVANTAGES

→ The number of exercises for a particular muscle group may be limited in order to moderate the volume of this technique.

PRESCRIPTION TABLE

Load	Number of repetitions per set	Number of sets per exercise	Number of exercises per muscle group	Rest between sets
74%, 83%	10, 6	5	1-4	2-3 minutes

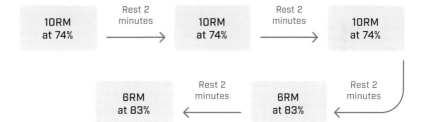

Technique #113

Perceived effort

▪▪▪▪▪▪

Effect on hypertrophy

▪▪▪▪▪▪

Effect on strength and power

▪▪▪▪▪▪

Effect on muscular endurance

▪▪▪▪▪▪

Experience required

▪▪▪

✓ Accumulation method

☐ Intensification method

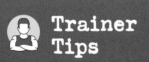

Trainer Tips

You can vary the repetitions for each stage. For example, you could use the following steps:

1. Stage 4RM-8RM
   (3 × 4RM + 2 × 8RM)
2. Stage 3RM-7RM
   (3 × 3RM + 2 × 7RM)
3. Stage 2RM-6RM
   (3 × 2RM + 2 × 6RM)
4. Stage 1RM-5RM
   (3 × 1RM + 2 × 5RM)

STAGE 6RM-10RM

HOW DOES IT WORK?

Complete 3 consecutive sets at 6RM and 2 consecutive sets at 10RM. Each set is separated by 2-3 minutes of rest and you can vary the number of reps in each stage. This technique must be done after stage 10RM-6RM (technique #112).

ADVANTAGES

→ Starting with heavier sets and moving to lighter sets allows you to benefit from muscular potentiation. You might be able to increase the load by 1%-2% compared to your actual 10RM.

DISADVANTAGES

→ The number of exercises for a particular muscle group may be limited in order to moderate the volume of this technique.

PRESCRIPTION TABLE

Load	Number of repetitions per set	Number of sets per exercise	Number of exercises per muscle group	Rest between sets
83%, 74%	6, 10	5	1-4	2-3 minutes

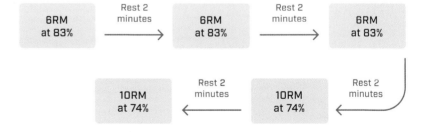

Technique #114

Perceived effort

■ ■ ▫ ▫ ▫

Effect on
hypertrophy

■ ■ ■ ▫ ▫

Effect on strength
and power

■ ■ ▫ ▫ ▫

Effect on muscular
endurance

■ ■ ▫ ▫ ▫

Experience required

■ ▫ ▫

✓ Accumulation
method

☐ Intensification
method

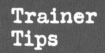

Trainer Tips

Depending on your muscle typology (ratio of fast- to slow-twitch fibers), your load may vary within 1 set. Don't hesitate to change it. For example, rowing experts may be able to perform their 12RM at 90% due to a high proportion of type I fibers in their back. Therefore, for them, the percentages should be higher than those mentioned.

INTERNAL PYRAMID METHOD

HOW DOES IT WORK?

This method involves varying the load from the lightest to the heaviest and vice versa in 1 set. For example, you may do 3 reps at 70%, followed by 2 reps at 75%, then 1 at 80%, followed by 2 at 75%, and finally 3 at 70%, for a total of 11 reps per set. You must keep the rest period as short as possible while changing the weight.

ADVANTAGES

→ This technique increases the intensity of an exercise throughout a single set because instead of doing 11 constant reps at 72% of your 1RM, you keep 72% of the load, but vary the intensity by 70%-80%. Compared to using a constant percentage, this method is better at recruiting higher threshold muscle fibers.

DISADVANTAGES

→ This technique should preferably be performed on selective plate devices.

PRESCRIPTION TABLE

Load	Number of repetitions per set	Number of sets per exercise	Number of exercises per muscle group	Rest between sets
70%-80%	11	2-5	1	1-3 minutes

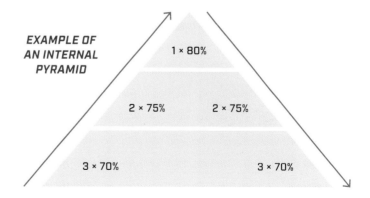

EXAMPLE OF AN INTERNAL PYRAMID

1 × 80%

2 × 75%   2 × 75%

3 × 70%   3 × 70%

Technique #115

Perceived effort

■■■□□□

Effect on
hypertrophy

■■■□□

Effect on strength
and power

■■■□□

Effect on muscular
endurance

■■■□□

Experience required

■■□

✓ Accumulation
method

☐ Intensification
method

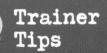
Trainer Tips

Feel free to create your own pyramid by changing the number of repetitions per level. For more advanced individuals, you can even incorporate other techniques inside the pyramid. For example, you could do 12RM, then a 10RM burn set (technique #118), then an 8RM maximal fatigue (technique #97), and so forth.

EXTERNAL PYRAMID METHOD

HOW DOES IT WORK?

This method involves moving from the heaviest load (high intensity) to the lightest (low intensity) or vice versa as you complete multiple sets.

Example 1 (half-pyramid): 7RM, 9RM, 11RM, 13RM, 15RM (5 sets)

Example 2 (full pyramid): 12RM, 10RM, 8RM, 6RM, 4RM, 6RM, 8RM, 10RM, 12RM (9 sets)

ADVANTAGES

→ It improves strength and hypertrophy while recruiting a high range of both slow- and fast-twitch muscle fibers.

→ It is easy to use with any exercise.

DISADVANTAGES

→ There is a risk of possible stagnation in hypertrophy gains if this technique is used for too long because few exercises are performed in the workout.

PRESCRIPTION TABLE

Load	Number of repetitions per set	Number of sets per exercise	Number of exercises per muscle group	Rest between sets
70%-90%	3-15	5-10	1	2-3 minutes

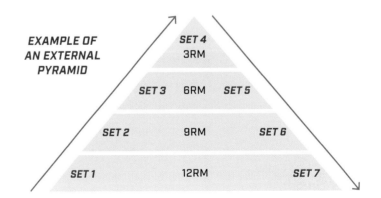

EXAMPLE OF AN EXTERNAL PYRAMID

SET 4 — 3RM
SET 3 — 6RM — SET 5
SET 2 — 9RM — SET 6
SET 1 — 12RM — SET 7

Technique #116

Perceived effort
▪▪▫▫▫

Effect on hypertrophy
▪▪▪▫▫

Effect on strength and power
▪▪▪▫▫

Effect on muscular endurance
▪▪▫▫▫

Experience required
▪▫▫

✓ Accumulation method

☐ Intensification method

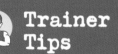

Trainer Tips

The best exercises for this technique are the dumbbell bench press (decline, horizontal, incline), dumbbell flys, seated presses, pull-downs, raises (front, side, back), rows, shrugs, lunges, lying elbow extensions, and curls (standing, sitting, inclined).

RACK PYRAMID METHOD

HOW DOES IT WORK?

This method is so named because it uses the standard dumbbells in a rack found in all weight rooms. It is a derivative of the external pyramid method (technique #115) using only dumbbells. Start with 10 warm-up reps and gradually increase the load with the available dumbbells (typically 1.25-2.5 kg per dumbbell per increase), doing as many reps as possible on each set until you can only accomplish 1 repetition. Then reverse the order and decrease the load until you reach your starting point again. The rest time between sets will be 1-2 minutes.

ADVANTAGES

→ It provides a large muscle stimulus and therefore allows excellent muscle growth.

DISADVANTAGES

→ It requires access to all dumbbells in the rack, making the technique impossible to accomplish during peak weight room hours.

→ Due to the high number of sets, it can be very time consuming.

PRESCRIPTION TABLE

Load	Number of repetitions per set	Number of sets per exercise	Number of exercises per muscle group	Rest between sets
72%-100%	1-10	2-15	1	1-2 minutes

EXAMPLE OF THE RACK PYRAMID METHOD

Set	Weight (kg)	Reps	Rest
1	20	10	1 minute
2	25	10	1 minute
3	30	10	1 minute
4	35	8	2 minutes
5	40	6	2 minutes
6	45	3	2 minutes
7	50	1	2 minutes
8	45	2	2 minutes
9	40	3	2 minutes
10	35	5	2 minutes
11	30	6	2 minutes
12	25	7	2 minutes
13	20	8	2 minutes

Technique #117

Perceived effort

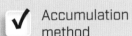

Effect on hypertrophy

Effect on strength and power

Effect on muscular endurance

Experience required

✓ Accumulation method

☐ Intensification method

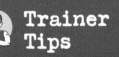

Trainer Tips

Beginners maintain the elastic energy in their muscles for about 0.25 seconds, whereas experienced athletes can maintain it for 2-3 seconds after letting go of the bar. Make sure you are taking a long enough pause!

PURE CONCENTRIC

HOW DOES IT WORK?

Start a movement at the beginning of its concentric phase. Once you have set the load back down, wait at least 2 seconds after letting go of the bar for the elastic energy to dissipate, then start the next rep. This technique can also be used in a strength gains plan by pairing it with partial reps with max effort (technique #30).

ADVANTAGES

→ This method lets you work only the concentric phase without prestretching the muscle.
→ It allows you to work shorter ranges of motion within a movement.
→ It is useful for building strength when maximizing acceleration.

DISADVANTAGES

→ It has less of an effect on hypertrophy than other methods because the eccentric phase is not maximized.
→ The lack of prestretching reduces the recruitment of fast-twitch fibers.

PRESCRIPTION TABLE

Load	Number of repetitions per set	Number of sets per exercise	Number of exercises per muscle group	Rest between sets
70%-85%	6-12	3-10	1	2-3 minutes

EXAMPLES OF PURE CONCENTRIC

Front squat, set the bar at the top 1/3 of the movement	Bench press, set the bar at the bottom 2/3 of the movement	Deadlift from floor
4 sets of 6 reps at 85%	5 sets of 6 reps at 75%	3 sets of 8 reps at 70%

Technique #118

Perceived effort

▆▆▆▢▢

Effect on hypertrophy

▆▆▆▢▢

Effect on strength and power

▆▆▢▢▢

Effect on muscular endurance

▆▆▆▢▢

Experience required

▆▢▢

✓ Accumulation method

☐ Intensification method

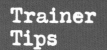

Trainer Tips

During partial reps, be sure to control the eccentric portion to avoid uncontrolled rapid movements that put more strain on your tendons and ligaments and increase your risk of injury.

BURN SET

HOW DOES IT WORK?

At the end of a set, perform max reps in a partial movement (1/4 or 1/2 of a rep).

ADVANTAGES

→ It is very effective at working the arms.

→ It can be used to fatigue all of the muscle groups involved in a movement (e.g., during a bench press, if your triceps fatigue prematurely, you can continue to do low half-reps at the end of the set to fatigue your pectorals).

→ It increases the time under tension, producing more muscle gains.

DISADVANTAGES

→ None.

PRESCRIPTION TABLE

Load	Number of repetitions per set	Number of sets per exercise	Number of exercises per muscle group	Rest between sets
70%-83%	6-12 + maximum partial reps	2-4	1-4	2-3 minutes

Leg extension		Leg extension
10 reps	**+**	*Maximum partial reps at the start of movement*

Technique #119

Perceived effort

Effect on hypertrophy

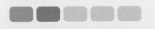

Effect on strength and power

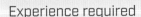

Effect on muscular endurance

Experience required

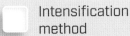

✓ Accumulation method

☐ Intensification method

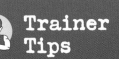

Trainer Tips

Take 2-4 seconds to complete the eccentric phase of each forced rep. This will help maximize muscular development while reducing your risk of injury.

FORCED SET

HOW DOES IT WORK?

At the end of a set, do 1-4 additional reps with the help of a partner. Your partner should provide just enough assistance so that you can finish the concentric part of the movement. Complete the eccentric part of the movement unassisted. When this technique is used without a partner, it is called a cheat set (technique #120).

ADVANTAGES

→ It is very effective at working the arms.

→ It makes it possible to achieve muscular failure in both the concentric and eccentric phases.

→ It causes more muscle microtears thanks to the extra time spent in the eccentric phase.

→ It causes an increase in growth hormone almost three times more than standard training.

DISADVANTAGES

→ It requires a partner in order to finalize the concentric phases of the additional repetitions.

PRESCRIPTION TABLE

Load	Number of repetitions per set	Number of sets per exercise	Number of exercises per muscle group	Rest between sets
70%-85%	6-12 + 1-4 additional reps	5-10	1	2-3 minutes

Standing barbell curl

8 max reps

+

Standing barbell curl

+ 1-4 reps

Set until failure

With partner assistance (concentric phase only)

Technique #120

Perceived effort

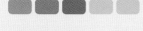

Effect on hypertrophy

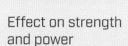

Effect on strength and power

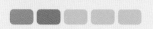

Effect on muscular endurance

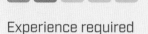

Experience required

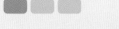

✓ Accumulation method

☐ Intensification method

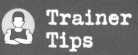

Trainer Tips

Cheating is recommended for improving efforts made in the eccentric phase at the end of a set. It should never be used for all the reps in a set, a mistake that is—in my opinion—all too common among beginners in strength training.

CHEAT SET

HOW DOES IT WORK?

At the end of a set, perform an additional 1-4 reps, using your body weight to create just enough momentum to help you finish the concentric part of the movement. The eccentric part of the movement is then performed under control. The partnered version of this technique is called the forced set (technique #119).

ADVANTAGES

→ It is very effective at working the arms.

→ It makes it possible to achieve muscular failure in both the concentric and eccentric phases.

→ It causes more muscle microtears thanks to the extra time spent in the eccentric phase.

DISADVANTAGES

→ There is a risk of injury if the compensating movement is performed incorrectly.

PRESCRIPTION TABLE

Load	Number of repetitions per set	Number of sets per exercise	Number of exercises per muscle group	Rest between sets
70%-85%	6-12 + 1-4 additional reps	5-10	1	2-3 minutes

Lat pull-down

8 max reps

+

Lat pull-down

+ 1-4 reps

Set until failure

With backswing
(concentric phase only)

Technique #121

Perceived effort

■ ■ ■ □ □

Effect on hypertrophy

■ ■ ■ □ □

Effect on strength and power

■ ■ □ □ □

Effect on muscular endurance

■ ■ □ □ □

Experience required

■ ■ ■

✓ Accumulation method

☐ Intensification method

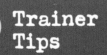

Trainer Tips

The heavier load and little rest used in this technique serve to increase blood flow to the targeted muscles.

SUPER-PUMP SET LONG VERSION

HOW DOES IT WORK?

Perform 15-18 sets of the same movement with 2-3 reps per set and 15 seconds rest between sets. For example, you might perform 16 sets of 3 reps at 70%, or 18 sets of 2 reps at 74%. This is similar to a very long cluster.

ADVANTAGES

→ It increases the density of your workout.
→ It is easy to use with any exercise.
→ It gives a rapid muscular pump.
→ It is perfect when you don't have much time to train.

DISADVANTAGES

→ It requires enough experience that your muscles are able to recover sufficiently in just 15 seconds between each set.
→ This technique can be monotonous when performed for several weeks in a row.

PRESCRIPTION TABLE

Load	Number of repetitions per set	Number of sets per exercise	Number of exercises per muscle group	Rest between sets
70%-80%	2-3	15-18	1	15 seconds

EXAMPLE OF A SET WITH 70% LOAD (15 SECONDS REST)

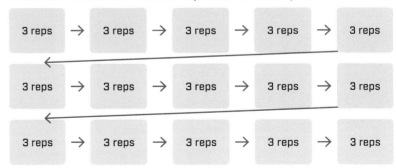

Technique #122

Perceived effort

Effect on hypertrophy

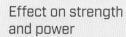

Effect on strength and power

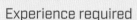

Effect on muscular endurance

Experience required

✓ Accumulation method

☐ Intensification method

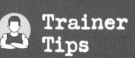

Trainer Tips

You can create your own rounds using any load. Just make sure to reach double the reps of your chosen RM, then split them into 4-6 rounds. For example:
- 6 × 2 with 6RM
- 4 × 4 with 8RM

Ⓢ

SUPER-PUMP SET SHORT VERSION

HOW DOES IT WORK?

Using a load equal to your 10RM, perform 5 rounds of 4 reps punctuated by 10 seconds of rest for 1 set (20 reps in all). Other options are also available (see Trainer Tips).

ADVANTAGES

→ It increases the density of your workout.
→ It is easy to use with any exercise.
→ It gives a rapid muscular pump.
→ It is perfect when you don't have much time to train.

DISADVANTAGES

→ It requires enough experience that your muscles are able to recover sufficiently in just 10 seconds between each round.
→ This technique can be monotonous when performed for several weeks in a row.

PRESCRIPTION TABLE

Load	Number of repetitions per set	Number of sets per exercise	Number of exercises per muscle group	Rest between sets
74%	4 + 4 + 4 + 4 + 4	2-4	1-3	2-3 minutes

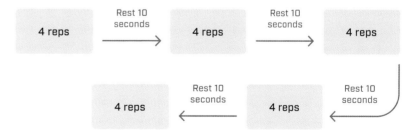

Technique #123

Perceived effort

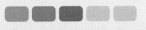

Effect on
hypertrophy

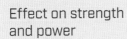

Effect on strength
and power

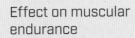

Effect on muscular
endurance

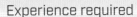

Experience required

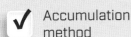

✓ Accumulation
method

☐ Intensification
method

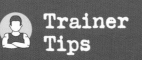

Trainer Tips

You can create your own rounds using any load. Just start with half the reps of your chosen RM, then complete the rounds until 1. For example, you can do 6, 5, 4, 3, 2, 1 with your 12RM.

Ⓢ

SUPER-PUMP SET REGRESSIVE VERSION

HOW DOES IT WORK?

Using a load equal to your 10RM, perform 5 regressive rounds separated by 10 seconds of rest to complete 1 set (15 reps in all). After each round, remove a rep to obtain the following order: 5, 4, 3, 2, 1. Other options are also available (see Trainer Tips).

ADVANTAGES

→ It increases the density of your workout.

→ It is easy to use with any exercise.

→ It gives a rapid muscular pump.

→ It is perfect when you don't have much time to train.

DISADVANTAGES

→ It is less efficient than the super-pump set short version (technique #122) because fewer total repetitions are accomplished with the same load. This technique can therefore be carried out before the short version in your planning.

PRESCRIPTION TABLE

Load	Number of repetitions per set	Number of sets per exercise	Number of exercises per muscle group	Rest between sets
74%	5 + 4 + 3 + 2 + 1	2-4	1-3	2-3 minutes

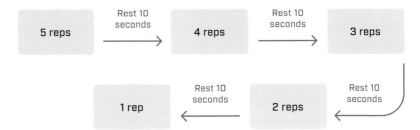

Technique #124

Perceived effort

▮▮▯▯▯

Effect on hypertrophy

▮▮▯▯▯

Effect on strength and power

▮▮▯▯▯

Effect on muscular endurance

▮▮▯▯▯

Experience required

▮▯▯

✓ Accumulation method

☐ Intensification method

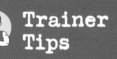

Trainer Tips

Use this technique for movements where your joints are sensitive (e.g., elbows, knees).

DOUBLE PROGRESSION METHOD

HOW DOES IT WORK?

This technique is divided into two parts. In the first part, considered a warm-up, reps increase but the load remains constant and there is very little rest (30-60 seconds). In the second part, reps decrease as the load and rest period increase (90 seconds to 3 minutes). For example, you might perform the following: 4 reps at 70%; 6 reps at 70%; 8 reps at 70%; 10 reps at 70%; 12 reps at 70%; 10 reps at 75%; 8 reps at 80%; 6 reps at 85%; and 4 reps at 90%.

ADVANTAGES

→ It combines submaximal and maximum training.
→ The first part serves as a warm-up (ideal for those who are less skilled at the exercise to which the technique is applied).

DISADVANTAGES

→ It is monotonous and may not provide a large enough stimulus for individuals advanced in bodybuilding.

PRESCRIPTION TABLE

Load	Number of repetitions per set	Number of sets per exercise	Number of exercises per muscle group	Rest between sets
70%-90%	4-12	4 warm-up + 5	1	30 seconds to 3 minutes

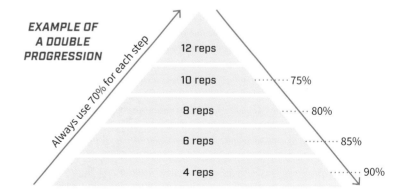

EXAMPLE OF A DOUBLE PROGRESSION

Always use 70% for each step

12 reps	
10 reps	75%
8 reps	80%
6 reps	85%
4 reps	90%

Technique #125

Perceived effort
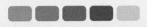

Effect on hypertrophy
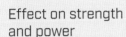

Effect on strength and power
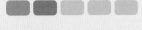

Effect on muscular endurance
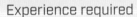

Experience required
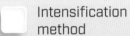

✓ Accumulation method

☐ Intensification method

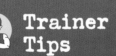
Trainer Tips

The experience required and the effect on hypertrophy, strength and power, and muscular endurance for this technique will vary according to the techniques used. However, the perceived exertion will be high because the body will never be able to adjust before the next week's schedule.

MUSCULAR CHAOS

HOW DOES IT WORK?
Change your routine each week to stress your body and prevent it from adapting. For example, choose 4 or 5 techniques you are familiar with and use them for 1 week each. Because you have already used these techniques, you should already know which loads to use. This technique is designed for more advanced athletes.

ADVANTAGES
→ This technique makes it difficult for the body to adapt to the stimulus week after week.
→ It promotes strong muscular adaptations (hypertrophy) if the right loads are used and if the training techniques are sufficiently varied.

DISADVANTAGES
→ It requires the completion of several techniques before being able to use this training technique.
→ It requires sufficient experience to properly use the training techniques required.

PRESCRIPTION TABLE

Load	Number of repetitions per set	Number of sets per exercise	Number of exercises per muscle group	Rest between sets
Dependent on the techniques used				

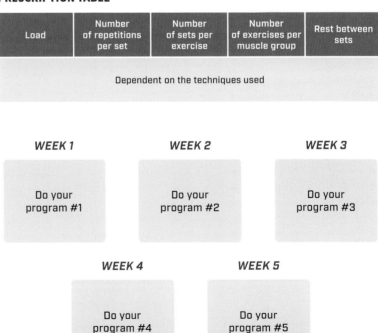

WEEK 1 — Do your program #1

WEEK 2 — Do your program #2

WEEK 3 — Do your program #3

WEEK 4 — Do your program #4

WEEK 5 — Do your program #5

Technique #126

Perceived effort

▪▪▪▫▫

Effect on
hypertrophy

▪▪▪▪▫

Effect on strength
and power

▪▪▫▫▫

Effect on muscular
endurance

▪▪▫▫▫

Experience required

▪▪▫

✓ Accumulation
method

☐ Intensification
method

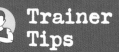

Trainer Tips

Slightly reduce your load compared to your traditional sets because the maximum contraction will exhaust your muscles more quickly. In hypertrophy, load is a tool, not a primary determinant (you don't have to use the heaviest load possible for gains).

MAXIMUM CONTRACTION

HOW DOES IT WORK?

Pause for 2 seconds at the end of the concentric phase of each repetition, during which time you will perform a maximum voluntary contraction of the primary muscle. This technique is the same as constant tension (technique #127), but with a slightly higher degree of difficulty due to the addition of a voluntary maximum contraction at the end of each repetition.

ADVANTAGES

→ By adding maximum isometric pauses, this technique lets you vary the tension within a set, further fatiguing muscle fibers and improving their development.

→ It improves the muscle–brain connection with the main agonist of the chosen movement.

DISADVANTAGES

→ It cannot be applied to certain exercises (e.g., lateral raise) without a partner to exert pressure at the end of the concentric phase in order to simulate a maximum voluntary contraction.

PRESCRIPTION TABLE

Load	Number of repetitions per set	Number of sets per exercise	Number of exercises per muscle group	Rest between sets
60%-83%	6-12	2-5	1-4	2-3 minutes

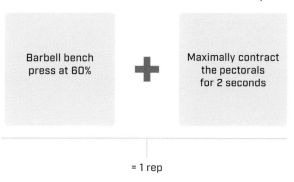

At the end of the repetition

Barbell bench press at 60% **+** Maximally contract the pectorals for 2 seconds

= 1 rep

Technique #127

Perceived effort

◼︎◼︎◼︎☐☐

Effect on
hypertrophy

◼︎◼︎◼︎☐☐

Effect on strength
and power

◼︎◼︎☐☐☐

Effect on muscular
endurance

◼︎◼︎◼︎☐☐

Experience required

◼︎◼︎◼︎

✓ Accumulation
method

☐ Intensification
method

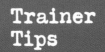

Trainer Tips

Be sure not to shorten your move or perform cheat moves in order to complete your reps. This technique is generally beneficial when using exercises with free weights in certain ranges of motion when working against gravity (e.g., beginning of a lateral raise; end of a Scott curl).

CONSTANT TENSION

HOW DOES IT WORK?

This technique involves performing a movement without resting between reps. For best results, combine constant tension and rest periods. Start the movement in constant tension and, once failure is reached, rest to allow for the evacuation of metabolic waste (such as H+ ions), leaving you able to execute 1-2 more reps.

ADVANTAGES

→ The muscle is put under constant strain without the ability to reoxygenate (by not locking the knees or elbows). Because of the accumulation of serum H+ ions, more growth hormone is released, thereby promoting muscle growth and recovery.

DISADVANTAGES

→ None.

PRESCRIPTION TABLE

Load	Number of repetitions per set	Number of sets per exercise	Number of exercises per muscle group	Rest between sets
70%-83%	6-12 + 1-2	2-5	1-4	2-3 minutes

Beginning and end of the concentric phase

Lateral raise, start at 30 degrees of shoulder abduction	**+**	Lateral raise, end at 90 degrees of shoulder abduction

= 1 rep

Technique #128

Perceived effort

■■■■□

Effect on hypertrophy

■■■□□

Effect on strength and power

■■□□□

Effect on muscular endurance

■■■□□

Experience required

■□□

✓ Accumulation method

☐ Intensification method

Trainer Tips

Don't let pain compromise your technique! Continue to control the eccentric phase for 2-3 seconds and be explosive during the concentric phase while controlling the rebound during the transition phase.

DESCENDING SETS 1

HOW DOES IT WORK?

After your last set of an exercise, perform, without rest, 1-3 additional clusters, decreasing the load by 10%-20% after each cluster. This is also known as the *multi-poundage system*.

ADVANTAGES

→ This technique fatigues more muscle fibers to a greater extent than a simple failure set (technique #69). It is considered a prerequisite for descending sets 2 and 3 (techniques #129-#130).

→ It is easy to apply to exercises using cables and free weights.

DISADVANTAGES

→ It is difficult to use with body-weight exercises (unless you use elastic straps to reduce the weight) and barbell exercises (which require about 10-15 seconds to remove weights).

PRESCRIPTION TABLE

Load	Number of repetitions per set	Number of sets per exercise	Number of exercises per muscle group	Rest between sets
70%-83% – 10%-20% – 10%-20% – 10%-20%	6-12 + max + max + max	1-5	1-4	2-3 minutes

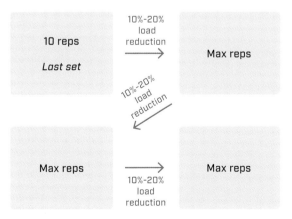

Technique #129

Perceived effort

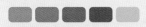

Effect on hypertrophy

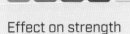

Effect on strength and power

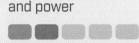

Effect on muscular endurance

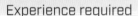

Experience required

✓ Accumulation method

☐ Intensification method

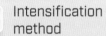

Trainer Tips

In order to facilitate the application of this technique, choose exercises that can be done on a selective plate apparatus. This will allow you to quickly change the load in order to do your descending sequences without monopolizing all the weights and bars at the training center.

DESCENDING SETS 2

HOW DOES IT WORK?

After performing a set to failure with your 6RM-12RM, add 1-3 extra clusters to an exercise using regressive loads. Decrease the weight by 10%-20% after each cluster.

ADVANTAGES

→ This method combines maximal strength work (first failure at 6RM-12RM) and strength endurance work (additional reps).

→ It can also be used to develop strength endurance with longer sets.

→ It is easy to apply to exercises using cables and free weights.

DISADVANTAGES

→ It is difficult to use with body-weight exercises (unless you use elastic straps to reduce the weight) and barbell exercises (which require about 10-15 seconds to remove weights).

PRESCRIPTION TABLE

Load	Number of repetitions per set	Number of sets per exercise	Number of exercises per muscle group	Rest between sets
70%-83% – 10%-20% – 10%-20% – 10%-20%	6-12 + max + max + max	2-6	1-4	2-3 minutes

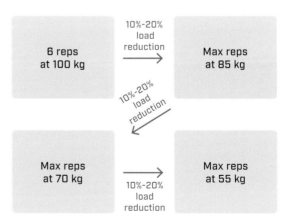

Technique #130

Perceived effort
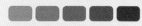

Effect on hypertrophy
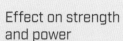

Effect on strength and power
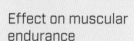

Effect on muscular endurance
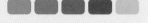

Experience required

✓ Accumulation method

☐ Intensification method

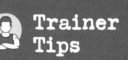

Trainer Tips

In order to increase general muscular work, difficulty, fatigue, and hypertrophy, you can apply the descending sets to both exercises of the superset.

DESCENDING SETS 3

HOW DOES IT WORK?

This is a postfatigue method (agonist superset, technique #71) with the addition of an isolation exercise. After performing a set to failure with your 6RM-12RM on a multijoint exercise, do a set to failure with your 6RM-12RM on an isolation exercise, then add 1-3 extra clusters on this exercise using regressive loads (decrease by 10%-20%).

ADVANTAGES

→ This method combines maximal strength work (first failure at 6RM-12RM) and strength endurance work (additional reps).
→ It can also be used to develop strength endurance with longer sets.
→ It is easy to apply to exercises using cables and free weights.

DISADVANTAGES

→ It is difficult to use with body-weight exercises (unless you use elastic straps to reduce the weight) and barbell exercises (which require about 10-15 seconds to remove weights).

PRESCRIPTION TABLE

Load	Number of repetitions per set	Number of sets per exercise	Number of exercises per muscle group	Rest between sets
70%-83% – 10%-20% – 10%-20% – 10%-20%	6-12 + 6-12 + max + max + max	2-6 supersets	1-3	2-3 minutes

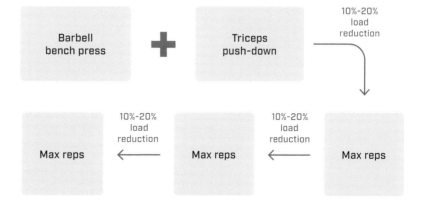

Technique #131

Perceived effort

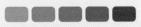

Effect on
hypertrophy

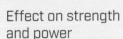

Effect on strength
and power

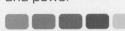

Effect on muscular
endurance

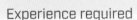

Experience required

✓ Accumulation
method

☐ Intensification
method

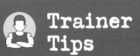

Trainer Tips

Prepare to suffer. This is one of the most painful techniques I have tried: My thighs were sore, I was nauseated, and my body wanted to stop, but I knew I had to push through. Are you fit enough to try it?

BREATHING SQUAT

HOW DOES IT WORK?

Using a load equal to your 10RM for the back squat, do double the reps (20). Once you have picked up the load, do not set it back down until the 20 reps have been completed, hence the need to rest for 5-10 seconds with the bar on your shoulders between reps. It is also known as the super squat and the rest period 10RM.

Before you begin, you will need to estimate the load with which you will be able to complete 20 reps 8 weeks from now. Start by figuring out your current 5RM, then subtract 40 kg. For example, if your 5RM is 100 kg, you would start your first workout of 20 reps with 60 kg (100 kg – 40 kg). After each subsequent workout, add 2.5 kg to the bar (1.25 kg/side). Therefore, if you work out twice a week (which I recommend), you will complete 16 workouts in 8 weeks, which explains the 40 kg subtracted at the beginning (16 × 2.5 kg = 40 kg). Thus, after 2 months of training, you will be able to do 20 reps with your old 5RM! Just try it and you will quickly understand why it is called a "breathing" squat!

ADVANTAGES

→ This method is fast (only 1 set) and can be used at the beginning of a workout for gains in strength or at the end of a workout for maximal fatigue of muscle fibers.

DISADVANTAGES

→ It is inappropriate for those who do not have good back squat technique or experience lower back pain. The only other exercises that can be used as an alternative with this technique are the leg press and hack squat (resting at 10RM during a bench press, for example, is impossible because the upper body is quicker to fatigue than the lower body).

PRESCRIPTION TABLE

Load	Number of repetitions per set	Number of sets per exercise	Number of exercises per muscle group	Rest between sets
70%-85%	20	1	1	N/A

Technique #132

Perceived effort

▪▪▪▪▫

Effect on
hypertrophy

▪▪▪▪▫

Effect on strength
and power

▪▪▪▫▫

Effect on muscular
endurance

▪▪▪▪▫

Experience required

▪▫▫

✓ Accumulation
method

☐ Intensification
method

Trainer Tips

Start by figuring out your 20RM before your first workout. Once this is done, rest for 3 minutes, then start this technique. Don't be surprised if you cannot complete all 10 sets of 10. It may look more like: 10, 10, 10, 10, 10, 10, 10, 9, 9, 8. Use the same load the following week until you can complete all 10 sets of 10. Only then should you increase the load.

GERMAN VOLUME PHASE 1

HOW DOES IT WORK?

Complete 10 sets of 10 reps with a load equal to your 20RM with 1 minute of rest between sets. This technique, also known as the 10 sets method, was the main technique used by Jacques Demers, the German-born Canadian powerlifter, to prepare for the 1984 Los Angeles Olympics, where he won a silver medal.

ADVANTAGES

→ For Olympic lifting, this technique allows you to use a moderate load (60%) for a large number of reps without compromising form, which is very important.

→ For traditional exercises, it allows you to complete a highly dense workout (100 reps) in just 15 minutes.

→ It is great for hypertrophy and very easy to apply.

DISADVANTAGES

→ None.

PRESCRIPTION TABLE

Load	Number of repetitions per set	Number of sets per exercise	Number of exercises per muscle group	Rest between sets
60%	10	10	1	1 minute

🕐 Rest 1 minute

If you can't complete 10 reps, do as many as you can, but never decrease the load.

10 reps	10 reps	10 reps	10 reps	10 reps
10 reps	10 reps	10 reps	10 reps	10 reps

Technique #133

Perceived effort

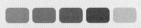

Effect on hypertrophy

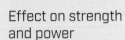

Effect on strength and power

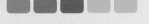

Effect on muscular endurance

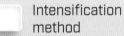

Experience required

✓ Accumulation method

☐ Intensification method

Trainer Tips

Start by figuring out your true 12RM before your first workout by performing a set. Use a load with which you think you will be able to complete 12RM and do as many reps as possible. If, for example, you do 14, increase the load slightly, rest for 3 minutes, then start your workout.

GERMAN VOLUME PHASE 2

HOW DOES IT WORK?

Complete 10 sets of 6 reps with a load equal to your 12RM with 1 minute of rest between sets.

ADVANTAGES

→ This method combines high workout density with high-intensity training, which results in gains in both strength and hypertrophy.

→ It is easy to apply because you stay at the same station with the same load for all 10 sets.

DISADVANTAGES

→ It requires at least 6 months of training experience so that your muscles are prepared for such high-volume and high-intensity work. Otherwise, you will simply not be able to complete the sets.

PRESCRIPTION TABLE

Load	Number of repetitions per set	Number of sets per exercise	Number of exercises per muscle group	Rest between sets
70%	6	10	1	1 minute

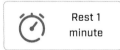 Rest 1 minute

If you can't complete 6 reps, do as many as you can, but never decrease the load.

6 reps	6 reps	6 reps	6 reps	6 reps
6 reps	6 reps	6 reps	6 reps	6 reps

Technique #134

Perceived effort

Effect on hypertrophy

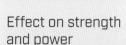

Effect on strength and power

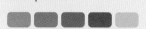

Effect on muscular endurance

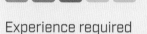

Experience required

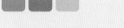

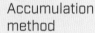

✓ Accumulation method

☐ Intensification method

Trainer Tips

Start by figuring out your true 12RM before your first workout by performing a set. Use a load with which you think you will be able to complete 12RM and do as many reps as possible. If, for example, you do 14, increase the load slightly, rest for 3 minutes, then start your workout.

GERMAN VOLUME PHASE 3

HOW DOES IT WORK?

Complete 10 sets of 6 reps with a load equal to your 12RM with 1 minute of rest between sets. For each new workout, increase the load by 4%-5% and subtract 1 rep per set to create two 3-week waves (see example).

ADVANTAGES

→ This method combines high workout density with high-intensity training, which results in gains in both strength and hypertrophy.

DISADVANTAGES

→ It requires at least 1 year of training experience to be sure that your muscles are prepared for such high-volume and high-intensity work. Otherwise, you will simply not be able to complete the sets.

PRESCRIPTION TABLE

Load	Number of repetitions per set	Number of sets per exercise	Number of exercises per muscle group	Rest between sets
70%-80%	4-6	10	1	1 minute

This technique is perfect for tracking your progress over 6 weeks of training (1 session per week), which would look like this if your 12RM is equal to 100 lb for an exercise:

→ **Workout 1:** 10 sets of 6 repetitions with 100 kg
→ **Workout 2:** 10 sets of 5 repetitions with 105 kg
→ **Workout 3:** 10 sets of 4 repetitions with 110 kg
→ **Workout 4:** 10 sets of 6 repetitions with 105 kg
→ **Workout 5:** 10 sets of 5 repetitions with 110 kg
→ **Workout 6:** 10 sets of 4 repetitions with 115 kg

At this point (workout 7), you would normally be able to do 10 sets of 6 reps with 110 kg, a 10% increase in strength after 6 workouts.

Technique #135

Perceived effort

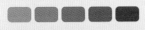

Effect on hypertrophy

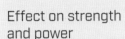

Effect on strength and power

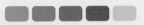

Effect on muscular endurance

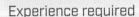

Experience required

☑ Accumulation method

☐ Intensification method

Trainer Tips

For this technique (which is actually one of my own adaptations), if you are unable to complete all 6 reps, decrease the load for the next set. The goal is to complete all 60 reps regardless of load variation. The reps are kept constant, but the intensity may vary. It is also more demanding than other methods given that you will reach muscular failure multiple times.

GERMAN VOLUME PHASE 4

HOW DOES IT WORK?

Complete 10 sets of 6 reps with a load equal to your 9RM, with 1 minute of rest between sets. Because the goal is to always do 6 reps for each set, you may decrease the load as you complete your sets.

ADVANTAGES

→ This technique uses heavy loads and little rest to create greater muscle fatigue. This combination prevents muscle fibers from fully recovering and forces the muscle to work in a position of partial recovery for 15 minutes. Loss of strength as a result of this technique varies from −15% to −25%, even 15 minutes after finishing.

DISADVANTAGES

→ It requires at least 1 year of training experience to be sure that your muscles are prepared for such high-volume and high-intensity work. Otherwise, you simply won't be able to complete your sets.

PRESCRIPTION TABLE

Load	Number of repetitions per set	Number of sets per exercise	Number of exercises per muscle group	Rest between sets
77%	6	10	1	1 minute

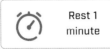 Rest 1 minute

Make sure you always complete 6 reps. If a series fails, then slightly decrease the load for the next series.

6 reps	6 reps	6 reps	6 reps	6 reps
6 reps	6 reps	6 reps	6 reps	6 reps

Technique #136

Perceived effort

■ ■ ■ ■ □

Effect on
hypertrophy

■ ■ ■ ■ □

Effect on strength
and power

■ □ □ □ □

Effect on muscular
endurance

■ ■ ■ □ □

Experience required

■ □ □

✓ Accumulation
method

☐ Intensification
method

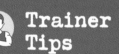
REGRESSIVE CONCENTRIC-ISOMETRIC

Ⓢ

HOW DOES IT WORK?

Alternate concentric and isometric reps using a load equivalent to 40%-60%. Do 5
reps followed by a 5-second isometric hold halfway through the movement, then
4 reps followed by a 4-second isometric hold halfway through the movement,
continuing this pattern until the last isometric hold, which you should maintain
until failure.

ADVANTAGES

→ This method traps blood in the muscle for the entire set, thereby creating an
accumulation of metabolic acidosis. This causes the release of growth hormone,
which helps rebuild muscle, promoting muscle gain.

→ It also promotes aerobic adaptations (e.g., capillarization).

DISADVANTAGES

→ Given the light load used, strength gains are minimal.

PRESCRIPTION TABLE

Load	Number of repetitions per set	Number of sets per exercise	Number of exercises per muscle group	Rest between sets
40%-60%	5 + 4 + 3 + 2 + 1	2-4	1-3	1-3 minutes

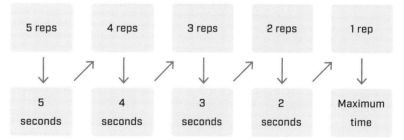

CONCENTRIC PHASES

| 5 reps | 4 reps | 3 reps | 2 reps | 1 rep |

| 5 seconds | 4 seconds | 3 seconds | 2 seconds | Maximum time |

ISOMETRIC PHASES

Technique #137

Perceived effort

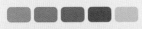

Effect on hypertrophy

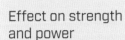

Effect on strength and power

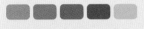

Effect on muscular endurance

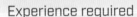

Experience required

✓ Accumulation method

☐ Intensification method

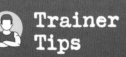

Trainer Tips

Using the provided percentages, calculate the best weight for the exercises you will apply this technique to before your workout so you do not lose time in the gym. You can also bring a percentage chart to rapidly figure out the best weight to use.

DROPSET WITH PROGRESSIVE REPS

HOW DOES IT WORK?

Do 1 rep at 95%, then 3 reps at 80%, then 5 reps at 65%, then 7 reps at 50%, and finally 9 reps at 35%. This technique is based on the dropset (technique #74), with heavy loads to light loads in a single set (4 dropsets total). You can use a rest time of 10 seconds or less between dropsets. It is also known as the intraset decreasing load method.

ADVANTAGES

→ This technique combines strength and volume work, fatiguing fast-twitch muscle fibers at the beginning and slow-twitch fibers near the end. Fatiguing more fibers helps maximize the potential for hypertrophy.

DISADVANTAGES

→ Because loads must be changed frequently, you should figure out the loads you will need before your workout.

PRESCRIPTION TABLE

Load	Number of repetitions per set	Number of sets per exercise	Number of exercises per muscle group	Rest between sets
95% + 80% + 65% + 50% + 35%	1 + 3 + 5 + 7 + 9	2-4	1-2	2-4 minutes

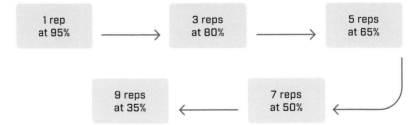

Technique #138

Perceived effort

■■□□□

Effect on
hypertrophy

■■□□□

Effect on strength
and power

■■■□□

Effect on muscular
endurance

■□□□□

Experience required

■□□

✓ Accumulation
method

☐ Intensification
method

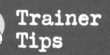

Trainer Tips

Once you are familiar with this method and are able to maintain good technique during repetitions, try using training accessories such as chains or superbands to increase resistance at the end of the movement.

Ⓢ

ECCENTRIC–CONCENTRIC CONTRAST

HOW DOES IT WORK?

This technique is actually a mix of the eccentric and pure concentric methods. Lower the load in a controlled manner in 5-10 seconds and, once the load reaches the end of the eccentric phase, rest for 3-5 seconds, during which time you should release the tension in your muscles (this is not an isometric pause). To do this, set the load on the ground (deadlift) or on the safety guards (squat, bench press). Then complete the concentric part of the movement with as much speed as possible.

ADVANTAGES

→ This combination method helps improve muscle power and involves more time under tension than the pure concentric method alone (technique #117).

DISADVANTAGES

→ The load used is too light to produce significant adaptations in hypertrophy.

PRESCRIPTION TABLE

Load	Number of repetitions per set	Number of sets per exercise	Number of exercises per muscle group	Rest between sets
60%-70%	6-10	2-5	1-3	1-2 minutes

Eccentric phase		Release the load		Explosive concentric phase
5-10 seconds	**+**	3-5 seconds	**+**	

Technique #139

Perceived effort

▪▪▪▪▫

Effect on
hypertrophy

▪▪▪▪▫

Effect on strength
and power

▪▪▪▪▪

Effect on muscular
endurance

▪▪▪▪▪

Experience required

▪▪▪

✓ Accumulation
method

☐ Intensification
method

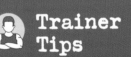

Trainer Tips

When you reach concentric failure, ask your partner to help you lift the load to complete 1-2 more reps in order to also reach eccentric failure.

ECCENTRIC–ISOMETRIC CONTRAST 1

HOW DOES IT WORK?

Also known as the static-dynamic method and the eccentric pause method, this technique incorporates isometric pauses of 3-6 seconds at various positions into the eccentric phase. The greater the range of motion, the more pauses should be included. Exercises with a large range of motion (squat, deadlift) should have 3-4 pauses; medium range-of-motion exercises (bench press, horizontal row) should have 2-3 pauses; and short range-of-motion exercises (calves, shrugs) should have only 2 pauses. This is a version of the postfatigue isometric (technique #98) that is used for each rep.

ADVANTAGES

→ This technique not only increases the amount of time spent under tension but also the amount of time spent in the eccentric phase. This results in greater muscle damage and therefore greater hypertrophy gains.

DISADVANTAGES

→ A spotter is required to monitor lifts where you may get stuck (e.g., bench press, squat).

PRESCRIPTION TABLE

Load	Number of repetitions per set	Number of sets per exercise	Number of exercises per muscle group	Rest between sets
60%-75%	1-5	2-4	1-3	1-2 minutes

5-second pause at 1/4 movement	**+**	5-second pause at halfway point	**+**	5-second pause at 3/4 movement

Technique #140

Perceived effort

■ ■ ■ □ □

Effect on hypertrophy

■ ■ ■ □ □

Effect on strength and power

■ ■ ■ □ □

Effect on muscular endurance

■ □ □ □ □

Experience required

■ ■ ■

✓ Accumulation method

☐ Intensification method

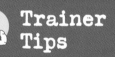

Trainer Tips

When you reach concentric failure, ask your partner to help you lift the load to complete 1-2 more reps in order to also reach eccentric failure.

ECCENTRIC–ISOMETRIC CONTRAST 2

HOW DOES IT WORK?

Also known as the static-dynamic method and the eccentric pause method, this technique is the strength version of the eccentric–isometric contrast 1 (technique #139) because it uses heavier loads. Insert several isometric pauses of 1-2 seconds into the eccentric phase of the movement. The greater the range of motion, the more pauses should be included. Exercises with a large range of motion (squat, deadlift) should have 3-4 pauses; medium range-of-motion exercises (bench press, horizontal row) should have 2-3 pauses; and short range-of-motion exercises (calves, shrugs) should have only 2 pauses.

ADVANTAGES

→ This technique not only increases the amount of time spent under tension but also the amount of time spent in the eccentric phase. This results in greater muscle damage and therefore greater hypertrophy gains.

DISADVANTAGES

→ A spotter is required to monitor lifts where you may get stuck (e.g., bench press, squat).

PRESCRIPTION TABLE

Load	Number of repetitions per set	Number of sets per exercise	Number of exercises per muscle group	Rest between sets
75%-90%	1-5	3-5	1-3	2-4 minutes

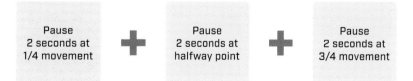

Pause 2 seconds at 1/4 movement **+** Pause 2 seconds at halfway point **+** Pause 2 seconds at 3/4 movement

Technique #141

Perceived effort

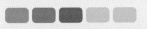

Effect on hypertrophy

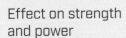

Effect on strength and power

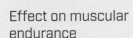

Effect on muscular endurance

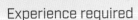

Experience required

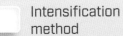

 ✓ Accumulation method

☐ Intensification method

Trainer Tips

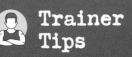

You can vary the position of the isometric pause if you wish. For example, you could alternate pausing at 1/4 movement, 1/2 movement, and 3/4 movement.

Ⓢ

CONCENTRIC STATIC-DYNAMIC

HOW DOES IT WORK?

This technique is like the explosive static-dynamic method (technique #182), but without the propulsion at the end of the movement. Include a pause of 2-3 seconds during the concentric part of the movement, generally at the halfway point, then quickly finish the concentric phase.

ADVANTAGES

→ This technique increases the time spent under tension during a classic set by adding an isometric phase to the middle of the concentric portion for each rep. Greater muscle fatigue will be felt compared to a failure set (technique #69).

DISADVANTAGES

→ None.

PRESCRIPTION TABLE

Load	Number of repetitions per set	Number of sets per exercise	Number of exercises per muscle group	Rest between sets
60%-85%	6-12	2-4	1-3	2-3 minutes

Start of the concentric phase		Pause 2 seconds halfway through the concentric phase		Quickly finish the concentric phase

Technique #142

Perceived effort

▮▮▯▯▯

Effect on
hypertrophy

▮▮▮▯▯

Effect on strength
and power

▮▮▯▯▯

Effect on muscular
endurance

▮▮▯▯▯

Experience required

▮▯▯

☑ Accumulation
method

☐ Intensification
method

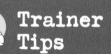

Trainer Tips

You can vary the number of fast
and slow reps during a set. For
example, you can do:
- 3 fast, 1 slow
- 3 fast, 3 slow
- 2 fast, 3 slow

TEMPO CONTRAST

HOW DOES IT WORK?

Alternate fast and slow reps during a single set (internal contrast method). Do 2 fast reps (1-0-1-0 tempo) followed by 2 slow reps (5-0-5-0 tempo) until muscle failure.

ADVANTAGES

→ This method stimulates fast-twitch fibers during high-speed movements by adding slow reps in order to increase the time spent under tension. More time spent under tension, coupled with fast-twitch muscle fiber fatigue, results in hypertrophy gains.

DISADVANTAGES

→ Strength gains will be less significant due to the inability to use heavy loads.

PRESCRIPTION TABLE

Load	Number of repetitions per set	Number of sets per exercise	Number of exercises per muscle group	Rest between sets
60%-85%	4-12	2-6	1-3	1-3 minutes

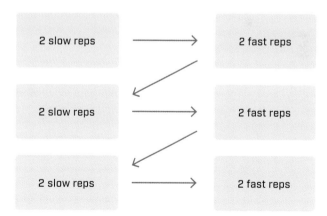

Technique #143

Perceived effort

■■□□□

Effect on hypertrophy

■■■□□

Effect on strength and power

■■■□□

Effect on muscular endurance

■■□□□

Experience required

■□□

- ✓ Accumulation method
- ☐ Intensification method

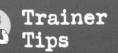

Trainer Tips

Over 6 weeks, this method will allow you to become stronger on the chosen exercises in addition to improving your technique. Always use a tempo of 2-3 seconds in the eccentric phase and 1 second in the concentric phase.

Ⓟ

6 × 6 × 6

HOW DOES IT WORK?

The objective of this technique is to use 6 sets of 6 repetitions on all exercises for a muscle group for a duration of 6 weeks. You will keep the same load on all sets; the ideal load will only lead you to muscle failure on the last set of each exercise. The goal is to be able to increase the load used in the last week of training, but if you can increase the weight sooner, do it. In fact, if in the last set you can do 8 reps instead of 6, increase the weight automatically the next week.

ADVANTAGES

→ It can be used with all exercises.

→ It increases hypertrophy and muscle strength.

→ It is very simple to apply by choosing only 1-3 exercises for each muscle group.

→ It can be done easily without a partner.

DISADVANTAGES

→ None.

PRESCRIPTION TABLE

Load	Number of repetitions per set	Number of sets per exercise	Number of exercises per muscle group	Rest between sets
75%-80%	6	6	1-3	2-3 minutes

EXAMPLE OF A 6 × 6 × 6 SESSION WITH PRESS EXERCISES

Exercises	Sets	Reps	Rest
Barbell bench press	6	6	2 minutes
Incline dumbbell bench press	6	6	2 minutes
Upright row with low pulley	6	6	2 minutes
Dumbbell lateral raise	6	6	2 minutes
Dip	6	6	2 minutes
Triceps push-down	6	6	2 minutes

Technique #144

Perceived effort

▪▪▪▪▫

Effect on hypertrophy

▪▪▪▪▫

Effect on strength and power

▪▪▪▪▫

Effect on muscular endurance

▪▪▫▫▫

Experience required

▪▫▫

☑ Accumulation method

☐ Intensification method

5 × 6

Ⓢ

HOW DOES IT WORK?

This method is simple: Using a load of 78%-80%, attempt to complete 5 sets of 6 repetitions with 1-minutes rest between sets. As soon as you get to a set where you are not able to do the required 6 repetitions, switch exercises and try to do more the following week. You should use the same weight each week until you are able to complete all 5 sets of 6 repetitions.

ADVANTAGES

→ It can increase muscle strength by 5%-10% in the space of 6 workouts.
→ It forces muscle recovery by handling heavy loads with short rest.

DISADVANTAGES

→ None.

PRESCRIPTION TABLE

Load	Number of repetitions per set	Number of sets per exercise	Number of exercises per muscle group	Rest between sets
78%-80%	6	2-5	1	1 minute

EXAMPLE OF A 5 × 6 TRAINING PLAN

Set	Session 1		Session 2		Session 3	
	Reps	Weight	Reps	Weight	Reps	Weight
1	6	100 kg	6	100 kg	6	100 kg
2	6	100 kg	6	100 kg	6	100 kg
3	6	100 kg	6	100 kg	6	100 kg
4	5	100 kg	6	100 kg	6	100 kg
5			4	100 kg	6	100 kg

Set	Session 4		Session 5		Session 6	
	Reps	Weight	Reps	Weight	Reps	Weight
1	6	105 kg	6	105 kg	6	105 kg
2	6	105 kg	6	105 kg	6	105 kg
3	4	105 kg	6	105 kg	6	105 kg
4			4	105 kg	6	105 kg
5					5	105 kg

Technique #145

Perceived effort

Effect on hypertrophy

Effect on strength and power

Effect on muscular endurance

Experience required

☑ Accumulation method

☐ Intensification method

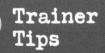 **Trainer Tips**

This method will allow you to accomplish, after 9 workouts, 10 repetitions at your current 5RM-8RM. It can be used both for beginners and for intermediate or advanced athletes in bodybuilding.

1-REP TO 1-SET METHOD

HOW DOES IT WORK?

This method structures your training for the next 9 weeks. You will start by performing 10 sets of a single repetition with 90 seconds of rest between sets. Each week, you'll decrease your rest time by 5-15 seconds until you will not have any rest, forcing you to do your 10 sets of 1 rep all at once (i.e., 1 set of 10 repetitions). In the first week, use a load that allows you to complete your 10 sets with 90 seconds of rest (about 78%-85% of your 1RM).

ADVANTAGES

→ It increases strength and muscle hypertrophy by amplifying training density (amount of work per unit of time).

DISADVANTAGES

→ None.

PRESCRIPTION TABLE

Load	Number of repetitions per set	Number of sets per exercise	Number of exercises per muscle group	Rest between sets
78%-85%	1, 10	10, 1	1	0-90 seconds

Week	Sets	Reps	Rest (in seconds)
1	10	1	90
2	10	1	75
3	10	1	60
4	10	1	45
5	10	1	30
6	10	1	15
7	10	1	10
8	10	1	5
9	1	10	0

Technique #146

Perceived effort

■ ■ ■ ■ □

Effect on hypertrophy

■ ■ ■ ■ □

Effect on strength and power

■ ■ ■ ■ □

Effect on muscular endurance

■ ■ ■ □ □

Experience required

■ □ □

☑ Accumulation method

☐ Intensification method

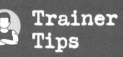

DENSITY TRAINING

HOW DOES IT WORK?

This method structures your workouts over several weeks so you can perform 12 reps with a targeted load. This will be accomplished by completing 24 total reps every workout in order to get there. You'll start by performing 12 sets of 2 reps in 12 minutes. Once this is accomplished, you will spend the next week doing 8 sets of 3 reps in 8 minutes; then 6 sets of 4 repetitions in 6 minutes; then 5 sets of 5 repetitions in 5 minutes; 4 sets of 6 repetitions in 4 minutes; 3 sets of 8 repetitions in 3 minutes; and to finish, a single set of 12 repetitions in 1 minute.

ADVANTAGES

→ It is easy to plan and execute.

→ It's very time efficient.

→ It increases strength rapidly.

DISADVANTAGES

→ None.

PRESCRIPTION TABLE

Load	Number of repetitions per set	Number of sets per exercise	Number of exercises per muscle group	Rest between sets
75%-85%	2-12	1-12	1	0-50 seconds

Week	Sets	Reps	Rest (in seconds)	Total time (in minutes)
1	12	2	50	12
2	8	3	45	8
3	6	4	40	6
4	5	5	35	5
5	4	6	30	4
6	3	8	25	3
7	1	12	0	1

Technique #147

Perceived effort

▪▪▪▫▫

Effect on
hypertrophy

▪▪▪▫▫

Effect on strength
and power

▪▪▪▫▫

Effect on muscular
endurance

▪▪▫▫▫

Experience required

▪▪▪

✓ Accumulation
method

☐ Intensification
method

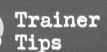

Trainer Tips

I frequently suggest using unilateral exercises to beginners to ensure they achieve equal strength in both arms and both legs. Use the same weight (the maximum weight for your weaker arm or leg) for both arms or both legs and increase the weight as your weaker arm or leg increases in strength. This will increase the strength in your weaker arm or leg while maintaining the strength in your stronger arm or leg until their strength is equal.

UNILATERAL EXERCISES

HOW DOES IT WORK?

This method does not split the workout between your right side and your left side like the unilateral split (technique #64) does; rather, it utilizes the training of your arms or your legs individually in order to use relatively higher loads. In fact, a study[10] on elbow curls for biceps training demonstrated that the force exerted when working with both biceps simultaneously was 10%-20% less than the sum of the forces produced by flexing the elbow on the left side and on the right side individually. In other words, according to the study, if you are able to lift 25 kg for 1 repetition on the barbell biceps curl (or 12.5 kg per hand), then you will be able to lift 15 kg in each hand, using one arm at a time.

ADVANTAGES

→ It allows the use of heavier loads than when working with two limbs.
→ It activates more fast-twitch fibers.

DISADVANTAGES

→ It requires a contraction of the stabilizing muscles and of the core on certain exercises. Because you are only as strong as your weakest link, you will not be able to use a greater load for some exercises because your stabilizing muscles will not be able to manage this weight.

PRESCRIPTION TABLE

Load	Number of repetitions per set	Number of sets per exercise	Number of exercises per muscle group	Rest between sets
70%-85%	6-12	2-4	1-3	1-3 minutes

Muscle groups	Examples of unilateral exercises
Chest	One-arm dumbbell bench press (horizontal, incline, decline)
	One-arm dumbbell fly (horizontal, incline, decline) or one-arm machine fly (pec deck, cross-over)
Shoulders	One-arm dumbbell shoulder press (seated or standing)
	Upright one-arm dumbbell row
	One-arm dumbbell or low-pulley raise (front, lateral, rear)
Triceps	One-arm dumbbell triceps extension (seated, lying)
	One-arm triceps push-down (high pulley)
Back	One-arm dumbbell or pulley row
Biceps	One-arm curl (pronation, neutral, supination) with pulley or with dumbbell (standing, with Scott curl)
Legs	One-leg squat (Bulgarian, lunge)
	One-leg isolation (press, extension, curl [seated, lying, standing])
	One-leg deadlift (Romanian, standard)

Technique #148

Perceived effort

▢▢▢▢▢

Effect on
hypertrophy

▢▢▢▢▢

Effect on strength
and power

▢▢▢▢▢

Effect on muscular
endurance

▢▢▢▢▢

Experience required

▢▢▢

✓ Accumulation
method

☐ Intensification
method

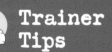

Trainer Tips

You can add load on your back during your push-ups, which is the only closed-chain exercise for chest training. However, although it is not a closed-chain exercise, you can use the barbell bench press as a substitute for push-ups if you have very high muscle strength.

ECO TRAINING METHOD

HOW DOES IT WORK?

This method consists of performing 3 different types of exercises separately (with 1-3 minutes rest between exercises) starting with an explosive exercise, followed by a closed-chain exercise, and then an open-chain exercise.

→ **Explosive exercise:** Plyometric exercise or ballistic exercise (technique #188)
→ **Closed-chain exercise:** Exercise where the hands or feet remain in a fixed position (e.g., squat, push-up, pull-up)
→ **Open-chain exercise:** Exercise where the hands and feet move freely (e.g., leg extension, most dumbbell exercises)

ADVANTAGES

→ It allows you to work the fast-twitch fibers in three ways: with an explosive movement when the nervous system is fresh, with a heavy load on the closed-chain exercise, and in isolation with the open-chain exercise.

DISADVANTAGES

→ None.

PRESCRIPTION TABLE

Load	Number of repetitions per set	Number of sets per exercise	Number of exercises per muscle group	Rest between sets
30%-50% + 83%-88% + 74%-78%	3 + 4-6 + 8-10	3 + 3 + 3	3	1-3 minutes

EXAMPLE OF AN ECO TRAINING METHOD WORKOUT

Muscle groups	Exercises
Chest	Explosive: Clap push-up
	Closed chain: Bench press
	Open chain: Pec deck
Shoulders	Explosive: Wall ball
	Closed chain: Handstand push-up
	Open chain: Dumbbell lateral raise
Quadriceps	Explosive: Jump squat
	Closed chain: Barbell front squat
	Open chain: Leg extension
Back	Explosive: Explosive inverted row with hand-position change (close and wide)
	Closed chain: Pull-up
	Open chain: Bent-over dumbbell row

Technique #149

Perceived effort

▪ ▪ ▪ ▫ ▫

Effect on
hypertrophy

▪ ▪ ▪ ▫ ▫

Effect on strength
and power

▪ ▪ ▪ ▫ ▫

Effect on muscular
endurance

▪ ▪ ▪ ▫ ▫

Experience required

▪ ▪ ▫

☑ Accumulation
method

☐ Intensification
method

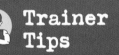

Trainer Tips

A 2006 Connecticut study demonstrated that this technique, which originated in the Eastern European bloc a few decades ago, could increase your 1RM on the squat and the bench press by more than 10% when performed over 4 weeks.[12]

OVERREACHING METHOD

HOW DOES IT WORK?

The objective of this technique is to reach a state of overreaching (in 2-4 weeks) in order to cause a supercompensation, which will cause greater gains in muscle strength. Overreaching is a state of overtraining without yet accumulating negative effects, and it must end just before significant changes in physiology take place. To do this, you will need to train all muscle groups 5 days a week, increasing the load used each week.

ADVANTAGES

→ It can provide strength gains of more than 10% within 5 weeks of training.[12]

DISADVANTAGES

→ There is a risk of overtraining if you perform this technique for too long. Therefore, watch for signs such as fatigue, loss of strength, loss of appetite, insomnia, or depression.

PRESCRIPTION TABLE

Load	Number of repetitions per set	Number of sets per exercise	Number of exercises per muscle group	Rest between sets
70%-88%	4-12	3	1	1-3 minutes

EXAMPLE OF AN OVERREACHING PLAN*

Week	Sets	Reps	Rest
1	3	10-12	2 minutes
2	3	8-10	2 minutes
3	3	6-8	2 minutes
4	3	4-6	2 minutes

*To be performed on all chosen exercises (1 per muscle group).

Technique #150

Perceived effort

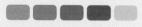

Effect on hypertrophy

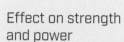

Effect on strength and power

Effect on muscular endurance

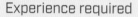

Experience required

✓ Accumulation method

☐ Intensification method

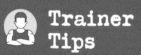

Trainer Tips

You do not have to complete 10 repetitions, as shown in the example. For instance, you can use the same concept to attempt to complete 5 sets of 8 or 12 reps with a load that you currently use to do only 4 sets in the same amount of time.

NUBRET PRO-SET

HOW DOES IT WORK?

This technique—named for Serge Nubret, a professional bodybuilder from France—involves increasing the density (the same amount or more work in less time) of a workout. For example, if you currently do 3 sets of 10 reps in 5 minutes of your chosen exercise, then your goal would be to try to accomplish 4 sets of 10 reps in 5 minutes by reducing the rest time between sets. You may not be able to complete all the reps right away, but keep trying until you can do them.

ADVANTAGES

→ This method increases muscle mass and strength by increasing the ability of muscles to recover between sets.

→ It is easy to use and can be applied to all exercises.

DISADVANTAGES

→ None.

PRESCRIPTION TABLE

Load	Number of repetitions per set	Number of sets per exercise	Number of exercises per muscle group	Rest between sets
70%-83%	6-12	3-4	1	30-120 seconds

EXAMPLE OF A NUBRET PRO-SET

Week	Sets	Reps	Duration
1	3	10	5 minutes
2	2	10	5 minutes
	1	9	
	1	7	
3	3	10	5 minutes
	1	8	
4	4	10	5 minutes

Technique #151

Perceived effort
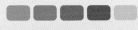

Effect on hypertrophy
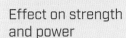

Effect on strength and power
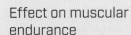

Effect on muscular endurance
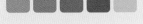

Experience required
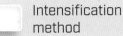

 ✓ Accumulation method

☐ Intensification method

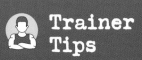

5-10-20 TRISET

HOW DOES IT WORK?

This method is a type of triset. Without rest between exercises, perform a multijoint exercise, preferably done with a barbell (pull-ups and dips are also good), for 5 repetitions (strength), then a multijoint exercise done with free weights or a machine for 10 repetitions (muscular hypertrophy), followed by an isolation exercise for 20 repetitions (muscular endurance and muscular hypertrophy). **Multijoint exercise with barbell + multijoint exercise with dumbbell or machine + isolation exercise**

ADVANTAGES

→ It helps to develop strength, muscular hypertrophy, and muscular endurance.

DISADVANTAGES

→ It may require the reservation of several pieces of equipment (bars, free weights) or weight machines.

→ It is very demanding on the body (space out the sessions for the same muscle group at least 5 days apart).

PRESCRIPTION TABLE

Load	Number of repetitions per set	Number of sets per exercise	Number of exercises per muscle group	Rest between sets
60%-85%	5 + 10 + 20	2-4	1-2 trisets	2-3 minutes

EXAMPLE OF A 5-10-20 TRISET

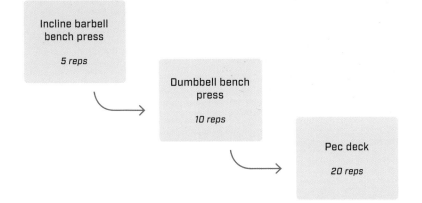

Incline barbell bench press — 5 reps → Dumbbell bench press — 10 reps → Pec deck — 20 reps

Technique #152

Perceived effort

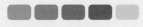

Effect on hypertrophy

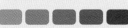

Effect on strength and power

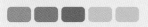

Effect on muscular endurance

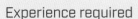

Experience required

✓ Accumulation method

☐ Intensification method

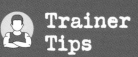

Trainer Tips

You can also use this technique as 4 individual sets. Choose your 4 exercises and perform 4 sets per exercise using the same pattern of repetitions (i.e., 4, 8, 12, 16) with 2 minutes of recovery between sets.

4-REP SYSTEM

HOW DOES IT WORK?

This method is a type of circuit training. You should complete, without rest, 4 reps of a multijoint exercise, followed by 8 reps of a multijoint or isolation exercise, 12 reps of an isolation exercise, then 16 reps of a multijoint or isolation exercise for the same muscle group.

Multijoint exercise + multijoint or isolation exercise + isolation exercise + multijoint or isolation exercise

ADVANTAGES

→ It provides a great stimulus for muscle growth.
→ It encourages biochemical changes in muscle that promote endurance.

DISADVANTAGES

→ It is very physically demanding.
→ It may take time to prepare and reserve all the needed equipment.

PRESCRIPTION TABLE

Load	Number of repetitions per set	Number of sets per exercise	Number of exercises per muscle group	Rest between sets
60%-85%	4 + 8 + 12 + 16	2-4	1	2-3 minutes

EXAMPLE OF A 4-REP WORKOUT FOR SHOULDERS

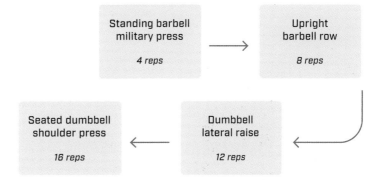

Technique #153

Perceived effort

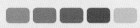

Effect on hypertrophy

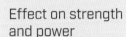

Effect on strength and power

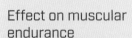

Effect on muscular endurance

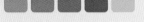

Experience required

☑ Accumulation method

☐ Intensification method

Trainer Tips

Avoid unilateral exercises for this technique because it will put too much stress on your stabilizers and your core muscles (abdominals, lower back) and technique can easily break down. I recommend the use of machines (e.g., squat on Smith machine, leg press) in order to facilitate explosive repetitions.

SPEED-SET TRAINING

HOW DOES IT WORK?

This method consists of performing 15 repetitions with three different speeds of movement within a set. You will perform reps 1-5 at an explosive pace, reps 6-10 at an ultra-slow pace (5 seconds concentric and 5 seconds eccentric), and reps 11-15 at a normal pace (1 second concentric and 2-3 seconds eccentric).

ADVANTAGES

→ It increases muscle strength and hypertrophy as well as reduces fat mass.
→ Fast reps increase power, slow reps increase time under tension, and normal reps increase muscle endurance.

DISADVANTAGES

→ None.

PRESCRIPTION TABLE

Load	Number of repetitions per set	Number of sets per exercise	Number of exercises per muscle group	Rest between sets
60%	5 fast + 5 slow + 5 normal	2-4	1-3	1-2 minutes

PHASE 1: FAST

Tempo: ‹1 second/rep

5 reps

PHASE 2: ULTRA SLOW

Tempo: 10 seconds/rep

5 reps

PHASE 3: STANDARD

Tempo: 1 second/concentric, 2-3 seconds/eccentric

5 reps

Technique #154

Perceived effort

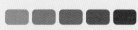

Effect on hypertrophy

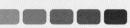

Effect on strength and power

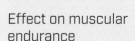

Effect on muscular endurance

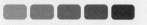

Experience required

✓ Accumulation method

☐ Intensification method

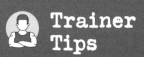

Trainer Tips

Be sure to determine your true 15RM-19RM before beginning this technique. A heavier load (<15RM) will not allow you to reach 60 repetitions, whereas a too-light load (>19RM) will allow you to reach 60 repetitions in less than 4 weeks.

4-MINUTE MUSCLE

HOW DOES IT WORK?

The objective of this technique is to try to complete as many repetitions as possible in 4 minutes with a load around your 15RM-19RM while taking short rest periods. You should be able to complete at least 40 reps in 4 minutes the first week. Your goal is to reach 60 repetitions in 4 minutes after 4-6 weeks of training with this technique.

ADVANTAGES

→ It can be performed on all exercises.
→ It is effective at increasing hypertrophy and muscular endurance as well as decreasing body fat.

DISADVANTAGES

→ None.

PRESCRIPTION TABLE

Load	Number of repetitions per set	Number of sets per exercise	Number of exercises per muscle group	Rest between sets
62%-66%	40-60	1	2-4	N/A

EXAMPLE OF A 4-MINUTE MUSCLE ROUTINE

Week	Reps	Total time
1	41	4 minutes
2	46	4 minutes
3	49	4 minutes
4	54	4 minutes
5	57	4 minutes
6	60	4 minutes

Technique #155

Perceived effort

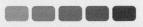

Effect on hypertrophy

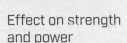

Effect on strength and power

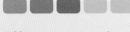

Effect on muscular endurance

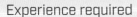

Experience required

✓ Accumulation method

Intensification method

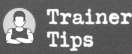 **Trainer Tips**

For this technique, it is a good idea to have a training partner who will time your 15 seconds per exercise and who can help you when you are close to muscle failure. During your 2 minutes of recovery, you will reverse roles.

POWER CIRCUIT TRAINING

HOW DOES IT WORK?

This technique consists of performing a circuit of 4-10 different exercises. You will perform 30 repetitions per exercise with a load of around 8RM-10RM, and each set will last 15 seconds. The goal is to complete as many reps as possible in those 15 seconds before moving on to the next exercise without rest. When you reach 30 repetitions on an exercise, it is then eliminated from the circuit and replaced by 15 seconds of rest. To make this circuit easier to set up, choose exercises using mostly barbells and free weights and limit machines to only 1-3 exercises. Also, alternate upper- and lower-body exercises to aid your recovery.

ADVANTAGES

→ It improves muscle strength and hypertrophy while decreasing fat mass.

DISADVANTAGES

→ It requires preparation of all your exercises before starting the circuit.

PRESCRIPTION TABLE

Load	Number of repetitions per exercise	Number of sets per exercise	Number of exercises per circuit	Rest between sets
74%-78%	30	2-5	4-10	1-2 minutes

Exercise	Set 1		Set 2		Set 3		Set 4	
	Time (s)	Reps	Time (s)	Reps	Time (s)	Reps	Time (s)	Reps
1. Dumbbell bench press	15	8	15	8	15	8	15	6
2. Leg press	15	8	15	8	15	8	15	6
3. Bent-over dumbbell row	15	8	15	8	15	8	15	6
4. Lying leg curl	15	10	15	8	15	6	15	6
5. Standing barbell curl	15	10	15	10	15	10	15	0
6. Lower back extension	15	10	15	10	15	10	15	0
7. Dumbbell military press	15	8	15	8	15	8	15	6
8. Seated calf	15	15	15	15	15	0	15	0
9. Lying barbell triceps extension	15	10	15	10	15	10	15	0
10. Alternating jump lunge	15	9	15	9	15	8	15	4
Rest	2 minutes		2 minutes		2 minutes		2 minutes	

Technique #156

Perceived effort

■■□□□

Effect on hypertrophy

■■■□□

Effect on strength and power

■■■□□

Effect on muscular endurance

■■□□□

Experience required

■□□

✓ Accumulation method

☐ Intensification method

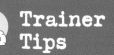

Trainer Tips

For lower-body exercises (e.g., leg extension, leg curl, squat, calf machine), you can vary the angle of work simply by adjusting the angle of your feet. For example, you could perform leg curl reps with your feet internally rotated, externally rotated, and in a neutral (parallel) position.

SMALL-ANGLE TRAINING

HOW DOES IT WORK?

This technique is actually a failure set (technique #69) except that, as the name suggests, it requires adjusting the angle of the movement as the sets progress. The goal is to maximize the recruitment of all muscle fibers by targeting all angles of a movement. You can adjust the height of the pulleys, the angle of your trunk, the width of your hands, the width of your feet, the position of your forearms, and so forth.

ADVANTAGES

→ It allows more muscle fibers to be used through the various working angles.
→ It can be applied to a wide variety of exercises.

DISADVANTAGES

→ None.

PRESCRIPTION TABLE

Load	Number of repetitions per set	Number of sets per exercise	Number of exercises per muscle group	Rest between sets
70%-83%	6-12	2-8	1-3	2-3 minutes

EXAMPLE SEQUENCE OF CHEST EXERCISE

Exercise	Set	Reps	Angle of exercise
Barbell bench press	1	6-12	Forearms perpendicular to floor
	2	6-12	Hands at shoulder width
	3	6-12	Hands at shoulder width + 5 cm
	4	6-12	Hands at shoulder width + 10 cm
	5	6-12	Hands at shoulder width + 15 cm
	6	6-12	Hands at shoulder width + 20 cm

EXAMPLE SEQUENCE OF SHOULDER EXERCISE

Exercise	Set	Reps	Angle of exercise
Dumbbell lateral raise	1	6-12	Front raise, neutral grip
	2	6-12	Front raise at 45 degrees
	3	6-12	Lateral raise
	4	6-12	Lateral raise, bent 15 degrees forward
	5	6-12	Lateral raise, bent 45 degrees forward
	6	6-12	Dumbbell rear delt fly

Technique #157

Perceived effort

▪▪▪▫▫

Effect on hypertrophy

▪▪▪▫▫

Effect on strength and power

▪▪▪▫▫

Effect on muscular endurance

▪▪▫▫▫

Experience required

▪▪▪

☑ Accumulation method

☐ Intensification method

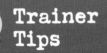

Trainer Tips

This technique makes it possible to evaluate the impact of your training session on muscle fatigue. If you accomplish 8 repetitions with 50 kg at the beginning and only 4 repetitions with the same load at the end of your training, we can say that your training session caused a 50% loss of strength. As a goal, aim for a minimum of 20% strength loss to maximize your future adaptations.

BOOKEND TRAINING

HOW DOES IT WORK?

This technique involves starting and ending your workout with the same exercise. For the first exercise, you will do 3 sets of 6-8 repetitions at 78%-83%. For the last exercise, you will perform 1 set of as many reps as possible using the same load you started with, followed by 2 sets of 12-15 repetitions at 66%-70%.

ADVANTAGES

→ It promotes strength gain with the first exercise and muscle growth with the last exercise by using a relatively heavy load on an exhausted muscle.

DISADVANTAGES

→ It requires a training partner on certain exercises (e.g., bench press, squat) during the first set of the last exercise because the number of repetitions is undetermined before starting.

PRESCRIPTION TABLE*

Load	Number of repetitions per set	Number of sets per exercise	Number of exercises per muscle group	Rest between sets
First: 78%-83% Last: 78%-83%, 66%-70%	First: 6-8 Last: Max reps, 12-15	First: 3 Last: 1 + 2	1	1-3 minutes

*First and last exercises only

EXAMPLE SEQUENCE OF CHEST EXERCISES

Exercises	Sets	Reps	Rest
Bench press	3	6-8	2 minutes
Incline dumbbell bench press	3	8-10	2 minutes
Dumbbell fly	3	10-12	1 minute
Pec deck	3	12-15	1 minute
Bench press	1	Maximum	1 minute
	2	12-15	1 minute

Technique #158

Perceived effort

Effect on hypertrophy

Effect on strength and power

Effect on muscular endurance

Experience required

✓ Accumulation method

☐ Intensification method

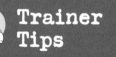

Trainer Tips

This is a useful method to be able to continue training while traveling (elastics are very easy to carry in a suitcase) or to start working out at home without investing too much money in weight training equipment.

ELASTICS TRAINING

HOW DOES IT WORK?

For this method your training sessions will only include exercises performed with elastic bands with handles or superbands. Depending on the bands available to you, you will be able to vary the number of repetitions as the weeks progress to allow for more hypertrophy and muscle strength gains. Perform exercises labeled with the same letter as supersets with no rest between them, then rest for 90 seconds between supersets (i.e., perform A1 and A2, 90-second rest; perform B1 and B2, 90-second rest; perform C1 and C2, 90-second rest; and perform D1 and D2, 90-second rest).

ADVANTAGES

→ It does not require a lot of equipment.

→ It is ideal for training at a hotel or at home.

→ It creates variation of tension, with the greatest resistance at the end of the movement.

DISADVANTAGES

→ Individuals with high muscular strength will not respond well to this type of training.

PRESCRIPTION TABLE

Load	Number of repetitions or seconds per set	Number of sets per exercise	Number of exercises per muscle group	Rest between sets
Elastic band only	6-20 reps or 40-80 seconds	2-3	3-4	1-2 minutes

EXAMPLE SEQUENCE OF UPPER-BODY EXERCISES (DAY 1)

Exercises	Sets	Reps	Rest
A1 Push-up	3	8-10	0 seconds
A2 Elastic fly	3	10-12	90 seconds
B1 Elastic row	3	10-12	0 seconds
B2 Elastic straight-arm pull-down	3	12-15	90 seconds
C1 Elastic biceps curl	3	12-15	0 seconds
C2 Elastic triceps extension	3	12-15	90 seconds
D1 Side plank	3	20-40 seconds/side	0 seconds
D2 Bicycle crunch	3	12-15/side	90 seconds

EXAMPLE SEQUENCE OF LOWER-BODY EXERCISES (DAY 2)

Exercises	Sets	Reps	Rest
A1 Jump squat	3	8-10	0 seconds
A2 Seated elastic leg curl	3	10-12	90 seconds
B1 Elastic leg extension	3	10-12	0 seconds
B2 Walking lunge	3	12-15/side	90 seconds
C1 Side walk with band	3	12-15/side	0 seconds
C2 Squat with band at knees	3	12-15	90 seconds
D1 One-leg hip thrust on floor	3	10-12/side	0 seconds
D2 Superman	3	12-15	90 seconds

Technique #159

Perceived effort

▪▪▪▪ ▪ ▪

Effect on
hypertrophy

▪▪▪ ▪ ▪ ▪

Effect on strength
and power

▪▪▪ ▪ ▪ ▪

Effect on muscular
endurance

▪▪▪ ▪ ▪ ▪

Experience required

▪▪▪

✓ Accumulation
method

☐ Intensification
method

Trainer Tips

Because they change the stability of the exercise, start by using training accessories (chains and superbands) without much weight on the bar during the first week to get used to them. From the second week, increase the load gradually.

VARIABLE RESISTANCE TRAINING

HOW DOES IT WORK?

This technique is the same as the failure set (technique #69), but with training aids such as chains or superbands attached to the bar.

ADVANTAGES

→ This method allows you to take advantage of the biomechanics of the muscle. When the muscles are in a lengthened position, there is greater passive tension (tendons) and less active tension (muscles). You are therefore weaker in these positions. Conversely, the more the muscle is shortened, the more the active tension increases and the stronger you are (to a certain degree). The overload created by the chains or superbands makes it possible to add resistance to the portion of the movement where you are stronger.

DISADVANTAGES

→ This technique is not possible in all weight rooms due to the required equipment and ground anchors (for the deadlift with superbands, for example).
→ This training technique requires prior experience with bands and chains.

PRESCRIPTION TABLE

Load	Number of repetitions per set	Number of sets per exercise	Number of exercises per muscle group	Rest between sets
60%-80%	6-12	2-5	1-2	3-5 minutes

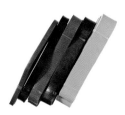

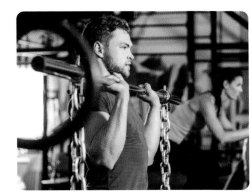

Technique #160

Perceived effort

▦ ▦ ▦ ▢ ▢

Effect on hypertrophy

▦ ▦ ▦ ▢ ▢

Effect on strength and power

▦ ▦ ▦ ▢ ▢

Effect on muscular endurance

▦ ▦ ▦ ▢ ▢

Experience required

▦ ▢ ▢

✓ Accumulation method

☐ Intensification method

👤 Trainer Tips

Although this method may seem ordinary, using it only with beginners would be a mistake. My advice is to choose 1-3 machine exercises per muscle group and combine them with another training technique in this book. You will never see machines the same way again!

MACHINE MUSCLE

HOW DOES IT WORK?

This method consists of using only machines during your training program. Try it for a week or two to change up your training structure.

ADVANTAGES

→ It is easy to use.

→ It is great when you don't have a lot of time to train.

→ It allows constant tension in the muscle (unlike dumbbells, which create variable tension according to gravity).

→ You can train to muscle failure without a training partner.

→ It allows the use of several techniques with load changes (e.g., dropset, technique #74).

→ It may be a good option for athletes who suffer from injuries.

DISADVANTAGES

→ The stabilizing muscles are not involved as much compared to free weights. Complementary work on these muscles (e.g., rotator cuff) is suggested.

PRESCRIPTION TABLE

Load	Number of repetitions per set	Number of sets per exercise	Number of exercises per muscle group	Rest between sets
66%-83%	6-15	2-4	3-5	1-2 minutes

EXAMPLES OF EXERCISES USING MACHINES

Incline chest press (chest)	Lateral raise machine (shoulders)	Seated row (back)
Pec deck (chest)	Upright row on Smith machine (shoulders)	Bent-over row on Smith machine (back)
Dip machine (triceps)	Seated press machine (shoulders)	Seated leg curl (hamstrings)
Overhead extension machine (triceps)	Hack squat (quadriceps)	Lying leg curl (hamstrings)
Crunches machine (abs)	Leg press (quadriceps)	Standing leg curl (hamstrings)
Leg raise on Roman chair (abs)	Leg extension (quadriceps)	Biceps curl machine (biceps)
Standing calf (calves)	Assisted pull-up (back)	Alternating biceps curl (biceps)

Technique #161

Perceived effort

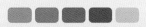

Effect on hypertrophy

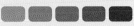

Effect on strength and power

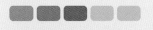

Effect on muscular endurance

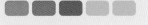

Experience required

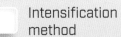

✓ Accumulation method

☐ Intensification method

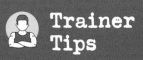

Trainer Tips

This technique is a must for everyone who has more than 1 year of training experience. All muscle fibers are recruited: type IIb (fast twitch) in the beginning, type IIa (fast twitch) in the middle, and type I (slow twitch) at the end.

HSS-100

HOW DOES IT WORK?

This method, created by my friend Christian Thibaudeau, is a workout plan for one muscle group.[38] You must complete the following, separately and in order:

1. **H:** Heavy, a maximum-strength exercise (see chapter 2)
2. **S:** Superset, the agonist superset (technique #71)
3. **S:** Special technique, any technique in chapter 3, 4, 5, 6, 7, or 8 of this book
4. **100:** 100 repetitions (technique #214)

An example HSS-100 program is included in chapter 10.

ADVANTAGES

→ It is an excellent training plan to gain muscle mass.

→ It is easy to use.

→ It increases the number of techniques for each workout.

DISADVANTAGES

→ None.

PRESCRIPTION TABLE

Load	Number of repetitions per set	Number of sets per exercise	Number of exercises per muscle group	Rest between sets
Dependent on the technique used	Dependent on the technique used	Dependent on the technique used	5	Dependent on the technique used

EXAMPLE OF HSS-100

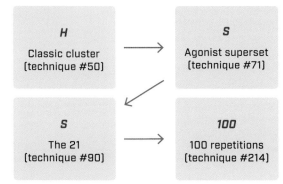

Technique #162

Perceived effort

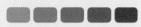

Effect on hypertrophy

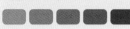

Effect on strength and power

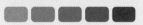

Effect on muscular endurance

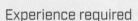

Experience required

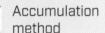 Accumulation method

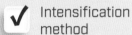 Intensification method

Trainer Tips

I love using layer system styles (HSS-100, technique #161, is a kind of layer system). An example of a layer system is: first exercise, strength technique (chapter 2); second exercise, emphasis on eccentric movement (chapter 5); third exercise, isometric position (chapter 4); and fourth exercise, metabolic style (rapid movements lasting less than 1 minute). All exercises are done separately.

THE LAYER SYSTEM

HOW DOES IT WORK?

This method, created by my friend Christian Thibaudeau, is a training plan for a muscle group using only one exercise.[39] Training with layers requires that you work on a muscular quality at each of the stages, or layers, of this system. You will have 5 layers to accomplish in each session:

1. **Layer 1: Activation and potentiation.** Perform an isometric exercise at maximum intensity (technique #165). Do 4 sets of 6 seconds each.

2. **Layer 2: Maximal strength.** Perform 5-7 sets of 2 repetitions, gradually increasing the load until you reach your 2RM. Start with 60%-70% load.

3. **Layer 3: Mechanical stress.** Perform a classic cluster (technique #50) at 90% of your 2RM determined at layer 2. Do 3 sets of 4-6 repetitions in the form of clusters.

4. **Layer 4: Slow eccentrics.** Complete 3 sets of 6-8 super slow eccentric reps (technique #106) at 70% of your 2RM.

5. **Layer 5: Growth hormone release.** Complete 1-2 sets of 45-75 seconds under tension at 50% of your 2RM. Use only a range of motion between 1/4 and 3/4 of the chosen movement to perform your repetitions under constant tension (technique #127).

PRESCRIPTION TABLE

Load	Number of seconds or repetitions per set	Number of sets per exercise	Number of exercises per muscle group	Rest between sets
50%-110%	6-75 seconds or 2-8 repetitions	1-7	1	1-3 minutes

4 sets of 6 seconds, rest 1 minute
5-7 sets of 2 reps (60%-100% of 2RM), rest 2 minutes
3 sets of 4-6 reps (90% of 2RM), rest 3 minutes
3 sets of 6-8 reps (70% of 2RM), rest 90 seconds
1-2 sets of 45-75 seconds (50% of 2RM), rest 90 seconds

CHAPTER 4

ISOMETRIC TRAINING

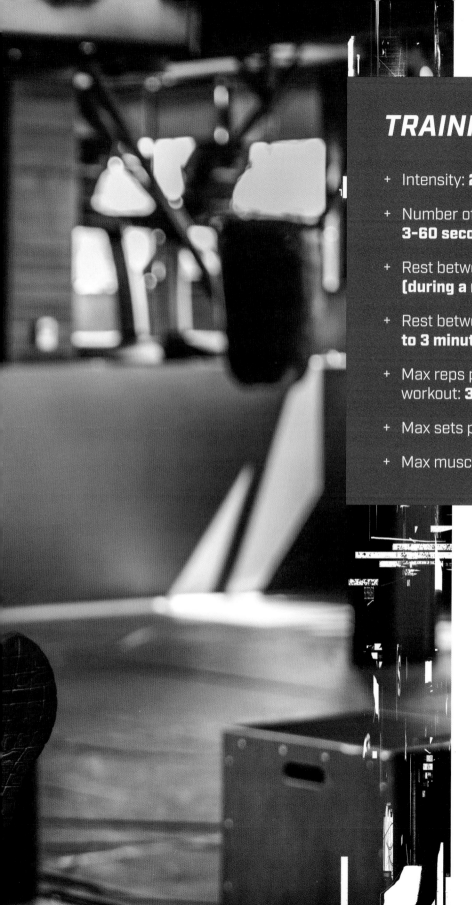

TRAINING PROGRAM

+ Intensity: **25%-110%**

+ Number of repetitions: **1-12 or 3-60 seconds of effort**

+ Rest between reps: **3-6 seconds (during a maximal effort)**

+ Rest between sets: **10 seconds to 3 minutes**

+ Max reps per muscle group per workout: **30**

+ Max sets per muscle group: **16**

+ Max muscle groups per workout: **2**

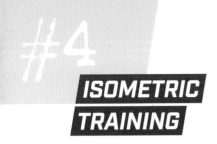

#4
ISOMETRIC TRAINING

Isometric training techniques, in my opinion, are underutilized and deserve special attention. They are known to allow 10%-15% higher force production than during the concentric phase of the same exercise and to intensify work in specific angles of movement.[2] Furthermore, in his book *A System of Multi-Year Training in Weightlifting*, Medvedyev stated that the recruitment of muscle motor units in isometric contractions was almost maximal, leading to strength and hypertrophy gains.[28] Strength gains, however, apply only to a working angle of +/−20 degrees, which is why it is important to vary the working angle when using these techniques.

Isometric training is not very representative of the typical movements used in everyday life or sport, which makes them all too easy to forget, even for trainers such as myself. The only sport that requires 100% isometric contractions is bodybuilding, from which one technique has been included in this book (posing, technique #163). Some other sports have a relatively high demand for isometric contraction, such as downhill skiing, snowboarding, and water skiing. However, these are primarily yielding isometric contractions or braking actions. For athletes who compete in these sports, it will be important to add quasi-isometric exercises to their training program.

It is rather ironic that we can improve a movement by training the body not to do that movement. Nevertheless, even in the absence of the movement, the muscle is placed under tremendous strain, resulting in subsequent transferable gains. Try it yourself! You will see that the following techniques are not easy and that they require concentration, motivation, and determination in order to extend the time spent under tension during each set. They will challenge you and introduce variety to your workouts.

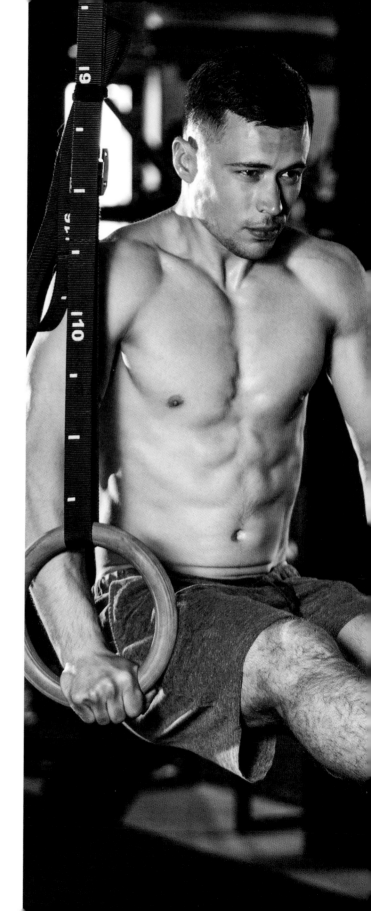

Perceived effort

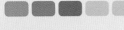

Effect on hypertrophy

Effect on strength and power

Effect on muscular endurance

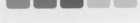

Experience required

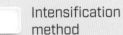

☑ Accumulation method

☐ Intensification method

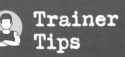

Trainer Tips

Personally, I like to use this technique as an agonist superset (technique #71). For example, try doing a front lat pull-down followed by an isometric front lat spread for 20-30 seconds.

POSING

HOW DOES IT WORK?

Hold bodybuilding poses for 10-60 seconds each. Choose 1-4 poses and do 8-12 isometric reps. This can constitute a 30-40 minute workout if you opt to hold each pose for 60 seconds, or you can insert the poses into your regular workout.

This technique is based on the premise that individuals who hold poses have better muscle density than those who do not. This muscle density stems from structural gains (and nonfunctional fibers, unless the isometric contractions are maximal) and increasing the number of components required for energy systems (creatine phosphate pool, capillarization, etc.).

ADVANTAGES

→ It requires no equipment and no external load.
→ It is simple and easy to perform, no matter where you are.

DISADVANTAGES

→ It requires a good muscle–brain connection in order to be able to contract the targeted muscle.
→ To get a great muscle contraction, you must know how to perform the poses.

PRESCRIPTION TABLE

Load	Number of repetitions per set	Number of sets per exercise	Number of exercises per muscle group	Rest between sets
50%-100% of your maximal muscle contraction capacity	8-12	1-3	1-4	2-3 minutes

Technique #164

Perceived effort

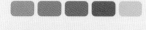

Effect on hypertrophy

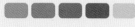

Effect on strength and power

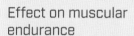

Effect on muscular endurance

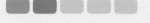

Experience required

✓ Accumulation method

☐ Intensification method

Trainer Tips

During an overcoming isometric contraction, moderate the amount of force produced to avoid an isometric contraction of maximum intensity (technique #165), which is not the goal here. Try to maintain constant tension in the muscle for 20-60 seconds.

MAXIMUM DURATION ISOMETRIC

HOW DOES IT WORK?

This technique, also known as total isometry, involves repeated efforts. You can use two types of isometry, overcoming and yielding. Overcoming isometry involves a push or pull against a stationary resistance. For example, in a squat cage, place the safety locks at the top of your bar so that they block your path in the concentric phase. Then exert sufficient pressure, with an empty bar, for the targeted time. If you are very strong, you can add weight on the bar to avoid lifting the squat cage.

Yielding isometry involves simply holding a load halfway through the movement to prevent it from descending with gravity (e.g., during a squat, pull-up, or bench press). One such example is the iso-max eccentric (technique #169).

Try to vary your workout by using at least three different positions.

ADVANTAGES

→ Because a muscle can produce 10%-15% more force during an isometric contraction than during a concentric contraction,[2] this method has the advantage of producing more overall tension in the muscle over a specific period of time compared to standard reps.

→ Reaching a time under tension of 20-60 seconds will create gains in hypertrophy. Therefore, yielding isometric will have better results on hypertrophy than overcoming isometric contractions because the loads will be higher.

DISADVANTAGES

→ This method requires good self-awareness in order to properly mediate the force generated to avoid premature exhaustion.

PRESCRIPTION TABLE

Load	Number of seconds per set	Number of sets per exercise	Number of exercises per muscle group	Rest between sets
60%-80%*	20-60 seconds	2-4 per position	1	1-2 minutes

*Meet this percentage range for the yielding isometric contraction phase, and try to meet this percentage range with the safety bars engaged during the overcoming isometric contraction phase (the percentage may be less). You are stronger during yielding isometric contraction, so even at the same percentage, the load will be greater.

Technique #165

Perceived effort

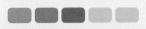

Effect on hypertrophy

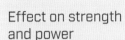

Effect on strength and power

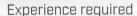

Effect on muscular endurance

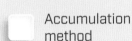

Experience required

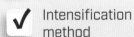

- [ ] Accumulation method
- [✓] Intensification method

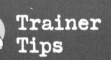

Trainer Tips

This technique requires some experience before attempting because it includes the manipulation of heavy loads (100%-110%) and therefore has a high risk of injury if you are not well prepared.

MAXIMUM INTENSITY ISOMETRIC

Ⓢ

HOW DOES IT WORK?

This method uses the same principle as the maximum duration isometric (technique #164), but with a shorter, maximum intensity effort. You can use two types of isometry, overcoming or yielding.

Overcoming isometry involves a push or pull against a stationary resistance. For example, in a squat cage, place the safety locks at the top of your bar so that they block your path in the concentric phase. Then exert sufficient pressure for the targeted time.

Yielding isometry involves simply holding a load halfway through the movement to prevent it from descending with gravity (e.g., during a squat, pull-up, or bench press).

Although overcoming isometric contractions are preferable, yielding isometric contractions may also be used. To do this, use 100%-110% of your 1RM. Don't forget to vary your workout by including at least three different positions.

ADVANTAGES

→ It increases muscle density.
→ It improves strength in specific angles of movement.

DISADVANTAGES

→ It has little impact on muscular hypertrophy.
→ It must be combined with dynamic movements.

PRESCRIPTION TABLE

Load	Number of seconds per set	Number of sets per exercise	Number of exercises per muscle group	Rest between sets
100%-110%*	3-6 seconds per position	3-6 (9-36 seconds total)	1	30-90 seconds

*during a yielding isometric contraction

Technique #166

Perceived effort

▮▯▯▯▯

Effect on hypertrophy

▮▯▯▯▯

Effect on strength and power

▮▮▮▯▯

Effect on muscular endurance

▮▯▯▯▯

Experience required

▮▮▮

☐ Accumulation method

☑ Intensification method

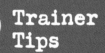

Trainer Tips

If your gym has strict rules regarding noise level, this technique may not be possible because it does produce a lot of noise when the barbell makes contact with the safety bars.

BALLISTIC ISOMETRIC

HOW DOES IT WORK?

In a squat cage, adjust the safety catches to a height that will prevent you from completing your concentric phase. Perform a very short, maximal effort isometric contraction (try to go from 0%-100% effort in 1-2 seconds). Be sure to vary the positions (use between 2 and 4) in order to work the muscle across the entire range of motion.

ADVANTAGES

→ This technique is very easy to use as long as you have access to a squat rack equipped with safety catches.

→ It helps improve recruitment speed from a state of complete relaxation to a state of maximal contraction.

DISADVANTAGES

→ Because so little time is spent under strain, gains in hypertrophy and endurance are negligible.

→ Given the maximum power generated by the muscle, it is important that anyone who tries this technique has a few months of prior training experience to prevent tendon or muscle injury.

PRESCRIPTION TABLE

Load	Number of seconds per set	Number of sets per exercise	Number of exercises per muscle group	Rest between sets
Body weight or barbell only	10-40 seconds (ideally 5-10 seconds per position)	5-10	1	10-30 seconds

Here are some examples of exercises you can do:

→ **Bench press** (chest)
→ **Squat** (legs)
→ **Barbell curl** (biceps)
→ **Lying barbell triceps extension** (triceps)
→ **Seated barbell shoulder press** (shoulders)
→ **Bent-over barbell row** (back)

Technique #167

Perceived effort

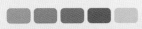

Effect on hypertrophy

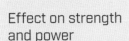

Effect on strength and power

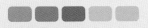

Effect on muscular endurance

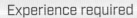

Experience required

☑ Accumulation method

☐ Intensification method

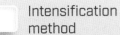
ISOMETRIC WITH PERTURBATIONS

Ⓢ

HOW DOES IT WORK?

Also known as pseudo-isometrics, this technique involves holding an isometric contraction for as long as possible while enduring perturbations of either the machine, the bar, or yourself caused by a partner.

This technique improves both intramuscular (inside the muscle) and intermuscular (between the muscles) coordination, which are useful and transferable to sports such as football, downhill skiing, and snowboarding. A good use of this technique is as part of an agonist superset (technique #71)—for example, a bench fly combined with an isometric bench press with the elbows at 90 degrees while a partner perturbs the bar with random pushing.

ADVANTAGES

→ This technique helps increase muscle recruitment by varying the tension in a set, thereby fatiguing a wider range of muscle fibers than during an isometric contraction with no perturbations.

DISADVANTAGES

→ It requires a partner to provide pressure variation while maintaining the isometric position.

PRESCRIPTION TABLE

Load	Number of seconds per set	Number of sets per exercise	Number of exercises per muscle group	Rest between sets
50%-80%	20-40 seconds	2-4 per position	1	60-90 seconds

Technique #168

Perceived effort

Effect on
hypertrophy

Effect on strength
and power

Effect on muscular
endurance

Experience required

✓ Accumulation
method

☐ Intensification
method

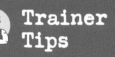

Trainer Tips

I recommend using this technique at the end of your workout for the targeted muscle group. This will promote muscular hypertrophy and help with your recovery by lengthening the muscle tissue postworkout.

QUASI-ISOMETRIC ECCENTRIC

HOW DOES IT WORK?

This technique involves performing eccentric reps very slowly—so slowly that the reps seem isometric, hence the name. Using light loads (25%-30%), start halfway through the movement. Hold this position as long as possible. The more time goes by, the more you will fatigue and slowly begin to drop the load. Continue the set until complete exhaustion.

This technique increases the flexibility of the muscle's series components (e.g., tendons, titin) more than conventional stretching, which stretches the parallel components (epimysium, perimysium, endomysium). This helps reduce the gap in stretching ability between series and parallel components, thereby reducing the risk of injury.

ADVANTAGES

→ It is easy to use and does not require heavy weight.

DISADVANTAGES

→ When this technique is accomplished alone, it provides very little adaptation. It should be used as the last exercise in your workout for a muscle group.

PRESCRIPTION TABLE

Load	Number of minutes per set	Number of sets per exercise	Number of exercises per muscle group	Rest between sets
Body weight or 25%-30%	1-4	1	1	N/A

Technique #169

Perceived effort

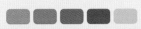

Effect on hypertrophy

Effect on strength and power

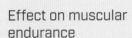

Effect on muscular endurance

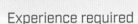

Experience required

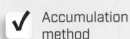

✓ Accumulation method

☐ Intensification method

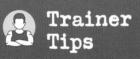

Trainer Tips

If you do not have a training partner, choose pulley or free weight exercises to make it easier to set down the load once muscle failure is achieved. Make sure you always have good control of the eccentric phase to avoid injury.

ISO-MAX ECCENTRIC

HOW DOES IT WORK?

Lower the bar to the point in the movement at which you are strongest and maintain this position for as long as possible. Once failure is reached, slowly lower the load to full range of motion and ask a partner to help you if you need to lift the bar again. Also referred to as eccentric–isometric contrast 3, this technique is similar to the maximal duration isometric method (technique #164) with the addition of a controlled eccentric phase following muscle failure.

ADVANTAGES

→ A muscle in isometric contraction can produce 10%-15% more force than during a concentric contraction.[2] This method has the advantage of producing more overall tension in the muscle over a specific period of time compared to standard reps.

→ The eccentric phase following failure causes further gains in hypertrophy.

DISADVANTAGES

→ Certain exercises require a spotter (e.g., bench press).

PRESCRIPTION TABLE

Load	Number of repetitions per set	Number of sets per exercise	Number of exercises per muscle group	Rest between sets
70%-90%	1	3-7	1-3	2-3 minutes

Maintain a load as long as possible until muscle failure Complete the eccentric phase following muscle failure

Technique #170

Perceived effort

Effect on hypertrophy

Effect on strength and power

Effect on muscular endurance

Experience required

☐ Accumulation method

☑ Intensification method

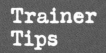

Trainer Tips

Electrostimulation activates fast-twitch fibers and therefore leads to fatigue only for these muscle fibers, which causes slight gains in strength and hypertrophy. It is useful for injured athletes to avoid early muscle wasting.

ELECTROSTIMULATION

HOW DOES IT WORK?

This technique was developed in the Soviet Union in the late 1960s and requires the use of an electrostimulation device. You must first apply the electrodes to the muscle group or region you want to work. Then, ideally adjust the frequency of the device to more than 2,500 Hz and the modulation to 50 Hz. You will then perform contractions lasting 10 seconds with a rest of 50 seconds, over a period of 10 minutes (10 cycles).

ADVANTAGES

→ This technique makes it possible to isolate muscle regions that are difficult to recruit (e.g., vastus medialis of the quadriceps).

DISADVANTAGES

→ It allows you to train only the muscles and not the neural components.

→ Research regarding electrostimulation is lacking, making it impossible to establish final recommendations; however, the prescription table is a good start if you want to use it.

PRESCRIPTION TABLE

Load	Number of seconds per contraction	Rest between contractions	Number of contractions per day	Number of days per week
100% of a maximal voluntary isometric contraction	10	50 seconds	10	5

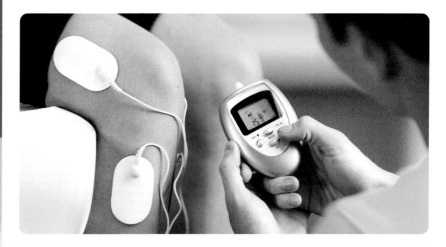

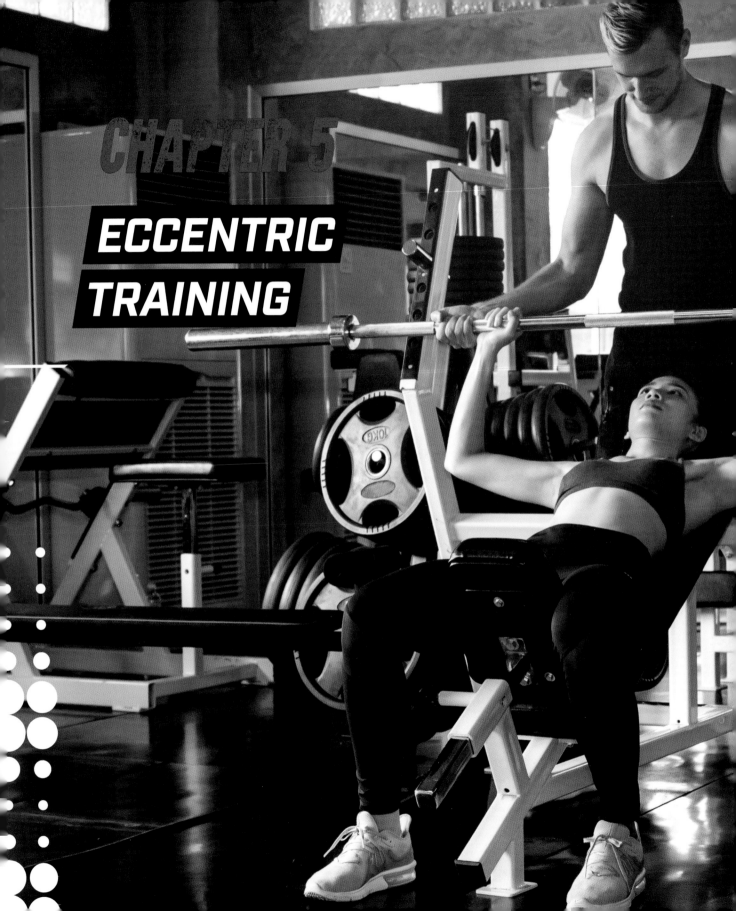

CHAPTER 5

ECCENTRIC TRAINING

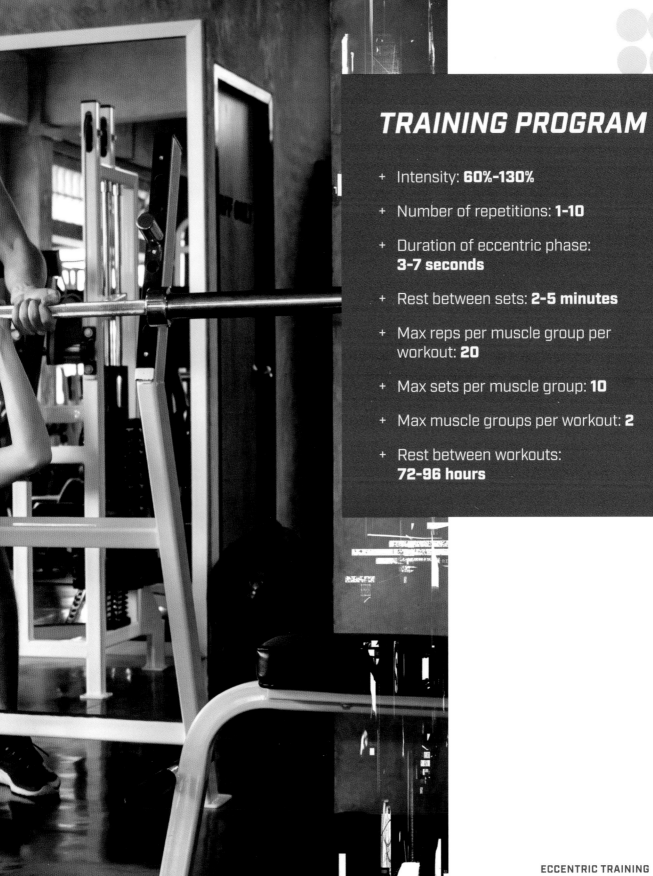

TRAINING PROGRAM

+ Intensity: **60%-130%**

+ Number of repetitions: **1-10**

+ Duration of eccentric phase:
  3-7 seconds

+ Rest between sets: **2-5 minutes**

+ Max reps per muscle group per
  workout: **20**

+ Max sets per muscle group: **10**

+ Max muscle groups per workout: **2**

+ Rest between workouts:
  72-96 hours

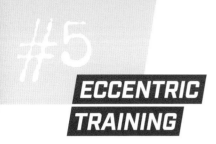

#5
ECCENTRIC TRAINING

Eccentric training has been found to be more effective than concentric and isometric training at improving strength and increasing muscle hypertrophy.[3,18,19] This is a result of several factors:

1. You use heavier loads than with concentric training.

2. You recruit fewer muscle fibers overall, thereby increasing the load supported by each individual fiber (mainly fast-twitch fibers conducive to hypertrophy).

3. The mechanical tension will be higher on each fiber.

4. Your nervous system has to make greater adaptations, leading to greater recruitment of motor units and better gains in strength.

The eccentric phase is therefore extremely important for muscle adaptation. However, it is still all too common for people to focus on the number of reps instead of prioritizing time spent under tension. I believe that we can teach people about the importance of the eccentric phase by including more of these techniques in training programs. The techniques in this section are very effective at improving strength and can even be an integral part of programs designed for building muscle mass, especially when used at the beginning of a workout. The difference between the eccentric contraction we

perform in all movements and the eccentric techniques in this chapter is that these techniques will permit us to use higher loads. However, because of the stress placed on joints and muscles, eccentric training techniques are reserved for individuals with strength training experience (>1.5 years). Moreover, you must always have someone nearby in case you get into trouble or just to help you during the concentric phase of the movements. Also, don't be surprised if you have more soreness in the days following the integration of these methods! The phrase "no soreness, no success" (a personal version derived from "no pain, no gain") then takes on its full meaning.

Strength Deficit
An eccentric–concentric strength deficit is the difference between your maximum eccentric strength and maximum concentric strength.[37] In order to evaluate your percentage of strength deficit, you will have to find your concentric 1RM on the chosen exercise, then your eccentric 1RM by increasing the load gradually. A successful eccentric rep is a rep that is descended (e.g., squat) under control for 3-5 seconds.[29] An ideal ratio of eccentric to concentric force should be approximately 1.2:1.0, which is equivalent to 15%-20% more eccentric force than concentric. If you notice a major strength deficit (e.g., an eccentric 1RM of 100 kg and concentric 1RM of 72 kg in the bench press, equivalent to a strength deficit of 28%), you will need to

integrate explosive training techniques (e.g., potentiation methods) to improve your neuromuscular activation. Conversely, if you have a small strength deficit (e.g., an eccentric 1RM of 105 kg—your body weight plus a 5-kg overload belt—and concentric 1RM of your body weight only in the pull-ups, equivalent to a 5% strength deficit), you will need to start hypertrophy techniques (chapter 3) quickly followed by maximal effort techniques (chapter 2), then eccentric work (chapter 5).

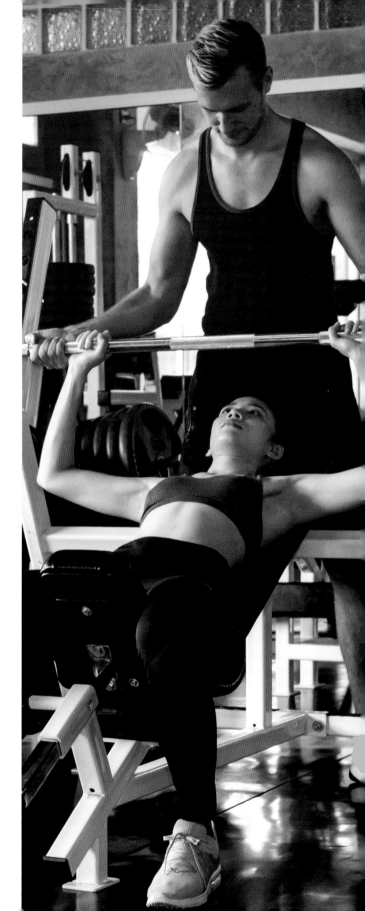

Technique #171

Perceived effort

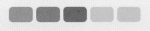

Effect on
hypertrophy

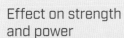

Effect on strength
and power

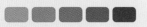

Effect on muscular
endurance

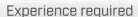

Experience required

☐ Accumulation
method

☑ Intensification
method

2/1 TECHNIQUE

Ⓢ

HOW DOES IT WORK?

This technique involves overloading a unilateral movement. To do this, execute the concentric phase explosively using both limbs, then control the eccentric phase for 3-5 seconds using only one limb.

ADVANTAGES

→ This technique is very easy to use with stationary machines (biceps curl, leg extension, leg curl, triceps extension, etc.) and cables.

→ It helps increase the eccentric work, which places more strain on fast-twitch fibers, leading to strength gains that transfer to the concentric phase of the same movement (one of the advantages of eccentric training).

DISADVANTAGES

→ It is impossible (or at least very difficult) to use with barbells and free weights.

PRESCRIPTION TABLE

Load	Number of repetitions per set	Number of sets per exercise	Number of exercises per muscle group	Rest between sets
100%-125%	1-6 per arm or leg	4-8	1-2	2-3 minutes

Concentric phase with both hands or legs	→	Controlled eccentric phase (3-5 seconds) with 1 arm or 1 leg

The following are sample exercises by muscle group:

Legs (two legs in concentric, one leg in eccentric): Leg press, leg extension, leg curl

Pectorals (two arms in concentric, one arm in eccentric):
Chest press or bench press in Smith machine

Back (pull with both arms in concentric, one arm in eccentric):
One-arm seated row with pulley

Shoulders (pull with both arms in concentric, one arm in eccentric):
One-arm lateral raise with low pulley

Triceps (pull with both arms in concentric, one arm in eccentric):
One-arm triceps kick-back

Biceps (two arms in concentric, one arm in eccentric): Curl machine

Technique #172

Perceived effort

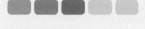

Effect on hypertrophy

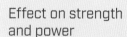

Effect on strength and power

Effect on muscular endurance

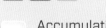

Experience required

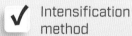

☐ Accumulation method

☑ Intensification method

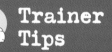

Trainer Tips

During certain exercises (e.g., lat pull-down), you can use a cheat set (technique #120) to complete the concentric phase. However, you will have to hold the load for at least 1 second at the end of the concentric phase in order to control it throughout the eccentric phase.

2-MOVEMENTS TECHNIQUE

HOW DOES IT WORK?

This technique is an alternative to the 2/1 technique (technique #171) for barbell and free weight exercises and involves overloading an isolation movement. Use a multijoint movement for the concentric phase and an isolation movement for the eccentric phase (3-5 seconds). The isolation movement focuses on a muscle group that is involved in the multijoint movement.

ADVANTAGES

→ It increases the amount of work and level of intensity in the eccentric phase, which places further strain on fast-twitch fibers, leading to gains in strength that can be transferred to the concentric phase of the isolation movement (one of the advantages of eccentric training).

DISADVANTAGES

→ It is impossible (or very difficult) to achieve with exercises on machines.

PRESCRIPTION TABLE

Load	Number of repetitions per set	Number of sets per exercise	Number of exercises per muscle group	Rest between sets
100%-125%	1-6	4-8	1-2	2-3 minutes

The following are sample exercises by muscle group:

Brachialis: Clean (concentric) + pronated barbell curl (eccentric)

Triceps: Close-grip bench press (concentric) + lying triceps extension (eccentric)

Shoulders: Clean and press (concentric) + front raise (eccentric)

Chest: Dumbbell bench press (concentric) + fly (eccentric)

Upper back: Bent-over dumbbell row to chest (concentric) + rear delt fly (eccentric)

Technique #173

Perceived effort

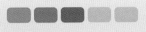

Effect on hypertrophy

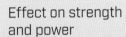

Effect on strength and power

Effect on muscular endurance

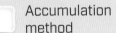

Experience required

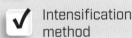

☐ Accumulation method

☑ Intensification method

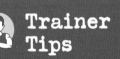

Trainer Tips

Make sure you are always able to control the load during the eccentric phase. If the load accelerates during this phase, stop the set or reduce the load immediately.

 Ⓢ

PURE ECCENTRIC (MAXIMAL AND SUPRAMAXIMAL)

HOW DOES IT WORK?

This technique involves performing only the eccentric phase of a movement for a given amount of time while a partner helps you execute the concentric phase. Weight releasers can be used to overload the eccentric phase if you do not have a partner.

ADVANTAGES

→ It is very demanding at the musculoskeletal and nervous system levels.

→ It encompasses all of the exercises that cannot be used with the 2/1 technique (technique #171) or the 2-movements technique (technique #172) to overload the eccentric phase of a movement. This includes the bench press, pull-up, standing curl, back squat (with 2 partners, 1 on each side of the bar), and so on.

DISADVANTAGES

→ It requires one or more partners or special equipment that is not usually found in most weight rooms (e.g., weight releasers).

PRESCRIPTION TABLE

Load	Number of repetitions per set	Number of sets per exercise	Number of exercises per muscle group	Rest between sets
90%-125%	1-4	4-8	1-2	2-3 minutes

The following are time and rep recommendations for various loads:

90%-95%: 5 seconds for 3-4 repetitions

95%-100%: 5 seconds for 2-3 repetitions

100%-105%: 7 seconds for 2 repetitions

105%-110%: 6 seconds for 2 repetitions

110%-115%: 5 seconds for 2 repetitions

115%-120%: 4 seconds for 2 repetitions

120%-125%: 4 seconds for 1 repetition

Technique #174

Perceived effort

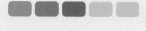

Effect on hypertrophy

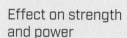

Effect on strength and power

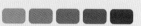

Effect on muscular endurance

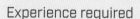

Experience required

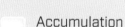

☐ Accumulation method

✓ Intensification method

Trainer Tips

Once you have developed your landing ability (when you are able to do 10 repetitions easily with your body weight without letting your hips go too deep in a squat position), you can then work on your ability to use the generated elastic force to increase your power during the following concentric phase (e.g., depth jump, technique #175).

DEPTH LANDING

HOW DOES IT WORK?

This technique helps improve your ability to absorb impacts. From a height of 0.75-1.25 meters, step off a box and land in a half- or quarter-squat (for general development) or in another position relevant to your sport.

ADVANTAGES

→ This is a shock training technique that helps develop your ability to absorb an external force.

DISADVANTAGES

→ This technique runs the risk of producing forces that range from 150%-200% of your concentric maximum (approximately 4-5 times your body weight). Slow and steady progress is therefore essential.
→ It may require several boxes to reach the desired height (inaccessible in some weight rooms).
→ It is very demanding on the muscular and nervous systems.

PRESCRIPTION TABLE

Load	Number of repetitions per set	Number of sets per exercise	Number of exercises per muscle group	Rest between sets
Body weight	3-10	3-5	1-2	2-3 minutes

The following are sample exercises by muscle group:

Chest: Depth landing push-up (drop between two boxes in a push-up position and land with your hands on the ground)

Legs: Depth landing squat (drop from a box and land in a quarter- or half-squat, or a depth that is relevant to your sport)

Back: Depth landing pull-up (drop from one pull-up bar to another just below)

Technique #175

Perceived effort

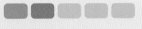

Effect on
hypertrophy

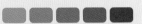

Effect on strength
and power

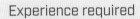

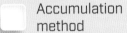

Effect on muscular
endurance

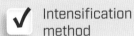

Experience required

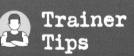

☐ Accumulation
method

☑ Intensification
method

Trainer Tips

To reduce the risk of injury caused by the extreme load placed on the joints and muscles using this kind of technique, do not exceed 40 ground contacts per workout. This also applies to depth landing (technique #174).

DEPTH JUMP

HOW DOES IT WORK?

This technique is the extension of the depth landing (technique #174). It requires you to harness the kinetic energy accumulated during ground impact and use it to enhance the power generated during the following concentric phase. You should therefore start from a height of 0.40-0.70 meters, quickly absorb the impact upon landing without letting your heels touch the ground, then propel yourself as high as possible. This constitutes 1 repetition.

ADVANTAGES

→ This technique improves your ability to utilize the kinetic energy accumulated by your tendons and connective tissue.
→ It is very effective at promoting power development.

DISADVANTAGES

→ This technique runs the risk of producing forces that range from 100%-160% of your concentric maximum.[11] Slow and steady progress is therefore essential.

PRESCRIPTION TABLE

Load	Number of repetitions per set	Number of sets per exercise	Number of exercises per muscle group	Rest between sets
Body weight	3-10	3-5	1-2	2-3 minutes

The following are sample exercises by muscle group:

Chest: Depth jump push-up (drop between two boxes in a push-up position, land with your hands on the ground, and push up as fast as possible to return to the boxes)

Legs: Depth jump squat (drop from a box, land in a squat position, and jump as high as possible)

Back: Depth jump pull-up (drop from one pull-up bar to another just below, land on the second bar, and pull up as fast as possible to the first bar)

Technique #176

Perceived effort

▣▣▣▣▢▢

Effect on hypertrophy

▣▣▣▢▢▢

Effect on strength and power

▣▣▣▣▢▢

Effect on muscular endurance

▣▢▢▢▢▢

Experience required

▣▣▣

☐ Accumulation method

☑ Intensification method

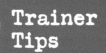

Trainer Tips

This technique is often used in Olympic weightlifting—either intentionally or unintentionally—due to the speed of the movement when the load is received. An introduction to Olympic weightlifting is a good avenue for learning this method.

OVERSPEED ECCENTRIC

HOW DOES IT WORK?

Perform the eccentric phase and the transition between the eccentric and concentric phases very quickly. Elastic bands (or superbands) and weight releasers may be used to create this overspeed. This technique is best used with barbell exercises.

ADVANTAGES

→ This technique is similar to a depth jump (technique #175), but for non-body-weight exercises (e.g., bench press, deadlift). The overload created is equal to about 100%-160% of your concentric maximum.[5,11] This increase in kinetic energy serves to trigger a greater adaptation of fast-twitch fibers, thereby promoting gains in strength and hypertrophy.

DISADVANTAGES

→ The risk of injury may be high for some exercises (e.g., bench press). Be careful when applying this technique to these exercises.

→ You need to be very proficient at technique and have a high level of body awareness to perform this technique safely.

PRESCRIPTION TABLE

Load	Number of repetitions per set	Number of sets per exercise	Number of exercises per muscle group	Rest between sets
50%-70%	3-10	3-5	1-2	2-3 minutes

The following are sample exercises by muscle group:

Chest: Overspeed eccentric bench press (bring the bar rapidly to your chest, stop it just before it touches your chest, and push it up as fast as possible)

Legs: Overspeed eccentric back squat (quickly lower yourself down from a standing position with a barbell on your shoulders, stop your descent when your glutes are close to your ankles, and rise up as fast as possible)

Back: Overspeed eccentric deadlift (lower the bar rapidly to the floor, briefly touch the bar to the floor, and rise up as fast as possible)

Technique #177

Perceived effort

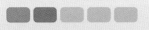

Effect on hypertrophy

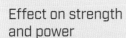

Effect on strength and power

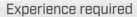

Effect on muscular endurance

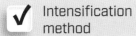

Experience required

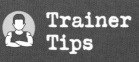

☐ Accumulation method

☑ Intensification method

Trainer Tips

If you cannot stop the weight immediately, the load is too heavy and should be reduced.

DROP AND CATCH

HOW DOES IT WORK?

This technique is similar to a depth landing (technique #174), except that it targets the upper body. It can be done with exercises such as the standing curl, barbell row, upright row, and dumbbell front raise. With each rep, let go of the bar with your hands, then immediately catch it, stopping the movement for 3-5 seconds by contracting your muscles as hard as you can.

ADVANTAGES

→ This is a shock training technique that helps develop your ability to absorb an external force. Once you have developed your landing ability, you can begin to work on your ability to use the generated elastic force to increase your power during the following concentric phase (e.g., drop, catch, and lift, technique #178).

→ It is great training for combat sports and high-contact sports such as football and rugby.

DISADVANTAGES

→ It requires good coordination in order to let go of and catch the bar.

PRESCRIPTION TABLE

Load	Number of repetitions per set	Number of sets per exercise	Number of exercises per muscle group	Rest between sets
Based on your ability to decelerate the load	3-10	3-5	1-2	2-3 minutes

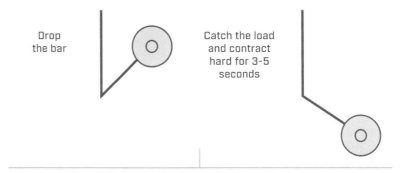

Drop the bar — Catch the load and contract hard for 3-5 seconds

Example: 1 rep of standing barbell curl

Technique #178

Perceived effort

■■□□□

Effect on
hypertrophy

■■□□□

Effect on strength
and power

■■■■■

Effect on muscular
endurance

■□□□□

Experience required

■■□

☐ Accumulation
method

✓ Intensification
method

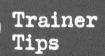

Trainer Tips

As with technique #177, if you cannot stop the weight immediately, it means that the load is too heavy.

DROP, CATCH, AND LIFT

HOW DOES IT WORK?

This technique is similar to a depth jump (technique #175), except that it targets the upper body. It can be done with exercises such as the standing curl, barbell row, upright row, and dumbbell front raise. With each rep, let go of the bar with your hands, then immediately catch it, accelerating it upward (concentric phase) as fast as possible.

ADVANTAGES

→ This technique improves your ability to utilize the kinetic energy accumulated by your tendons and connective tissue. You can also use it to improve strength-speed.

DISADVANTAGES

→ This technique runs the risk of producing forces that surpass your concentric maximum. Slow and steady progress with your loads is therefore essential.

→ It requires good coordination in order to let go of and catch the bar.

PRESCRIPTION TABLE

Load	Number of repetitions per set	Number of sets per exercise	Number of exercises per muscle group	Rest between sets
Based on your ability to decelerate the load	3-10	3-5	1-2	2-3 minutes

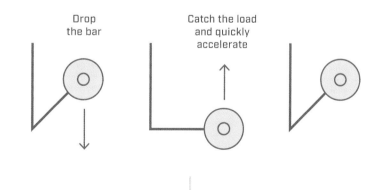

Example: 1 rep of standing barbell curl

Technique #179

Perceived effort

Effect on hypertrophy

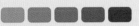

Effect on strength and power

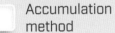

Effect on muscular endurance

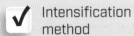

Experience required

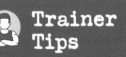

☐ Accumulation method

✓ Intensification method

SUPRAMAXIMAL CLUSTER

HOW DOES IT WORK?

This method is similar to a cluster (techniques #49-#56), but is included in this section given its entirely eccentric nature. Use supramaximal loads (100%-115%) and only perform the eccentric part of the movement. A partner will have to help you during the concentric phase. A set consists of 5 reps separated by 10-20 seconds of rest. Make sure to always control the eccentric phase for 3-5 seconds.

ADVANTAGES

→ It produces great gains in strength and hypertrophy.
→ It improves confidence by allowing you to handle loads above your actual maximum.

DISADVANTAGES

→ Certain exercises either require a partner to lift the bar (e.g., bench press) or safety locks to place the load at the end of the movement (e.g., bottom position in squat).
→ This technique carries a very high risk of injury. It is only recommended for well-trained individuals.

PRESCRIPTION TABLE

Load	Number of repetitions per set	Number of sets per exercise	Number of exercises per muscle group	Rest between sets
100%-115%	5	2-4	1	3-5 minutes

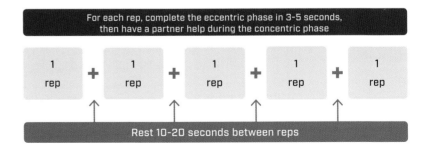

For each rep, complete the eccentric phase in 3-5 seconds, then have a partner help during the concentric phase

1 rep + 1 rep + 1 rep + 1 rep + 1 rep

Rest 10-20 seconds between reps

Technique #180

Perceived effort

Effect on hypertrophy

Effect on strength and power

Effect on muscular endurance

Experience required

☐ Accumulation method

☑ Intensification method

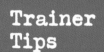

Trainer Tips

Start by familiarizing yourself with weight releasers using a lighter load (on your bar and the weight releasers) to avoid taking too much time to remove the brackets. At first, they may not release at the same time. Make sure you are comfortable before increasing the loads.

Ⓢ

CONTRAST WITH WEIGHT RELEASERS

HOW DOES IT WORK?

The purpose of this technique is to make the load as difficult in the eccentric phase as it is in the concentric phase. If you want to use your 85% for 5 reps, you will first have to figure out your maximums in the concentric and eccentric phases (the eccentric phase must be controlled for 5 seconds). Rerack the weight after each rep for 7-12 seconds to replace the brackets on the bar (weight releasers). If two partners place them while you hold the bar, the chances that they are not set at the same time are increased and so is the risk of injury.

ADVANTAGES

→ This technique lets you reach maximal fatigue in both the concentric and eccentric phases, which is not common with traditional techniques.

DISADVANTAGES

→ It can only be performed on a very small variety of exercises.
→ It needs frequent adjustment of loads (repositioning the weight releasers on the bar) and a good knowledge of your own limits.

PRESCRIPTION TABLE

Load	Number of repetitions per set	Number of sets per exercise	Number of exercises per muscle group	Rest between sets
70%-95% (of concentric and eccentric)	1-10	3-6	1	2-3 minutes

An example of this technique for the bench press might be the following: If you lift 120 kg eccentric and 100 kg concentric (1RM), the weight on the weight releasers will be calculated as 96 kg (120 × 80%) – 80 kg (100 × 80%) = 16 kg, so 8 kg on each weight releaser.

Perceived effort

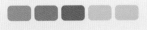

Effect on hypertrophy

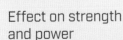

Effect on strength and power

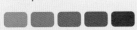

Effect on muscular endurance

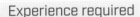

Experience required

☐ Accumulation method

✓ Intensification method

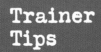

Trainer Tips

Start by familiarizing yourself with weight releasers using a lighter load (on your bar and the weight releasers) to avoid taking too much time to remove the brackets. At first, they may not release at the same time. Make sure you are comfortable before increasing the loads.

120/80 METHOD

HOW DOES IT WORK?

Use 120% of your max concentric load during the eccentric phase and 80% during the concentric phase immediately thereafter. This can be done in one of the following two ways:

1. Use weight releasers like in contrast with weight releasers (technique #180)
2. Have a partner press on the bar during the eccentric phase in order to overload (although this is not quantifiable)

ADVANTAGES

→ This technique combines a heavy eccentric phase with a concentric phase. Pure eccentric methods do not have a concentric phase because the partner is the one who lifts the bar. In the 120/80 version, you manage both phases on a muscular level, thereby increasing nervous and muscular fatigue.

DISADVANTAGES

→ It can only be performed on a very small variety of exercises.
→ It needs frequent adjustment of loads (repositioning the weight releasers on the bar) and a good knowledge of your own limits.

PRESCRIPTION TABLE

Load	Number of repetitions per set	Number of sets per exercise	Number of exercises per muscle group	Rest between sets
120% (of concentric) + 80% (of concentric)	2-5	2-5	1	3-5 minutes

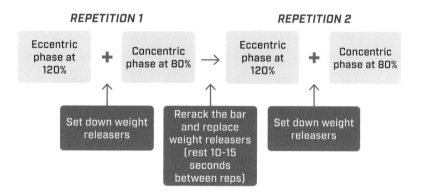

REPETITION 1

Eccentric phase at 120% **+** Concentric phase at 80% →

Set down weight releasers

Rerack the bar and replace weight releasers (rest 10-15 seconds between reps)

REPETITION 2

Eccentric phase at 120% **+** Concentric phase at 80%

Set down weight releasers

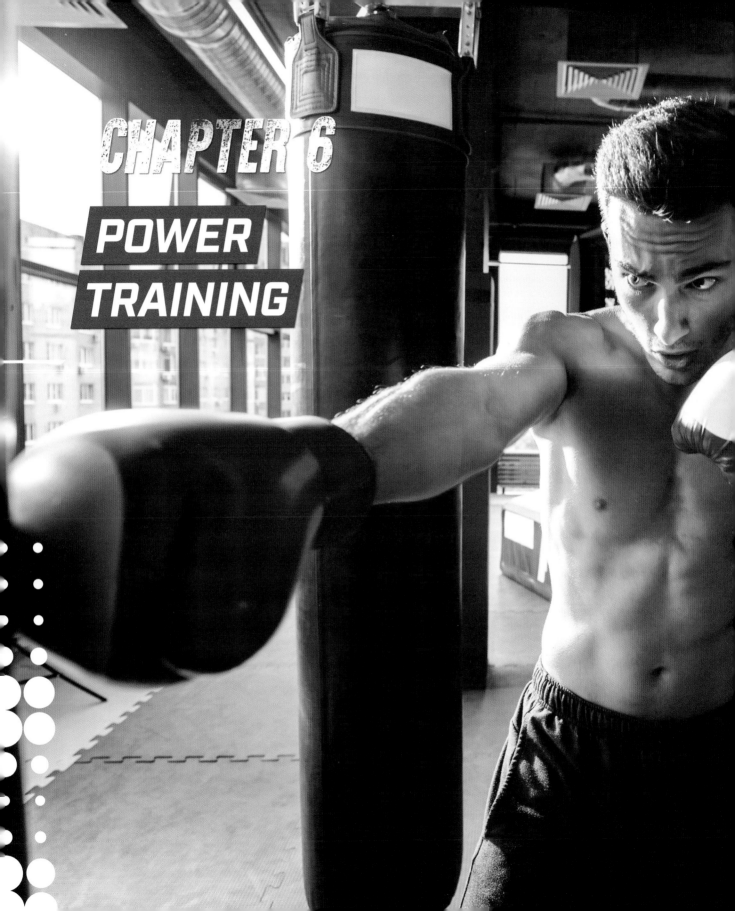

CHAPTER 6

POWER TRAINING

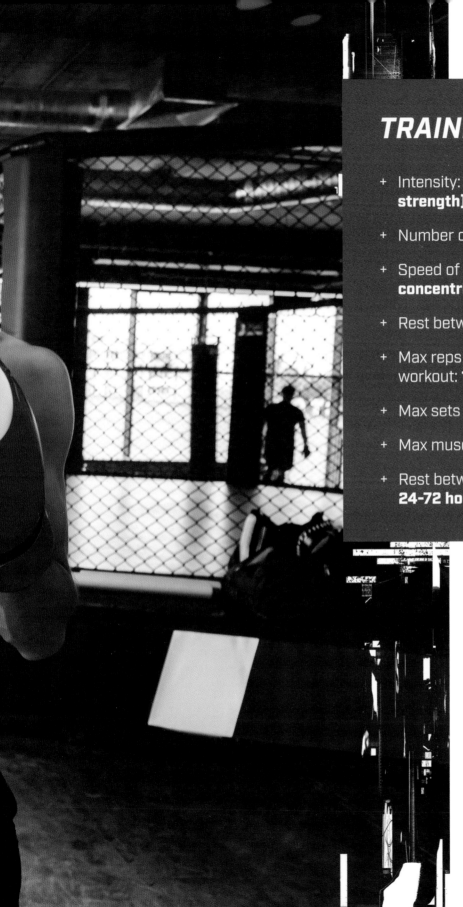

TRAINING PROGRAM

+ Intensity: **50%-120% (power-strength), 10%-50% (power-speed)**

+ Number of repetitions: **1-10**

+ Speed of execution: **Maximal in concentric and/or eccentric phase**

+ Rest between sets: **1-5 minutes**

+ Max reps per muscle group per workout: **120**

+ Max sets per muscle group: **15**

+ Max muscle groups per workout: **3**

+ Rest between workouts: **24-72 hours**

#6

POWER TRAINING

This section presents various strength-speed training techniques (so called because power is expressed as strength multiplied by speed or force multiplied by velocity) that help increase muscle contraction speed using both light (power-speed) and heavy (power-strength) loads. These techniques are vital to an athlete's training because they are one of the best ways to increase power, a muscle quality that is often a major determinant of performance. They also promote strength gains through nervous system adaptations such as improved intramuscular and intermuscular coordination. They are therefore great for athletes looking to increase power without gaining 5-10 kg in muscle mass.

However, before starting to integrate techniques from chapter 5 involving depth landings (technique #174) or depth jumps (technique #175), you must first be able to do a back squat with an equivalent load, or 1.5-2.0 times your body weight, to limit the risk of injury.[37] Remember that the basis of power is muscle strength and that the optimal percentage to develop maximum power is 80% of your 1RM for hang power clean or hang power snatch, 40%-60% for bench press throw, and 50%-70% for squat.[17,20] Also, the optimal percentage for the jump squat is when you are handling a load between 20%-50% of your 1RM.[9] Therefore, if you lift twice your body weight in the back squat, this will mean that working with your body weight will be about 33% of your 1RM (weight of the body/[body weight + 2 times your body weight supported on your shoulders]).

The most effective way to train power is with high-intensity exercises. If you are not able to do a back squat with 1 to 2 times your body weight, you should either work

on muscular strength before integrating depth landings or depth jumps (plyometrics at high intensity), or work on machines (e.g., powered leg press) in order to reduce the load to the level of your current muscular strength. However, the latter option should only be temporary—in order to excel in sport, all athletes must have the power to manage their own body weight. Therefore, reaching a 1RM in the back squat of 1 to 2 times the athlete's body weight is almost an obligatory passage for implementation of high-intensity plyometrics while limiting the risk of injury. However, this is not a prerequisite for low-intensity plyometric work (e.g., long jump, hurdle jumping, hopping), which should also be integrated into the physical preparation of any athlete.

If you are not an athlete and train instead for hypertrophy, you may still want to try these techniques to add variety to your workouts and optimize your gains in muscle mass. According to Newton's second law, force is equal to mass multiplied by acceleration ($F = m \times a$). By performing reps at high velocity, you increase the power of the movement ($P = force \times velocity$). However, in order to develop speed of movement, you will have to produce significant acceleration.

As acceleration increases, more force will be generated by the muscles. The more force that must be generated by a muscle, the higher the number of fast-twitch fibers it must recruit. Increased recruitment of muscle fibers leads to greater fatigue and equally greater gains in hypertrophy.

It is no secret that I am a big fan of including explosive methods in muscle-building programs not only to increase lean mass but also to make the person more functional.

What is the point of being a bodybuilder if you can't jump on a box or do a clap push-up? You can do these things; you simply need to train your ability to execute power moves. For hypertrophy purposes, you can use the methods in this chapter during your workouts or refer to chapter 3 for techniques that include potentiation exercises (techniques #84, #85, #93, #94, and #96).

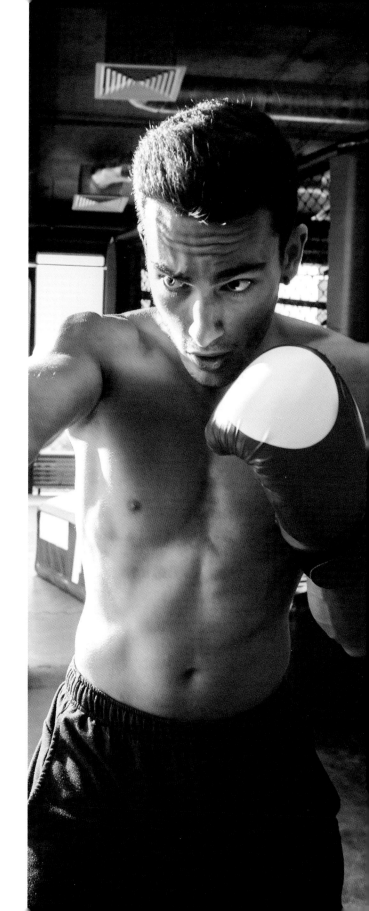

Technique #182

Perceived effort

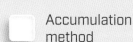

Effect on hypertrophy

Effect on strength and power

Effect on muscular endurance

Experience required

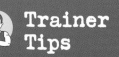

- [ ] Accumulation method
- [✓] Intensification method

EXPLOSIVE STATIC-DYNAMIC

HOW DOES IT WORK?

Also known as the concentric pause method, this technique is similar to the concentric static-dynamic technique (technique #141). Include a pause of 2-3 seconds during the concentric part of the movement, generally at the halfway point, then explosively finish the concentric phase (for example, jumping as high as you can). You can also do it on the Smith machine for the bench press by pausing for 2-3 seconds at the halfway point and throwing the bar explosively at the end. The same thing can be done in a push-up position by pushing yourself as high as possible.

This technique helps develop the speed component of power in the form of pure concentric movement. This feature is very representative of, for example, a football player's legs as he waits for his opponent for a few seconds in a flexed position, then leaps to intercept. This also applies to rugby players, hockey players, and other similar athletes. This technique is also good for hypertrophy training using heavier loads in order to increase the amount of time spent under tension.

ADVANTAGES

→ It is easy to use with any exercise.
→ It is representative of muscular movements in several sports (e.g., hockey, judo).

DISADVANTAGES

→ None.

PRESCRIPTION TABLE

Load	Number of repetitions per set	Number of sets per exercise	Number of exercises per muscle group	Rest between sets
30%-50%	3-6	3-6	1-2	60-90 seconds

Technique #183

Perceived effort

■■■□□

Effect on
hypertrophy

■■□□□

Effect on strength
and power

■■■■■

Effect on muscular
endurance

■■□□□

Experience required

■□□

☐ Accumulation
method

☑ Intensification
method

Trainer Tips

Before using Olympic weight-lifting exercises, I strongly suggest you have your form assessed by a trainer who is certified in this technique.

OLYMPIC WEIGHTLIFTING VARIATIONS

Ⓢ

HOW DOES IT WORK?
This technique uses Olympic weightlifting exercises to develop power. These include the clean, the snatch, and the jerk, as well as their variants.

ADVANTAGES
→ Because Olympic weightlifting exercises are high-velocity movements that require great general and muscular coordination, they are great training for sports that emphasize strength-speed.
→ This type of effort is similar to that required during sports, unlike working out on a machine using controlled movements.

DISADVANTAGES
→ These exercises are technically complex and if performed incorrectly, they may limit your progress or cause injury.

PRESCRIPTION TABLE

Load	Number of repetitions per set	Number of sets per exercise	Number of exercises per muscle group	Rest between sets
70%-90%	1-6	4-10	1-3	1-4 minutes

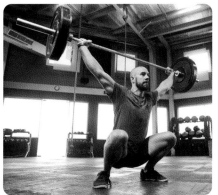
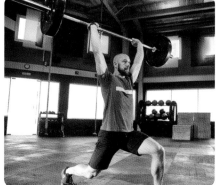

Technique #184

Perceived effort

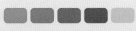

Effect on
hypertrophy

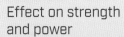

Effect on strength
and power

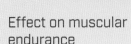

Effect on muscular
endurance

Experience required

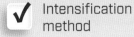

☐ Accumulation
  method

☑ Intensification
  method

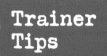

Trainer Tips

For your upper body, you can try push-ups and the inverted row with a variation in grip width. For example, alternate a push-up with a close and a wide grip and an inverted row with a close and a wide grip in a dynamic and continuous way.

PLYOMETRICS WITH OR WITHOUT LOAD

Ⓢ

HOW DOES IT WORK?

Plyometrics involve an explosive concentric contraction preceded by a prestretch phase (fast eccentric). This includes exercises such as depth jumps (technique #175), single-leg jumps, jumps with feet together, long jumps, forward lunge jumps, side jumps, backward jumps, and so on.

ADVANTAGES

→ Plyometrics develop power via structural (muscles and tendons) and nervous (intra- and intermuscular coordination, elastic energy recovery) modifications. The benefits of plyometrics are numerous and there are many books dedicated to presenting a wide range of possible plyometric exercises in order to help trainers apply this method. Books published by the National Strength and Conditioning Association (NSCA) are good examples.

DISADVANTAGES

→ They sometimes require special equipment (e.g., hurdles).

PRESCRIPTION TABLE

Load	Number of repetitions per set	Number of sets per exercise	Number of exercises per muscle group	Rest between sets
Body weight + 0%-13%	6-10	2-10	3-4	2-3 minutes

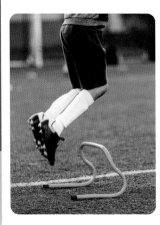

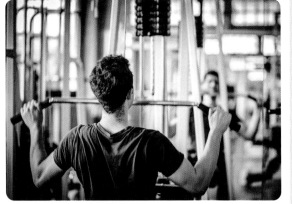

Technique #185

Perceived effort

Effect on hypertrophy

Effect on strength and power

Effect on muscular endurance

Experience required

☐ Accumulation method

✓ Intensification method

Trainer Tips

One study[1] showed that a 6-week program combining a squat with plyometric exercises increased power gains more on a vertical jump (+10.67 cm) compared to training only with the squat (+3.30 cm) or only with plyometric exercises (+3.81 cm).

COMPLEX TRAINING

HOW DOES IT WORK?

In this training technique, you select exercises according to your sport. Execute a strength movement targeting the part of the body required for the sport, followed by an explosive exercise (often with plyometric features similar to the movements involved in the sport) for a superset. Keep the rest between exercises as short as possible (<10 seconds).

ADVANTAGES

→ This technique works both components of power: the first exercise increases strength, whereas the second helps develop muscle contraction speed.

→ It takes advantage of postactivation potentiation.

→ It is easy to use.

DISADVANTAGES

→ It may require some special equipment (e.g., hurdles, plyometric boxes).

PRESCRIPTION TABLE

Load	Number of repetitions per set	Number of sets per exercise	Number of exercises per muscle group	Rest between sets
80%-90% + body weight	1-6 + 1-6	2-5 supersets	2-6	3-5 minutes

EXAMPLE FOR A BASKETBALL PLAYER

EXERCISE IN MAXIMAL STRENGTH	PLYOMETRIC EXERCISE
Front squat *6 reps*	Jump over hurdles *6 reps*

Technique #186

Perceived effort

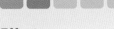

Effect on hypertrophy

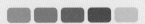

Effect on strength and power

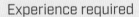

Effect on muscular endurance

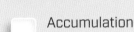

Experience required

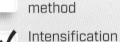

☐ Accumulation method

☑ Intensification method

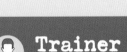

Trainer Tips

Do each rep at high speed. End the set as soon as you notice a decrease in speed in one of your reps. You want to prioritize power over muscle failure.

Ⓢ

TRADITIONAL EXERCISES WITH MAX POWER

HOW DOES IT WORK?

Perform a traditional exercise using a load of 40%-65%. Control the eccentric phase, but be as explosive as possible during the concentric phase without propelling the object or your body. This is a variation of the eccentric–concentric contrast (technique #138), but without the pause between the two phases.

ADVANTAGES

→ This technique improves the speed with which muscle fibers are recruited and acts primarily on the recruitment of fast-twitch muscle fibers. It helps your nervous system adapt to recruiting fibers more quickly (by decreasing their activation threshold slightly) while promoting alactic anaerobic adaptations (increasing the creatine and phosphate pool).

DISADVANTAGES

→ None.

PRESCRIPTION TABLE

Load	Number of repetitions per set	Number of sets per exercise	Number of exercises per muscle group	Rest between sets
40%-65%	1-6	4-10	1-3	1-2 minutes

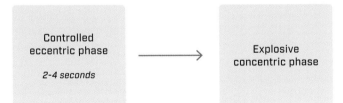

Controlled eccentric phase

2-4 seconds

→

Explosive concentric phase

Technique #187

Perceived effort

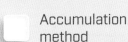

Effect on
hypertrophy

Effect on strength
and power

Effect on muscular
endurance

Experience required

☐ Accumulation
method

☑ Intensification
method

Trainer Tips

Many cage squat racks already have lower supports to place your bands when you do a squat or bench press, but if yours does not, a good way to set up the bands is to put one band on each end of the bar and attach each one to a heavy dumbbell on the floor. You can also perform an exercise with a superband only (for example, place both feet on one end of the band, grasp the other end with both hands, and perform a squat).

VARIABLE RESISTANCE WITH BANDS

HOW DOES IT WORK?

Using superbands, perform a traditional exercise explosively (concentric and eccentric phases) without propelling the object or your body. Use a load that ranges from 40%-65%, including the tension of the bands. To calculate the tension of the band, put it on the bar and attach a dumbbell to the other end of the band. Add more weight to the dumbbell until it touches the floor; this weight is the resistance of the band.

ADVANTAGES

→ This technique improves the speed with which muscle fibers are recruited. It helps your nervous system adapt to recruiting fibers more quickly (by decreasing their activation threshold slightly).

→ Your antagonist muscles will not need to contract strongly to stop the high-speed movement because this function is performed by the superbands. Your agonist muscle will therefore develop more power.

DISADVANTAGES

→ It requires superbands, which you may need to buy if your weight room does not have them.

PRESCRIPTION TABLE

Load	Number of repetitions per set	Number of sets per exercise	Number of exercises per muscle group	Rest between sets
40%-65%	1-6	4-10	1-3	1-2 minutes

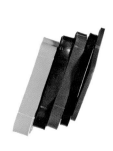
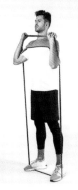
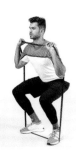

Technique #188

Perceived effort
■■□□□

Effect on hypertrophy
■□□□□

Effect on strength and power
■■■□□

Effect on muscular endurance
■□□□□

Experience required
■□□

- ☐ Accumulation method
- ☑ Intensification method

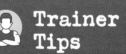

Trainer Tips

For an upper-body ballistic move, try propelling the bar during a bench press on the Smith machine. Because the bar is guided, you can ensure that it will fall back into your hands! Another variation is the popular clap push-up.

BALLISTIC EXERCISES

HOW DOES IT WORK?
Ballistic exercises involve propelling an object or your own body through space. This technique therefore includes plyometrics, jumps, and all exercises that require the projection of an object (such as hard or soft medicine balls).

ADVANTAGES
→ These exercises increase the speed of the movement and allow for the expression of maximal power.
→ It is easy to use and has a large impact on power gains.

DISADVANTAGES
→ It may require specific equipment (e.g., medicine ball, Smith machine, plyo boxes).

PRESCRIPTION TABLE

Load	Number of repetitions per set	Number of sets per exercise	Number of exercises per muscle group	Rest between sets
10%-25%	5-10	3-6	1-3	1-2 minutes

The following are some examples of ballistic movements:

→ Standing and overhead medicine ball throw

→ Slam ball on the floor

→ Wall ball as high as possible

→ Vertical medicine ball throw from a lying position

→ Kneeling medicine ball throw with trunk rotation

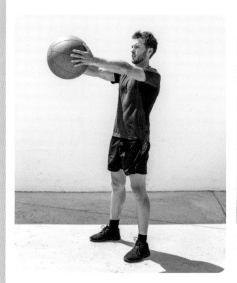 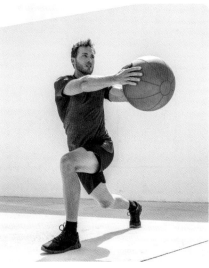

Technique #189

Perceived effort

Effect on hypertrophy

Effect on strength and power

Effect on muscular endurance

Experience required

☐ Accumulation method

☑ Intensification method

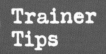

Trainer Tips

To improve your sprint speed, try running on synthetic turf while pulling a sled. For outdoor runs, you may also use a parachute or tire (see techniques #6 and #7).

Ⓢ

SPORT-SPECIFIC MOVEMENT WITH OVERLOAD

HOW DOES IT WORK?

This technique generally uses the tools specific to the sport practiced by the athlete. Simply increase the weight of the manipulated object (e.g., javelin, baseball bat, boxing gloves) by a maximum of 10% to promote power gains without compromising form.

ADVANTAGES

→ This technique promotes power gains that are directly transferable to competition by using a movement that is common in the sport.

→ It is best used for a short period of time at the end of an off-season.

DISADVANTAGES

→ Care must be taken not to change the movement's motor pattern with the introduction of a heavier load (increase the load by 2% each week up to a maximum of 10%). Should this happen, the technique would become counterproductive.

PRESCRIPTION TABLE

Load	Number of repetitions per set	Number of sets per exercise	Number of exercises per muscle group	Rest between sets
Object weight + 0%-10%	5-10	3-6	1-3	1-2 minutes

The following are some examples:

→ A shot putter could use a heavier weight for her shots.

→ A baseball player could use a heavier bat.

→ A firefighter in the FireFit Games could use a heavier dummy for the final sprint during his more technical workouts.

Technique #190

Perceived effort

▣▣▢▢▢

Effect on
hypertrophy

▣▢▢▢▢

Effect on strength
and power

▣▣▣▣▢

Effect on muscular
endurance

▣▢▢▢▢

Experience required

▣▣▢

☐ Accumulation
method

☑ Intensification
method

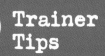

Trainer Tips

Starting strength training is uncommon in gyms because it involves throwing the body a distance or throwing a medicine ball against a wall. A performance center or functional training center is usually more appropriate for this type of training.

STARTING STRENGTH

HOW DOES IT WORK?

This method consists of executing movements from a stationary position and trying to produce maximum speed, distance, or height in the shortest time possible. In terms of progression through the training programs, you can start by working on your starting strength and then work on your starting strength endurance (in the same format as repeated jumps, impulses, and throws, technique #192). Starting strength requires high levels of muscle strength (see chapter 2) and speed of contraction (which is developed with this technique).

ADVANTAGES

→ It is very useful for sports requiring rapid movement, jumping, or pulling, such as badminton, volleyball, and judo.

DISADVANTAGES

→ It requires special equipment such as boxes or hurdles.
→ It may require a free distance of 20-30 meters for bounding strides or hopping.

PRESCRIPTION TABLE

Load	Number of repetitions per set	Number of sets per exercise	Number of exercises per muscle group	Rest between sets
Body weight	2-10	3-6	1-3	1-2 minutes

EXAMPLES OF STARTING STRENGTH EXERCISES

Jump from a bench, seated start (as high as possible)	Alternate leaping stride	Jump onto a box with one foot

Technique #191

Perceived effort

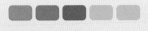

Effect on hypertrophy

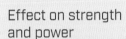

Effect on strength and power

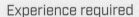

Effect on muscular endurance

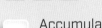

Experience required

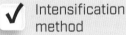

☐ Accumulation method

☑ Intensification method

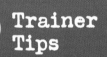

Trainer Tips

This technique is recommended for advanced athletes only because the load may exceed your maximum concentric muscle capacity once the weight releasers are engaged. The risk of injury is high and you must have control over the eccentric speed of your bar at all times.

OVERSHOOT (WITH WEIGHT RELEASERS)

Ⓢ

HOW DOES IT WORK?

This method takes advantage of the neurological overload caused by the first rep (potentiation). First, place approximately 50% of your concentric maximum on the bar, then add 30%-70% of your 1RM on the weight releasers. Lower the load in 2-4 seconds, then lift it as quickly as possible after the weight releases. Continue the set by quickly lowering the load (always keeping it under control) and explosively lifting it again. The goal is to maintain as much acceleration as possible for the next 2-5 reps.

ADVANTAGES

→ This technique promotes significant production of power because the first rep preactivates fast-twitch fibers.

DISADVANTAGES

→ It is limited only to the bench press and the squat because other exercises do not have a range of motion far enough from the ground to allow the use of weight releasers.

PRESCRIPTION TABLE

Load	Number of repetitions per set	Number of sets per exercise	Number of exercises per muscle group	Rest between sets
50%-120%	1 + 2-5	4-8	1-2	2-3 minutes

EXAMPLE FOR 1RM SQUAT OF 200 KG

100 KG + 50 KG PER WEIGHT RELEASER

100 KG TOTAL ON THE BAR

1 eccentric rep at 100% → 2-5 explosive reps at 50%

Technique #192

Perceived effort

▪▪▪▫▫

Effect on
hypertrophy

▪▪▫▫▫

Effect on strength
and power

▪▪▪▪▪

Effect on muscular
endurance

▪▪▫▫▫

Experience required

▪▪▫

☐ Accumulation
method

☑ Intensification
method

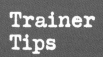

REPEATED JUMPS, IMPULSES, AND THROWS

HOW DOES IT WORK?

This technique includes:

1. **Jumps:** These are necessary in sports such as basketball and volleyball. Options include jumps (vertical, box, long) and Olympic weightlifting movements.

2. **Impulses:** These are necessary in sports such as swimming, kayaking, and boxing. An impulse is a fast movement of your body created by your upper-body strength used for push-ups, pull-ups, and inverted rows. Options include clap push-ups, Smith machine inverted rows with hand-position changes (underhand, overhand, close grip, wide grip), and explosive pull-ups.

3. **Throws or strikes:** These are necessary in sports such as baseball, tennis, and golf. Medicine ball throws (sitting, kneeling, standing, advancing, with a jump, in a straight line, with rotation of the trunk) are the most effective option.

In all three cases, you will complete a circuit of 6-8 exercises, performing 6-8 repetitions per exercise with 10-40 seconds of recovery between stations. The difference between these three elements lies in the selection and nature of the exercises.

PRESCRIPTION TABLE

Load	Number of repetitions or seconds per set	Number of sets per exercise	Number of exercises per circuit	Rest between sets
Body weight or medicine ball	6-8 reps or 5-10 seconds	2-5	6-8	4-5 minutes

EXAMPLE OF A REPEATED JUMPS CIRCUIT

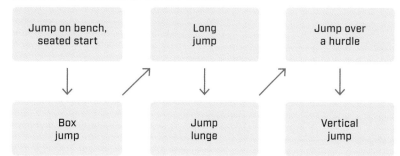

Technique #193

Perceived effort

Effect on hypertrophy

Effect on strength and power

Effect on muscular endurance

Experience required

☐ Accumulation method

☑ Intensification method

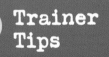

Trainer Tips

An ascending example might be a depth landing for 5 repetitions (shock exercise); box jumps for 8 repetitions (ballistic exercise); an explosive box squat at 70% with a 2-second drop sitting on the box for 8 repetitions (strength-speed exercise); and a leg press for 5 repetitions (strength exercise at slow speed).

CANADIAN ASCENDING– DESCENDING TRAINING

HOW DOES IT WORK?

This is a modified version of Bulgarian complex training (technique #197); the difference is that this technique includes two workouts per muscle group. The first workout is done in ascending form (lightest to heaviest), and the second workout, performed 72 hours later, is done in descending form (heaviest to lightest). The order of exercises is shown in the example. It should be noted that, unlike with the Bulgarian complex training technique, all the sets of an exercise must be completed before moving on to the next.

ADVANTAGES

→ This method is the best type of plan for working strength-speed from all angles with different levels of fatigue at each workout.

DISADVANTAGES

→ None.

PRESCRIPTION TABLE

Load	Number of repetitions per set	Number of sets per exercise	Number of exercises per muscle group	Rest between sets
Shock and ballistic exercises: Body weight or 15%-50% Strength-speed and slow strength exercises: 70%-95%	1-10	1-3	4	2-4 minutes

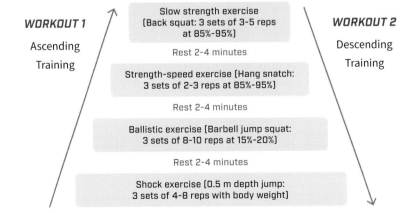

WORKOUT 1 Ascending Training

WORKOUT 2 Descending Training

Slow strength exercise (Back squat: 3 sets of 3-5 reps at 85%-95%)

Rest 2-4 minutes

Strength-speed exercise (Hang snatch: 3 sets of 2-3 reps at 85%-95%)

Rest 2-4 minutes

Ballistic exercise (Barbell jump squat: 3 sets of 8-10 reps at 15%-20%)

Rest 2-4 minutes

Shock exercise (0.5 m depth jump: 3 sets of 4-8 reps with body weight)

Technique #194

Perceived effort

■ ■ ■ ▢ ▢

Effect on hypertrophy

■ ■ ■ ▢ ▢

Effect on strength and power

■ ■ ■ ■ ■

Effect on muscular endurance

■ ■ ▢ ▢ ▢

Experience required

■ ■ ▢

☐ Accumulation method

☑ Intensification method

Trainer Tips

This technique is very effective for all athletes who wish to improve their physical and athletic abilities. It works both the force and speed components that make up power.

RUSSIAN COMPLEX TRAINING

HOW DOES IT WORK?

Alternate 2 exercises with 2-4 minutes of rest in between. One should emphasize strength (3-5 reps at 85%-95%) and the other should emphasize speed (8-10 reps at 15%-20%). Both exercises should target the same movement pattern and muscle groups. The superset versions (emphasis on strength, technique #195, and emphasis on speed, technique #196) are derivatives of this technique, but performed without rest between exercises to save time (and provide slightly lesser results).

ADVANTAGES

→ Because the rest time between exercises is longer than for techniques #195 and #196, this technique allows full recovery of phosphagens (ATP-PC), thus providing better power gains.

DISADVANTAGES

→ None.

PRESCRIPTION TABLE

Load	Number of repetitions per set	Number of sets per exercise	Number of exercises per muscle group	Rest between sets
85%-95% + 15%-20%	3-5 + 8-10	4-8	1-3	2-4 minutes

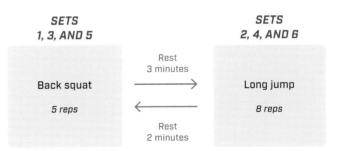

SETS 1, 3, AND 5

Back squat

5 reps

Rest 3 minutes →

← Rest 2 minutes

SETS 2, 4, AND 6

Long jump

8 reps

Technique #195

Perceived effort

■ ■ ■ ▢ ▢

Effect on hypertrophy

■ ■ ■ ▢ ▢

Effect on strength and power

■ ■ ■ ■ ▢

Effect on muscular endurance

■ ■ ▢ ▢ ▢

Experience required

■ ■ ▢

☐ Accumulation method

☑ Intensification method

👤 Trainer Tips

Despite the small loss of capacity, I consider this technique to be very effective at maintaining a good degree of efficiency and muscular adaptations while making training sessions shorter.

RUSSIAN COMPLEX TRAINING (EMPHASIS ON STRENGTH)

Ⓢ

HOW DOES IT WORK?

Perform 2 exercises in a superset without rest. The first should emphasize strength and the second should emphasize speed, and both should target the same movement pattern. This technique is identical to postpotentiation (technique #85), but performed with a focus on developing power (including the first exercise with repetitions in the strength range).

ADVANTAGES

→ This technique saves time compared to the standard version (technique #194).

DISADVANTAGES

→ It is somewhat less effective at developing power than the standard version.

PRESCRIPTION TABLE

Load	Number of repetitions per set	Number of sets per exercise	Number of exercises per muscle group	Rest between sets
85%-95% + 15%-20%	3-5 + 6-10	2-5	1-3 supersets	2-4 minutes

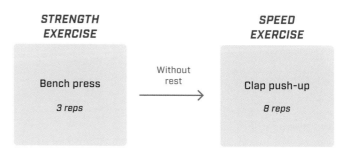

STRENGTH EXERCISE		SPEED EXERCISE
Bench press 3 reps	Without rest →	Clap push-up 8 reps

Technique #196

Perceived effort

■ ■ ■ ▢ ▢

Effect on hypertrophy

■ ■ ■ ▢ ▢

Effect on strength and power

■ ■ ■ ■ ▢

Effect on muscular endurance

■ ■ ▢ ▢ ▢

Experience required

■ ■ ▢

☐ Accumulation method

☑ Intensification method

Trainer Tips

Despite the small loss of capacity, I consider this technique to be very effective at maintaining a good degree of efficiency and muscular adaptations while making training sessions shorter.

RUSSIAN COMPLEX TRAINING (EMPHASIS ON SPEED)

HOW DOES IT WORK?

Perform 2 exercises in a superset without rest. The first should emphasize speed and the second should emphasize strength, and both should target the same movement pattern. This technique is identical to prepotentiation (technique #84), but performed with a focus on developing power (including the second exercise with repetitions in the strength range).

ADVANTAGES

→ This technique saves time compared to the standard version (technique #194).

DISADVANTAGES

→ It is somewhat less effective at developing power than the standard version.

PRESCRIPTION TABLE

Load	Number of repetitions per set	Number of sets per exercise	Number of exercises per muscle group	Rest between sets
15%-20% + 85%-95%	6-10 + 3-5	2-5	1-3 supersets	2-4 minutes

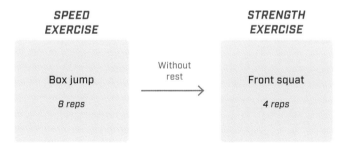

SPEED EXERCISE

Box jump

8 reps

Without rest →

STRENGTH EXERCISE

Front squat

4 reps

Technique #197

Perceived effort

▪▪▪▫▫

Effect on
hypertrophy

▪▪▪▫▫

Effect on strength
and power

▪▪▪▪▪

Effect on muscular
endurance

▪▪▫▫▫

Experience required

▪▪▫

☐ Accumulation method

☑ Intensification method

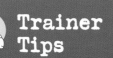

Trainer Tips

This technique develops power through a very wide range of parameters. We start by developing strength, then speed. The further the exercises progress, the more the load will decrease and the speed of the movement will increase. Give it a try!

BULGARIAN COMPLEX TRAINING

(S)

HOW DOES IT WORK?

This technique is an extended version of Russian complex training (technique #194). Instead of a complex of 2 exercises, complete a complex of 4-5 exercises, going from the heaviest exercise to the lightest. You will do (in order) a slow strength exercise, a strength-speed exercise, a ballistic exercise, and a shock exercise, resting for 2-4 minutes in between each exercise.

ADVANTAGES

→ This technique trains the muscles to move loads of different intensities at high velocity.

→ This technique is very effective at promoting power gains, while adequate rest maximizes the quality of the work.

DISADVANTAGES

→ This is a very advanced technique and isn't appropriate for someone without the requisite strength levels.

PRESCRIPTION TABLE

Load	Number of repetitions per set	Number of sets per exercise	Number of exercises per muscle group	Rest between sets
Slow strength and strength-speed exercises: 70%-95% Ballistic and shock exercises: Body weight or 15%-50%	1-10	1-3	4-5	2-4 minutes

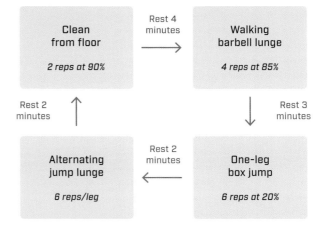

Clean from floor — 2 reps at 90%
Rest 4 minutes →
Walking barbell lunge — 4 reps at 85%
↓ Rest 3 minutes
One-leg box jump — 6 reps at 20%
← Rest 2 minutes
Alternating jump lunge — 6 reps/leg
↑ Rest 2 minutes

Technique #198

Perceived effort

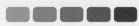

Effect on hypertrophy

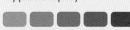

Effect on strength and power

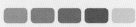

Effect on muscular endurance

Experience required

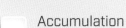

☐ Accumulation method

✓ Intensification method

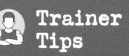

Trainer Tips

This is one of my favorite techniques that doesn't take too long to accomplish—especially on weight machines—and causes a lot of muscle fatigue. You will experience this in the slow reps you complete as the sets progress.

BIG KAHUNA

HOW DOES IT WORK?

This technique, designed by Christian Thibaudeau,[31] was inspired by the film *Back to the Beach.* It is an internal contrast method that involves doing 2 reps with 85%-90%, then 3 explosive reps with 60%, followed by slow reps (3-1-3-0 tempo) until failure with the same load (60%). You don't take any rest during this sequence.

ADVANTAGES

→ This technique is very effective in helping you gain muscle mass due to the high fatigue of fast-twitch fibers combined with the high time under tension.

→ It improves strength and power through high-intensity loads and explosive repetitions.

DISADVANTAGES

→ It requires a change in load, so it is less practical for exercises with a barbell (e.g., bench press, squat, deadlift).

→ This is a very advanced technique and isn't appropriate for someone without the requisite strength levels.

PRESCRIPTION TABLE

Load	Number of repetitions per set	Number of sets per exercise	Number of exercises per muscle group	Rest between sets
85%- 90% + 60% + 60%	2 + 3 + maximum	3-5	1-3	2-4 minutes

EXAMPLE OF A BIG KAHUNA SEQUENCE

REPETITIONS 1-2: Heavy at 85%-90%	2 × 100 kg
REPETITIONS 3-5: Explosive at 60%	3 × 70 kg
REPETITIONS 6 TO FAILURE: Slow at 60%	Maximum × 70 kg

Perceived effort

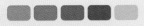

Effect on hypertrophy

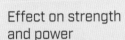

Effect on strength and power

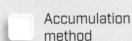

Effect on muscular endurance

Experience required

☐ Accumulation method

☑ Intensification method

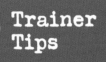
Trainer Tips

This technique is best practiced on weight machines so that loads can be changed quickly and fluidly. I hate applying this technique on exercises with weighted bars—it's up to you to experience it!

BIG KAHUNA REGRESSION

HOW DOES IT WORK?

This is an easier version of the big Kahuna (technique #198). Do 2 reps at 80%, followed by 2 explosive reps at 50%, then 2 reps at 80%, followed by 2 explosive reps at 50%, for a total of 8 reps per set.

ADVANTAGES

→ This method is effective at promoting simultaneous mass and strength gains.

DISADVANTAGES

→ Like all internal contrast techniques, it requires that you change loads within a set. You will need to calculate your loads ahead of time or enlist the help of a partner to unload the barbell.

PRESCRIPTION TABLE

Load	Number of repetitions per set	Number of sets per exercise	Number of exercises per muscle group	Rest between sets
80% + 50% + 80% + 50%	2 + 2 + 2 + 2	3-5	2-4	2-3 minutes

EXAMPLE OF A BIG KAHUNA REGRESSION SEQUENCE

REPETITIONS 1, 2, 5, AND 6:
Heavy at 80%

2 × 80 kg

REPETITIONS 3, 4, 7, AND 8:
Explosive at 50%

3 × 50 kg

Technique #200

Perceived effort

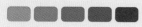

Effect on hypertrophy

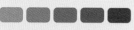

Effect on strength and power

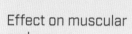

Effect on muscular endurance

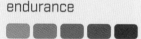

Experience required

☐ Accumulation method

✓ Intensification method

 Trainer Tips

This is one of my favorite techniques that doesn't take too long to accomplish—especially on weight machines—and causes a lot of muscle fatigue. You will come to failure several times in this technique, which requires good pain management on your part.

 Ⓢ

BIG KAHUNA PROGRESSION

HOW DOES IT WORK?

This is an extended version of the big Kahuna (technique #198). Do 2 reps with 85%-90%, then 3 explosive reps with 60%, followed by slow reps (3-1-3-0 tempo) until failure with 60%, then 3 explosive reps with 30%, followed by slow reps (3-1-3-0 tempo) until failure with 30%, and finally an isometric contraction at your weak point until failure with 30%.

ADVANTAGES

→ This technique is very effective in helping you gain muscle mass due to the high fatigue of fast-twitch fibers combined with the high time under tension.

→ It improves strength and power through high-intensity loads and explosive repetitions.

DISADVANTAGES

→ It requires a change in load, so it is less practical for exercises with a barbell (e.g., bench press, squat, deadlift).

→ This is a very advanced technique and isn't appropriate for someone without the requisite strength levels.

PRESCRIPTION TABLE

Load	Number of repetitions per set	Number of sets per exercise	Number of exercises per muscle group	Rest between sets
85%-90% + 60% + 60% + 30% + 30% + 30%	2 + 3 + maximum + 3 + maximum + isometric	1-3	1-3	2-4 minutes

EXAMPLE OF A BIG KAHUNA PROGRESSION SEQUENCE

REPETITIONS 1-2:
Heavy at 85%-90%

2 × 100 kg

REPETITIONS 3-5 + TO FAILURE:
Explosive at 60% + maximum with a slow tempo

3 + maximum × 70 kg

REPETITIONS 13-15 (EXAMPLE) + TO FAILURE:
Explosive at 30% + maximum with a slow tempo + isometric hold

3 + maximum + isometric × 40 kg

CHAPTER 7

POWER ENDURANCE TRAINING

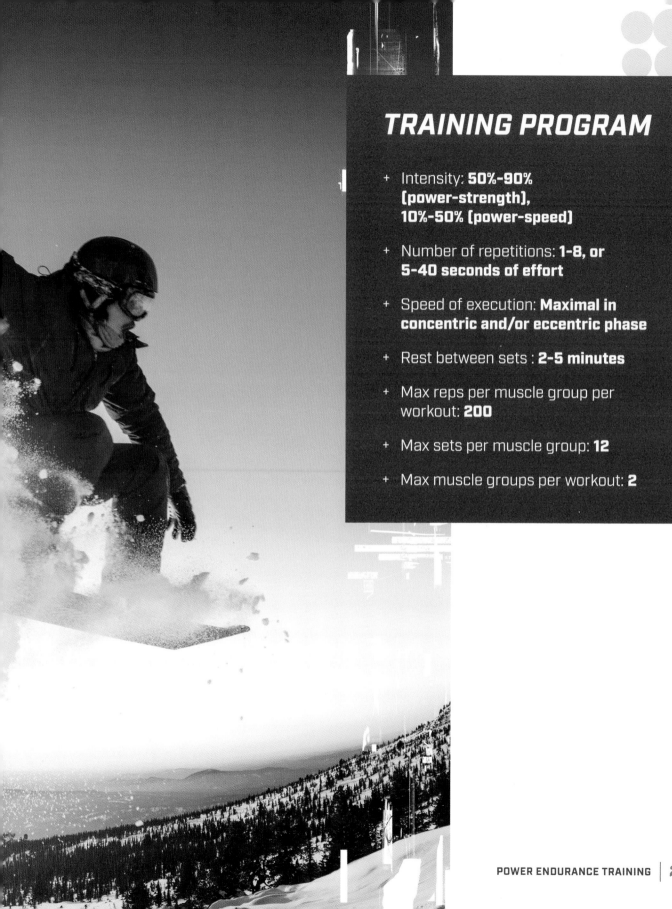

TRAINING PROGRAM

+ Intensity: **50%-90% (power-strength), 10%-50% (power-speed)**

+ Number of repetitions: **1-8, or 5-40 seconds of effort**

+ Speed of execution: **Maximal in concentric and/or eccentric phase**

+ Rest between sets : **2-5 minutes**

+ Max reps per muscle group per workout: **200**

+ Max sets per muscle group: **12**

+ Max muscle groups per workout: **2**

POWER ENDURANCE TRAINING

Power endurance training is primarily reserved for individuals who practice a sport that requires this particular muscular quality, such as hockey players, downhill skiers, snowboarders, and volleyball players. These athletes need to be able to generate a large amount of muscular power from the beginning of the game to the end (e.g., a volleyball player near the net must be able to jump as high at the end of the match as at the beginning in order to make the necessary blocks or plays for her team). The techniques in this category are not often used for hypertrophy or brute strength in the general population. However, you may choose to include them in your workouts for variety or to test them out before prescribing them to your clients. This will give you a better understanding of the difficulty of each technique and allow you to adjust the details of your prescription based on your client.

Power endurance training requires equipment that is not often found in traditional fitness centers, such as hurdles and plyometric boxes. You will need access to this equipment in order to get the most out of your workouts. Moreover, this type of training requires space for continuous jumps, multiple stations, and a combination of strength and cardio equipment. It will be up to you to find times when your gym is the least busy in order to maximize your workout and the exercises done at each station (e.g., squat rack).

I must also stress that before implementing these methods, you will first have to develop your strength (chapter 2), which is the basis of power, and then your power (chapter 6), which is the basis of strength-speed endurance techniques. This progression is essential; otherwise you will not have acquired the skills needed to develop power in a short period of time. Using the techniques in this chapter alone will in no way improve your ability to perform explosive actions with proper form: You will simply survive your workout. Be smart in your approach and start with the basics depending on your level.

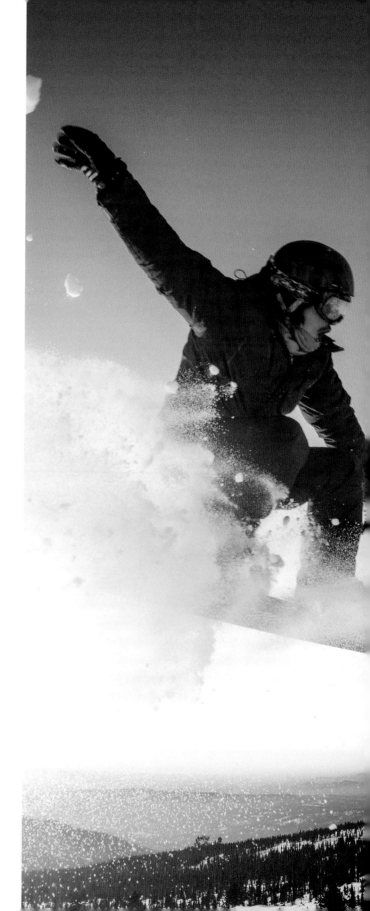

STEP 1

Strength

↓

STEP 2

Power

↓

STEP 3

Power
endurance

Technique #201

Perceived effort

■ ■ ■ ☐ ☐

Effect on hypertrophy

■ ■ ■ ■ ■

Effect on strength and power

■ ■ ■ ■ ☐

Effect on muscular endurance

■ ■ ■ ☐ ☐

Experience required

■ ■ ☐

☐ Accumulation method

☑ Intensification method

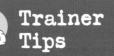

Trainer Tips

A good prerequisite would be the ability to perform 5 clap push-ups or 5 explosive inverted rows in less than 5 seconds. For demonstrations of upper- and lower-body exercises in plyometrics, I highly recommend the book *High-Powered Plyometrics* (Human Kinetics).

Ⓢ

INTERMITTENT PLYOMETRIC CIRCUIT

HOW DOES IT WORK?

Complete a set of 6-8 plyometric exercises (for 5-10 seconds of continuous effort) with 20-50 seconds of rest between exercises. Ideally, use this technique for the same muscle group or movement pattern.

ADVANTAGES

→ This method can be used to train the lower body (depth jump [technique #175], long jump, etc.) and the upper body (explosive push-up, explosive row, etc.).
→ It is easy to use.

DISADVANTAGES

→ It requires prior development of strength and power. You must be able to handle your own body weight during exercises such as push-ups and rows.

PRESCRIPTION TABLE

Load	Number of seconds per exercise	Number of sets per exercise	Number of exercises per muscle group	Rest between sets
Body weight	5-10	2-8	6-8	3-5 minutes

Rest 20-50 seconds between exercises		
Clap push-up	Superman push-up	Side-to-side push-up on a block
Hip tap push-up	Wide- vs. close-grip push-up on a block	Explosive push-up on a bench
Rest 3-5 minutes between sets		

Technique #202

Perceived effort

▪▪▪▪▫

Effect on hypertrophy

▪▪▫▫▫

Effect on strength and power

▪▪▪▪▫

Effect on muscular endurance

▪▪▪▫▫

Experience required

▪▪▫

✓ Accumulation method

✓ Intensification method

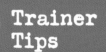

Trainer Tips

Incorporate a variety of different jumps into your circuit to vary the stimulation and adaptations (side jumps, low hurdles, high hurdles, single-leg jumps, jumps with more flexion, etc.).

CONTINUOUS PLYOMETRIC CIRCUIT

Ⓢ

HOW DOES IT WORK?

Complete an obstacle course of hurdles or jumps for 20-40 seconds without rest. Ideally, the course will represent the duration of the event. For example, to train for a downhill snowboarding race lasting about 30 seconds, plan a 30-second continuous plyometric circuit.

ADVANTAGES

→ This technique is great for recreating the muscle contraction requirements of the athlete's sport.

DISADVANTAGES

→ It requires a high level of preparation and the prior acquisition of strength-speed in order to properly perform the circuit with the best possible form. It is therefore reserved for more advanced individuals and is often used with athletes (skiers, snowboarders, etc.).
→ This method is used exclusively for lower-body workouts.

PRESCRIPTION TABLE

Load	Number of seconds per set	Number of sets per exercise	Number of exercises per muscle group	Rest between sets
Body weight	20-40	4-6	1	3-5 minutes

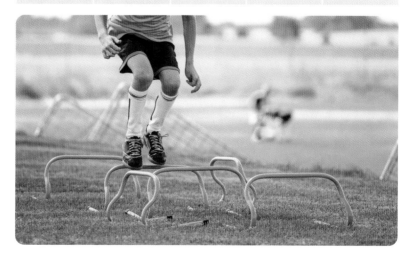

Technique #203

Perceived effort

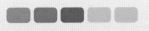

Effect on hypertrophy

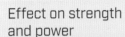

Effect on strength and power

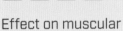

Effect on muscular endurance

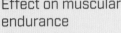

Experience required

✓ Accumulation method

✓ Intensification method

INTERMITTENT STRENGTH-SPEED ⓢ

HOW DOES IT WORK?

Complete 3-4 clusters of 6-8 reps of a dynamic exercise, ideally a ballistic exercise (technique #188) with a load of 10%-30%, with 10-15 seconds of rest between clusters. This represents a single set.

ADVANTAGES

→ This technique is a good option for a strength-speed endurance workout because it does not require a number of different stations or equipment that is not commonly found in traditional fitness centers (hurdles, tall boxes, etc.).

DISADVANTAGES

→ The individual must be able to handle her own body weight during exercises such as push-ups and rows. A good prerequisite would be the ability to perform 5 clap push-ups or 5 explosive inverted rows in less than 5 seconds.

PRESCRIPTION TABLE

Load	Number of repetitions per set	Number of sets per exercise	Number of exercises per muscle group	Rest between sets
10%-30%	6-8 + 6-8 + 6-8 + 6-8	2-3	1-3	3-5 minutes

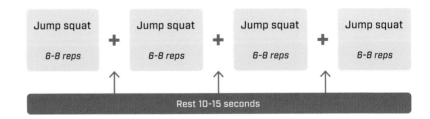

Technique #204

Perceived effort

■■■■□

Effect on hypertrophy

■■■□□

Effect on strength and power

■■■■□

Effect on muscular endurance

■■■□□

Experience required

■■□

☐ Accumulation method

✓ Intensification method

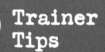

Trainer Tips

As a variant, this technique is a classic to end a hypertrophy session. Try it! Do your workout for one muscle group and incorporate this technique as the last component.

45-SECOND CIRCUIT

HOW DOES IT WORK?

Complete 6 exercises in a circuit to target both components of power: strength and speed. Start with a strength-speed exercise that primarily focuses on strength (e.g., a powerlifting movement at 70%-90%), followed by one that primarily focuses on speed (e.g., low plyometrics for 8-10 seconds), then perform a strength exercise (3RM-5RM). Repeat the same round a second time, using different exercises to target the same muscles and qualities, for a total of 6 exercises. After each exercise, rest for 45 seconds before moving on to the next.

ADVANTAGES

→ This technique allows you to work on the qualities of power-strength, power-speed, and strength within a single set. It is often used to train athletes (e.g., football, rugby, or hockey players) because it is highly effective.

DISADVANTAGES

→ Before introducing Olympic weightlifting exercises (technique #183) into this type of circuit, ensure that you have mastered the technique.

→ This is an advanced method and would be very difficult to perform in most gyms.

PRESCRIPTION TABLE

Load	Number of repetitions or seconds per set	Number of sets per exercise	Number of exercises per muscle group	Rest between sets
70%-90% + body weight + 70%-90%	3-6 reps or max reps in 5-10 seconds	3-4	6	3-5 minutes

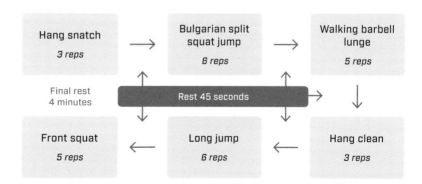

Technique #205

Perceived effort

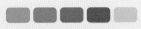

Effect on hypertrophy

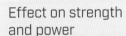

Effect on strength and power

Effect on muscular endurance

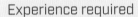

Experience required

☐ Accumulation method

☑ Intensification method

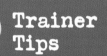

Trainer Tips

You can vary the muscle groups worked within the circuit. For example, the first 3 could be pushing exercises working the chest, shoulders, and triceps, and the last 3 could be pulling exercises working the back, upper back, and biceps.

LANDMINE CIRCUIT

HOW DOES IT WORK?

Complete 6 exercises in a circuit to target both components of power: strength and speed. Start with a strength-speed exercise using a landmine that primarily focuses on strength (e.g., 3-5 heavy landmine reps), followed by one that primarily focuses on speed (e.g., a dynamic body-weight exercise), then perform a strength exercise that works both the upper and lower body (e.g., barbell thrusters). Repeat the same round a second time, using different exercises to target the same muscles and qualities, for a total of 6 exercises. After each exercise, rest for 45 seconds before moving on to the next.

ADVANTAGES

→ The landmine circuit is similar to the 45-second circuit (technique #204) except that it works the upper and lower body simultaneously (great for athletes) while focusing a bit more on the upper body.

DISADVANTAGES

→ It requires a landmine.

PRESCRIPTION TABLE

Load	Number of repetitions or seconds per set	Number of sets per exercise	Number of exercises per muscle group	Rest between sets
70%-90% + body weight + 70%-90%	3-6 reps or max reps in 5-10 seconds	3-4	6	3-5 minutes

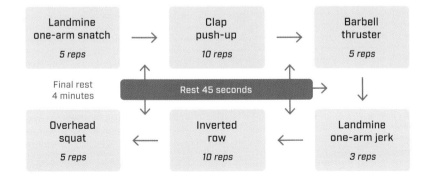

Technique #206

Trainer Tips

I like to use this technique to maximize time when developing an athlete who has time constraints for training. It is also ideal for training a muscle for a second time in the training week, but with a lower volume.

ANTAGONIST RUSSIAN COMPLEX ⓢ

HOW DOES IT WORK?

This method is actually a superset of two Russian complexes with an emphasis on strength (technique #195). Perform 4 consecutive exercises that work two antagonist muscle groups (push/pull), alternating 1 exercise focused on maximum load (3RM-5RM) and 1 exercise focused on movement speed (plyometrics) for each targeted muscle group.

ADVANTAGES

→ This method targets the qualities of strength and speed over time for two muscle groups and saves time when using Russian complexes.

DISADVANTAGES

→ It is less effective for improving the power endurance of a specific muscle compared to the previous techniques in this chapter, but rather acts on general power endurance.

PRESCRIPTION TABLE

Load	Number of repetitions or seconds per set	Number of sets per exercise	Number of exercises per muscle group	Rest between sets
85%-90% + body weight	3-5 reps + 5-10 seconds	2-4	2-4	3-5 minutes

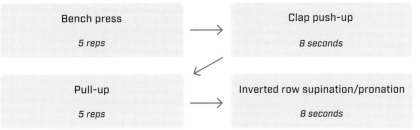

PUSH EXERCISES

Bench press	→	Clap push-up
5 reps		8 seconds
Pull-up	→	Inverted row supination/pronation
5 reps		8 seconds

PULL EXERCISES

Technique #207

Perceived effort

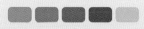

Effect on hypertrophy

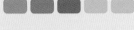

Effect on strength and power

Effect on muscular endurance

Experience required

✔ Accumulation method

✔ Intensification method

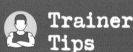

Trainer Tips

This type of training is great for combat sports. Start by performing 6-minute circuits and try to complete them in under 5 minutes, improving your time each week. CrossFit-style group workouts are good examples of the application of metabolic training.

METABOLIC TRAINING

HOW DOES IT WORK?

This method is basically a series of sustained high-speed contractions that promote metabolic acidosis. It consists of performing 1-5 sets of 2-5 exercises in a circuit with incomplete rest (work-to-rest ratio of 3:1). For example, if you do 5 exercises in a row (each exercise is done as fast as possible) and it takes you 3 minutes to accomplish, you must take 1 minute of rest at the end (3 minutes of work to 1 minute of rest) and repeat that for 1-5 sets. The whole circuit should be more than 30 seconds in duration—it can even be longer than 5 minutes! This is best used at the end of a workout.

For the sake of progression, you must move from shorter circuits (2-3 exercises) to longer circuits (4-5 exercises), shorter work periods to longer work periods, and from fast to very fast movement speed.

ADVANTAGES

→ The acidosis created allows for the more effective release of growth hormone, which is great for fat loss and hypertrophy.
→ The difficulty of this technique helps assess your ability to self-motivate.

DISADVANTAGES

→ This method needs to start conservatively and progress as fitness improves.

PRESCRIPTION TABLE

Load	Number of seconds or repetitions per set	Number of sets per exercise	Number of exercises per muscle group	Rest between sets
Body weight + elastic bands	>30 seconds or >10 reps per exercise	1-5	2-5	Work : rest 3 : 1

The following are sample exercises by muscle group (perform as fast as possible, use 3:1 work-to-rest ratio):

1. **Lower body:** 5 sets of 20 speed squats + 20 jump squats + 15 burpees + 10 long jumps
2. **Back:** 3 sets of 20 standing rows with band + 20/side alternating lat pull-downs with band + 20 swim pulls with band + 10 kipping pull-ups
3. **Chest:** 3 sets of 10/side one-arm medicine-ball push-ups + 10 side-to-side medicine-ball push-ups + 15 medicine-ball push-ups

Technique #208

Perceived effort

■ ■ ■ □ □

Effect on hypertrophy

■ ■ ■ ■ □

Effect on strength and power

■ ■ ■ ■ □

Effect on muscular endurance

■ ■ ■ □ □

Experience required

■ ■ ■

☐ Accumulation method

☑ Intensification method

Trainer Tips

Metabolic exercises accomplished with a band are not often present in gyms because bodybuilders are not big fans of this method, but they are a great tool to create good power development. As an example, I often use them with my boxing athletes.

POTENTIATION + METABOLIC (S)

HOW DOES IT WORK?

This technique is considered a superset. Perform, without rest, a potentiation movement followed by a metabolic movement targeting the same muscle group. The potentiation exercise may be done with a load (e.g., Olympic weightlifting, technique #183) or without (e.g., clap push-ups) for 3-8 reps, whereas the second exercise is done using elastic bands or your body weight. The duration of the latter will vary between 20 and 40 seconds depending on the difficulty of the movement.

ADVANTAGES

→ This technique will develop your power-strength (potentiation exercise) and your power-speed (metabolic exercise).

DISADVANTAGES

→ This technique requires elastic bands.

PRESCRIPTION TABLE

Load	Number of repetitions or seconds per set	Number of sets per exercise	Number of exercises per muscle group	Rest between sets
50%-90% (for Olympic lifts) or body weight + elastic bands	3-8 reps + 20-40 seconds	3-6	1-3 supersets	2-3 minutes

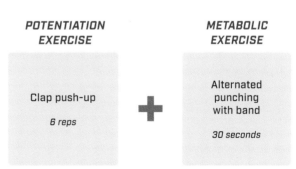

POTENTIATION EXERCISE

Clap push-up

6 reps

+

METABOLIC EXERCISE

Alternated punching with band

30 seconds

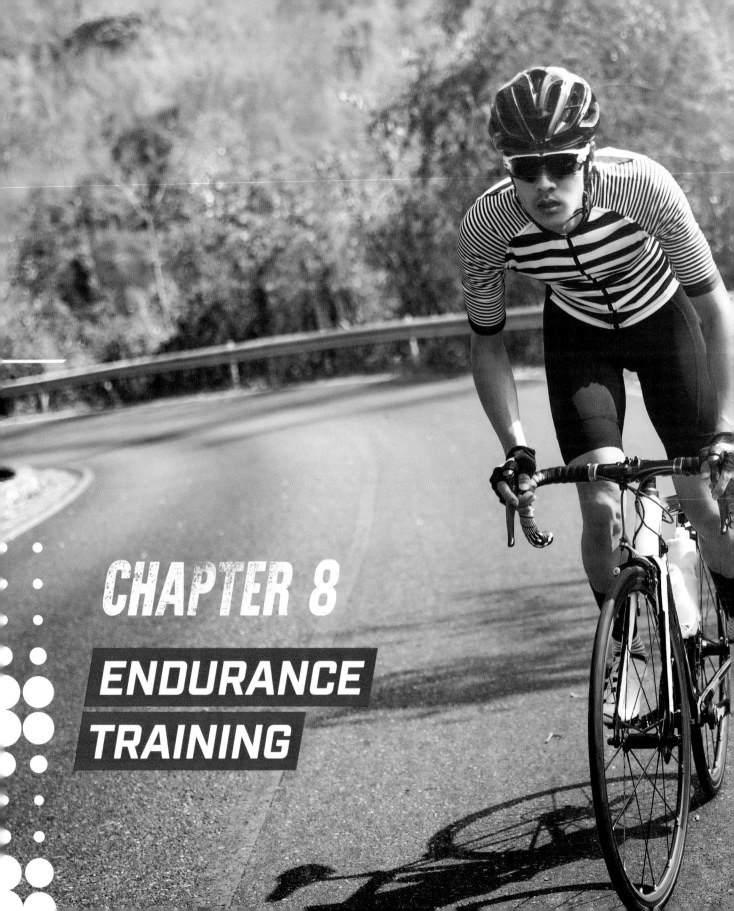

CHAPTER 8
ENDURANCE
TRAINING

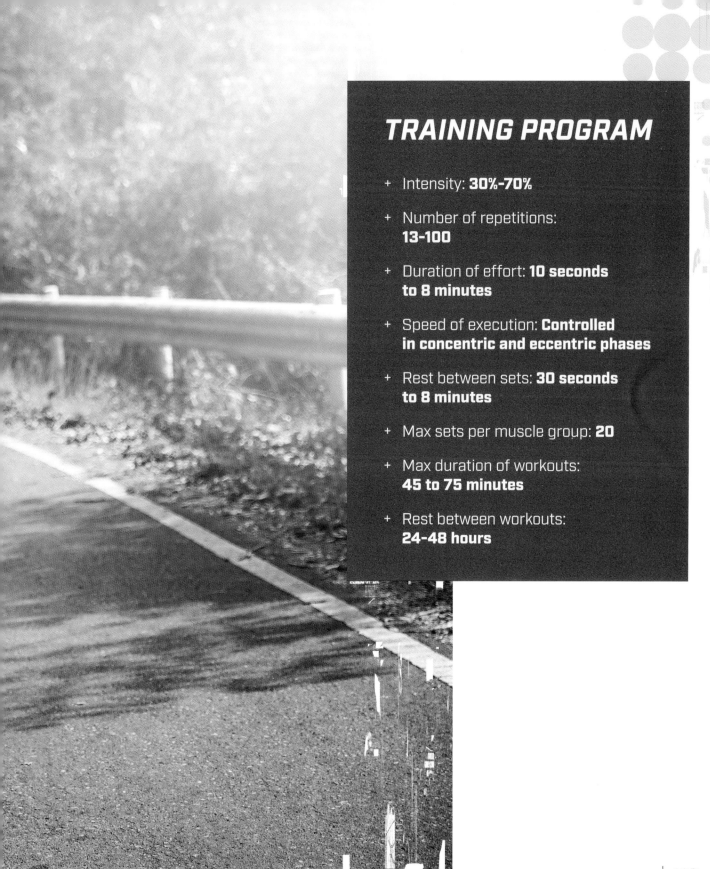

TRAINING PROGRAM

+ Intensity: **30%-70%**

+ Number of repetitions:
  13-100

+ Duration of effort: **10 seconds
  to 8 minutes**

+ Speed of execution: **Controlled
  in concentric and eccentric phases**

+ Rest between sets: **30 seconds
  to 8 minutes**

+ Max sets per muscle group: **20**

+ Max duration of workouts:
  45 to 75 minutes

+ Rest between workouts:
  24-48 hours

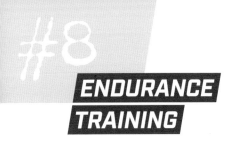

ENDURANCE TRAINING

Strength endurance training improves multiple muscle components in order to extend low-intensity effort. This involves mainly aerobic adaptations that help oxygenation, which in turn results in the following improvements:

1. An increase in the number of mitochondria

2. An increase in capillarization

3. A slight hypertrophy of type I fibers

4. Better form in movement execution

5. An improvement in the body's ability to store and use various energy substrates

This type of training is primarily reserved for muscles that are rich in slow-twitch fibers, such as stabilizing muscles (abs, lower back, rotator cuff, etc.). A common mistake made by athletes who engage in endurance sports is that they go to the gym to work on . . . their endurance! This makes sense at first, but in fact, muscular endurance is already stimulated to a large degree during their sport; it is unnecessary to stimulate it further. Cyclists, for example, work on their endurance while riding, and therefore time in the gym should be devoted to the improvement of less-stimulated cycling skills, such as muscular strength and power, which are crucial for hills and sprints. Strength endurance training for long-distance runners, on the other hand, should focus on the muscles involved in running, such as the abs and lower back.

I like to use strength endurance techniques to promote hypertrophy gains in my clients via the stimulation of type I fibers. Some muscles will react more strongly to these methods than others, depending on the type of muscle. The quadriceps, for example, are composed of 50% fast-twitch fibers and 50% slow-twitch fibers. Consequently, adding strength endurance techniques will have a significant impact on their development. Some studies[7] show better strength gains when strength endurance methods are included at the end of a workout, which is why I generally use them at this time, one at a time. My favorite is 100 repetitions (technique #214), which I alternate with my training partner.

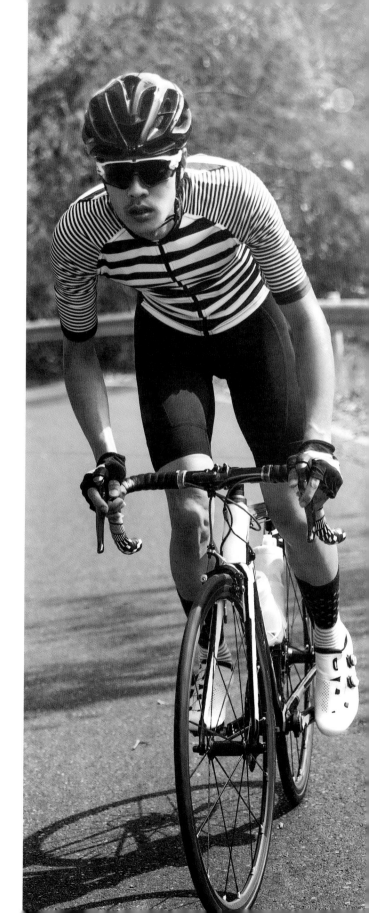

Technique #209

Perceived effort

■ ■ ■ ■ ■

Effect on
hypertrophy

■ ■ ■ ■ ■

Effect on strength
and power

■ ■ ■ ■ ■

Effect on muscular
endurance

■ ■ ■ ■ ■

Experience required

■ ■ ■

✓ Accumulation
method

☐ Intensification
method

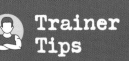

Trainer Tips

You can play with the density of your workouts by varying the amount of rest on a weekly basis. For example:

Week 1: 90 seconds
Week 2: 80 seconds
Week 3: 70 seconds

You can also start your workouts with submaximal sets to further facilitate your initiation into this form of training.

GENERAL STANDARDS 13RM-30RM

HOW DOES IT WORK?

Do 13-30 maximum repetitions.

ADVANTAGES

→ This basic technique provides an introduction to strength endurance training.

DISADVANTAGES

→ None.

PRESCRIPTION TABLE

Load	Number of repetitions per set	Number of sets per exercise	Number of exercises per muscle group	Rest between sets
50%-70%	13-30	3-8	1-3	45-120 seconds

EXAMPLES OF GENERAL STANDARDS 13RM-30RM WORKOUTS

WORKOUT 1	4 × 15RM, rest 90 seconds
WORKOUT 2	6 × 20RM, rest 60 seconds
WORKOUT 3	8 × 30RM, rest 45 seconds

Technique #210

Perceived effort

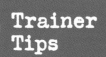

Effect on hypertrophy

Effect on strength and power

Effect on muscular endurance

Experience required

✓ Accumulation method

☐ Intensification method

Trainer Tips

You can vary the size and number of the stages and the number of reps for each set as long as you stay between 13 and 30 reps. For example:
1. 15 + 15 + 20 + 20 + 30 + 30
2. 15 + 15 + 15 + 25 + 25 + 25
3. 13 + 13 + 13 + 20 + 20

STAGES 20RM-20RM-20RM-30RM-30RM

Ⓢ

HOW DOES IT WORK?
Complete 3 sets of 20 max repetitions, followed by 2 sets of 30 max repetitions.

ADVANTAGES
→ This technique makes use of stages. Although it is not a groundbreaking technique, it does stimulate and fatigue a wider range of slow-twitch fibers than doing constant reps.
→ It is a basic introduction to strength endurance techniques.

DISADVANTAGES
→ None.

PRESCRIPTION TABLE

Load	Number of repetitions per set	Number of sets per exercise	Number of exercises per muscle group	Rest between sets
60%, 50%	20, 30	5	1-3	45-75 seconds

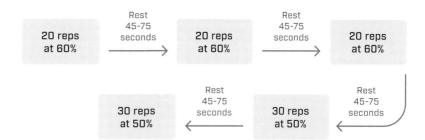

Technique #211

Perceived effort

■■■□□□

Effect on
hypertrophy

■■□□□

Effect on strength
and power

■□□□

Effect on muscular
endurance

■■■■□

Experience required

■■■

☑ Accumulation
method

☐ Intensification
method

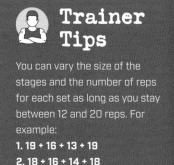

Trainer Tips

You can vary the size of the
stages and the number of reps
for each set as long as you stay
between 12 and 20 reps. For
example:

1. 19 + 16 + 13 + 19
2. 18 + 16 + 14 + 18
3. 17 + 15 + 13 + 17
4. 16 + 14 + 12 + 16

STAGES 20RM-15RM-12RM-20RM

(S)

HOW DOES IT WORK?

Start with 20RM, then 15RM, followed by 12RM. Increase the load as you complete each set. For the last set, return to 20RM. The more sets you complete, the more rest you will need between sets.

ADVANTAGES

→ This technique uses the principle of potentiation, but on a small scale. Although your nervous system will not be maximally activated (given loads that are far from maximal), you will still notice a difference between your 12RM and your 20RM, possibly resulting in a slight increase of your 20RM during your fourth set compared to the first.

DISADVANTAGES

→ None.

PRESCRIPTION TABLE

Load	Number of repetitions per set	Number of sets per exercise	Number of exercises per muscle group	Rest between sets
60%, 65%, 70%, 61%-63%	20, 15, 12, 20	4	1-3	45-120 seconds

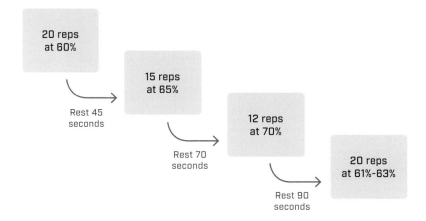

20 reps at 60%

Rest 45 seconds

15 reps at 65%

Rest 70 seconds

12 reps at 70%

Rest 90 seconds

20 reps at 61%-63%

Technique #212

Perceived effort

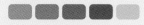

Effect on hypertrophy

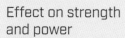

Effect on strength and power

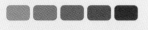

Effect on muscular endurance

Experience required

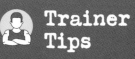

✓ Accumulation method

☐ Intensification method

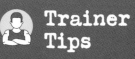

Trainer Tips

You can use this technique with beginners, but avoid plyometric exercises. Ideally, alternate a basic exercise, an abdominal or lumbar exercise, then a cardiovascular exercise (in any order).

CIRCUIT

HOW DOES IT WORK?

Complete 2-3 circuits of 6-12 consecutive exercises without rest. The number of reps per exercise should be between 6 and 12 for plyometric exercises or between 13 and 30 for all other exercises. In each circuit, you can target different muscle groups or focus on a single group (e.g., legs). You can also vary the type of exercise in a circuit by introducing plyometric and cardiovascular exercises (e.g., jump rope).

ADVANTAGES

→ This technique stimulates multiple muscular qualities (strength, power, endurance) one after another, thereby increasing muscle fatigue and energy expenditure. It is therefore great for fat loss.

DISADVANTAGES

→ It may be difficult to use if you choose exercises that require multiple machines. Try using barbells or free weights to make the circuit smoother.

PRESCRIPTION TABLE

Load	Number of repetitions per set	Number of sets per exercise	Number of exercises per muscle group	Rest between sets
30%-70% or body weight	13-30 or 6-12 (plyometric) or 30-90 seconds (cardio)	3-6	1-12	45-120 seconds

EXAMPLE OF A CIRCUIT WITH 8 EXERCISES

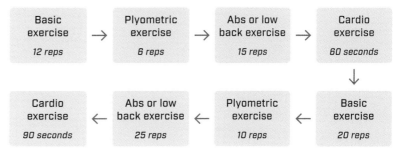

Technique #213

Perceived effort

Effect on hypertrophy

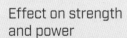

Effect on strength and power

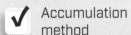

Effect on muscular endurance

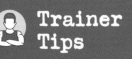

Experience required

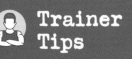

✓ Accumulation method

☐ Intensification method

Trainer Tips

You can use this technique with beginners, but avoid plyometric exercises. Ideally, alternate a basic exercise, an abdominal or lumbar exercise, then a cardiovascular exercise (in any order).

MINICIRCUIT

HOW DOES IT WORK?

Complete 2-3 circuits of 4-5 consecutive exercises without rest. The number of reps per exercise should be between 6 and 12 (load of 30%-60%) for plyometric exercises or between 13 and 20 (load of 60%-70%) for all other exercises. In each circuit, you can target different muscle groups or focus on a single group (e.g., legs). You can also vary the type of exercise (plyometrics, cardio, etc.).

ADVANTAGES

→ Because it employs fewer exercises than the circuit (technique #212), the intensity of the loads is increased (to a maximum of 20RM compared to 30RM in circuits), thereby increasing the exhaustion of many type I fibers.

DISADVANTAGES

→ It may be difficult to use if you choose exercises that require multiple machines. Try using barbells or free weights to make the minicircuit smoother.

PRESCRIPTION TABLE

Load	Number of repetitions per set	Number of sets per exercise	Number of exercises per muscle group	Rest between sets
30%-70% or body weight	13-20 or 6-12 (plyometric) or 30-90 seconds (cardio)	2-4	1-5	45-120 seconds

EXAMPLE OF A MINICIRCUIT FOR LEGS WITH 4 EXERCISES

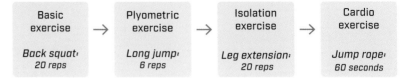

Basic exercise — Back squat: 20 reps → Plyometric exercise — Long jump: 6 reps → Isolation exercise — Leg extension: 20 reps → Cardio exercise — Jump rope: 60 seconds

Technique #214

Perceived effort

■ ■ ■ ■ □

Effect on
hypertrophy

■ ■ □ □ □

Effect on strength
and power

■ ■ □ □ □

Effect on muscular
endurance

■ ■ ■ ■ □

Experience required

■ □ □

✓ Accumulation
method

☐ Intensification
method

 Trainer Tips

This is one of my favorite techniques for hypertrophy because it stimulates slow-twitch fibers, which are often less fatigued by the end of previous exercises. It is also very effective for the legs. Try it with the leg press or back squat during your next lower-body workout!

100 REPETITIONS

 (S)

HOW DOES IT WORK?

With a partner, take turns completing 100 total reps in as few sets as possible with a starting load of 20RM-40RM. Only rest during your partner's reps. When your partner is unable to do another rep, it is your turn (and vice versa) until one of you reaches 100 reps. At first, you may need 10 sets to complete 100 reps, but as the weeks go by, the number of sets required will decrease. Once you can complete 100 reps in less than 4 sets, increase the load by 5%-7% for the next workout.

ADVANTAGES

→ This is a very challenging and motivating technique because, as long as you are using the same load, you and your partner are competing! It is an excellent addition at the end of hypertrophy and strength programs.

DISADVANTAGES

→ It requires a partner.
→ Because of the high volume required, you should develop a base level of muscular endurance with other endurance techniques before attempting this technique.

PRESCRIPTION TABLE

Load	Number of repetitions per exercise	Number of sets per exercise	Number of exercises per muscle group	Rest between sets
40%-60%	100	Minimum to reach 100 repetitions	1	Depending on your partner

EXAMPLE OF POSSIBLE SEQUENCES WITH YOUR 20RM-40RM

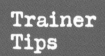

YOU

| 32 reps |
| 57 reps |
| 80 reps |
| 100 reps |

YOUR PARTNER

| 26 reps |
| 50 reps |
| 70 reps |
| 86 reps |

Technique #215

Perceived effort

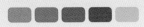

Effect on hypertrophy

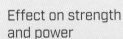

Effect on strength and power

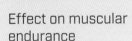

Effect on muscular endurance

Experience required

✓ Accumulation method

☐ Intensification method

Trainer Tips

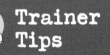

This is one of my favorite techniques at the end of hypertrophy training to stimulate the slow-twitch fibers, which are often less fatigued by the end of previous exercises. It is more difficult than 100 repetitions (technique #214) and can be done with a training partner.

70 REPETITIONS

HOW DOES IT WORK?

This method consists of performing 70 repetitions with your 20RM in as few sets as possible with 2 minutes of rest between each set. You'll probably hit 70 reps in 6-8 sets in the first week. Your goal is to complete 70 reps in 4 sets or less. When you are successful, then increase the load by 5%-10%.

ADVANTAGES

→ It improves endurance, strength, and muscle hypertrophy by altering the biochemical pathways in the muscle fibers (the fibers will become more efficient to create energy for muscle contractions).

→ It is easy to use with any exercise.

DISADVANTAGES

→ None.

PRESCRIPTION TABLE

Load	Number of repetitions per exercise	Number of sets per exercise	Number of exercises per muscle group	Rest between sets
60%	70	Minimum to reach 70 repetitions	1-2	2 minutes

EXAMPLE OF A 70-REPETITION SEQUENCE

Set	Weight	Rest	Number of reps completed			
			Week 1	Week 2	Week 3	Week 4
1	50 kg	2 minutes	20	22	23	24
2	50 kg	2 minutes	17	17	18	19
3	50 kg	2 minutes	13	13	14	15
4	50 kg	2 minutes	8	9	9	12
5	50 kg	2 minutes	6	7	6	
6	50 kg	2 minutes	4	2		
7	50 kg	2 minutes	2			
Total number of reps			70	70	70	70

Technique #216

Perceived effort

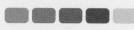

Effect on hypertrophy

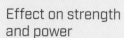

Effect on strength and power

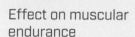

Effect on muscular endurance

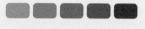

Experience required

✓ Accumulation method

☐ Intensification method

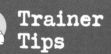

Trainer Tips

You can increase the number of exercises to perform in the strength part (superset, triset) in order to increase the difficulty. Similarly, for upper-body strength intervals, you can swap out the bike for the rower, arm bike machine, or ski machine.

STRENGTH INTERVALS (CARDIOACCELERATION)

Ⓢ

HOW DOES IT WORK?

Complete, without rest, a 6-8 minute circuit composed of 4 phases:

1. Active rest on a cardio machine (10-45 seconds)
2. Sprint on a cardio machine (e.g., increase the resistance or speed on your bike) (10-30 seconds)
3. Active rest on a cardio machine (10-45 seconds)
4. Strength exercise on a weight machine or with barbells or free weights (6RM-12RM)

Complete 2-4 rounds (sets) before taking 3-5 minutes of rest.

ADVANTAGES

→ This technique combines strength and strength endurance training.
→ Its variable loads and partial recovery help stimulate a wide range of fibers.

DISADVANTAGES

→ It may be difficult to use if the cardio section in your gym is far from the weight room.

PRESCRIPTION TABLE

Load	Number of repetitions per set	Number of sets per exercise	Number of exercises per muscle group	Rest between sets
Body weight, 30%-70% (endurance), 70%-83% (hypertrophy)	30-120 seconds (cardio), 13-30 (endurance), 6-12 (hypertrophy)	2-4	2-4	No rest between sets and 3-5 minutes at the end of the 2-4 sets

EXAMPLE OF A STRENGTH INTERVAL

Active rest on cardio machine	→	Sprint on cardio machine	→	Active rest on cardio machine	→	Strength exercise
Spinning + low resistance: 45 seconds		*Spinning + high resistance: 15 seconds*		*Spinning + low resistance: 45 seconds*		*Leg press: 10 reps*

Technique #217

Perceived effort

▮▮▮▯▯

Effect on
hypertrophy

▮▮▯▯▯

Effect on strength
and power

▮▮▮▯▯

Effect on muscular
endurance

▮▮▮▮▯

Experience required

▮▮▮

☑ Accumulation
method

☐ Intensification
method

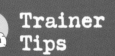

Trainer Tips

If you are using this technique for the development of power, stop the set as soon as rep speed decreases. If you want to focus on strength endurance, you can continue even at low speed until failure. For example, if you begin to lose power after 4 rounds, you may stop if your goal is to develop power or continue if you want to develop your endurance, but the next round will be less explosive.

SHORT INTERVALS AT 60%

HOW DOES IT WORK?

Execute repetitions as quickly as possible using a load of 60%. One set consists of 4-6 rounds of 6-8 reps. The rest time between rounds is equal to the working time.

ADVANTAGES

→ The explosive nature of this technique develops both strength endurance and strength-speed endurance.

→ This technique can be used to increase power as long as the emphasis is put on the speed of the movement instead of the number of repetitions (volume).

DISADVANTAGES

→ None.

PRESCRIPTION TABLE

Load	Number of repetitions per set	Number of sets per exercise	Number of exercises per muscle group	Rest between sets
60%	24-48 (4-6 rounds × 6-8 reps)	2-5	2-3	2-3 minutes

EXAMPLE OF 1 SET

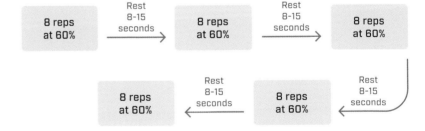

Technique #218

Perceived effort

■ ■ ■ □ □

Effect on
hypertrophy

■ ■ □ □ □

Effect on strength
and power

■ ■ ■ □ □

Effect on muscular
endurance

■ ■ ■ ■ □

Experience required

■ □ □

✓ Accumulation
method

☐ Intensification
method

Trainer Tips

If you are using this technique for the development of power, stop the set as soon as rep speed decreases. If you want to focus on strength endurance, you can continue even at low speed until failure.

LONG INTERVALS AT 60%

Ⓢ

HOW DOES IT WORK?
Execute repetitions as quickly as possible using a load of 60%. One set consists of 3-4 rounds of 12-15 reps. The rest time between rounds is equal to the working time.

ADVANTAGES
→ The explosive nature of this technique develops both strength endurance and strength-speed endurance.
→ This technique can be used to increase power as long as the emphasis is put on the speed of the movement instead of the number of repetitions (volume).

DISADVANTAGES
→ None.

PRESCRIPTION TABLE

Load	Number of repetitions per set	Number of sets per exercise	Number of exercises per muscle group	Rest between sets
60%	36-60 (3-4 rounds × 12-15 reps)	2-5	2-3	2-3 minutes

EXAMPLE OF 1 SET

15 reps at 60% → Rest 15-25 seconds → 15 reps at 60% → Rest 15-25 seconds → 15 reps at 60% → Rest 15-25 seconds → 15 reps at 60%

Technique #219

Perceived effort

■■■□□

Effect on
hypertrophy

■□□□□

Effect on strength
and power

■■■□□

Effect on muscular
endurance

■■■□□

Experience required

■■■

✓ Accumulation
method

☐ Intensification
method

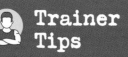 **Trainer
Tips**

This technique is the same as
the 100 repetitions method
(technique #214), but can be
used without a partner. Try to
beat your max number of reps
each workout! If working for
strength-speed, end the set
once speed begins to decrease.
If trying to improve strength
endurance, continue even at low
speed until muscle failure.

CONTINUOUS WORK AT 40%

HOW DOES IT WORK?
Using 40% of your 1RM, do as many reps as possible as quickly as possible until muscle failure.

ADVANTAGES
→ Although this technique develops strength endurance, it also stimulates strength-speed endurance adaptations due to the explosive nature of the reps. This technique can therefore be used for the latter purpose as long as the emphasis is put on the speed of the movement.

DISADVANTAGES
→ None.

PRESCRIPTION TABLE

Load	Number of repetitions per set	Number of sets per exercise	Number of exercises per muscle group	Rest between sets
40%	Maximum	3-4	1-3	2-3 minutes

Achieving a high number of reps using this technique depends on both your physical ability and mental capacity to handle your body's pain signals due to metabolic acidosis.

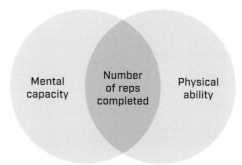

Technique #220

Perceived effort
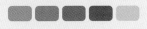

Effect on hypertrophy
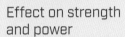

Effect on strength and power
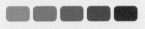

Effect on muscular endurance
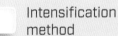

Experience required
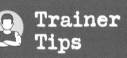

 ✓ Accumulation method

☐ Intensification method

Trainer Tips

I often use this technique to work the calves with a rest of 2-3 seconds at the end of the eccentric phase to release the elastic energy accumulated in the Achilles tendon. This will give you better results!

REST PERIOD 15RM

 (S)

HOW DOES IT WORK?

Do 30 reps with your 15RM. You will need to break up your set with pauses of 5-10 seconds (rack the bar during the pauses). If your goal is hypertrophy, try using this technique at the end of your workout.

ADVANTAGES

→ This technique increases the volume of work while maintaining a higher intensity load than with a true 30RM. The minibreaks allow blood to enter the muscles (reactive hyperemia), causing internal muscle pressure that can lead to hypertrophy gains.

→ The combined fatigue of both slow- and fast-twitch muscle fibers is very effective for training muscles that are composed equally of both (e.g., quadriceps).

DISADVANTAGES

→ This is a very intense technique similar to the breathing squat (technique #131), so a minimum of 6 months of training experience is necessary.

PRESCRIPTION TABLE

Load	Number of repetitions per set	Number of sets per exercise	Number of exercises per muscle group	Rest between sets
65%	30	3-5	1-3	1-2 minutes

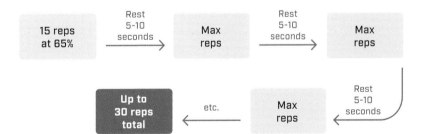

Technique #221

Perceived effort

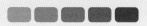

Effect on hypertrophy

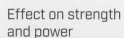

Effect on strength and power

Effect on muscular endurance

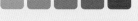

Experience required

✓ Accumulation method

☐ Intensification method

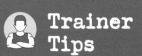
TABATA METHOD

HOW DOES IT WORK?

This technique consists of using the Tabata concept for cardiovascular training, but with muscular exercises. Tabata intervals use a 2:1 work-to-rest ratio, typically comprising 20 seconds of effort and 10 seconds of rest per rep accomplished over 8 reps, for a total duration of 4 minutes. The goal in this workout is to increase the number of total reps completed in 4 minutes or to increase the load used. A good start would be to find a load that allows you to complete the first six 20-second reps but causes difficulty completing reps 7 and 8.

ADVANTAGES

→ It improves muscular endurance.
→ It allows you to burn more fat mass.
→ It increases muscle capillarization (i.e., the number of blood vessels that supply your muscles).

DISADVANTAGES

→ None.

PRESCRIPTION TABLE

Load	Number of seconds per set	Number of sets per exercise	Number of exercises per muscle group	Rest between sets
40%	20 (effort) + 10 (rest) × 8	1-3	1-2	1-2 minutes

EXAMPLE OF FULL-BODY TABATA WORKOUT*

Exercises	Reps	Duration of effort	Rest
Dumbbell thruster	8	20 seconds	10 seconds
Deadlift	8	20 seconds	10 seconds
Leg press	8	20 seconds	10 seconds
Walking lunge	8	20 seconds	10 seconds
Bench press	8	20 seconds	10 seconds
Bent-over barbell row	8	20 seconds	10 seconds
Dumbbell lateral raise	8	20 seconds	10 seconds
Bicycle crunch	8	20 seconds	10 seconds

*After each exercise (1 set = 8 × [20 + 10]), take 1-2 minutes of rest before going to the next exercise.

Technique #222

Perceived effort

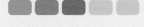

Effect on
hypertrophy

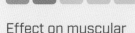

Effect on strength
and power

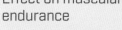

Effect on muscular
endurance

Experience required

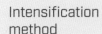

✓ Accumulation
method

☐ Intensification
method

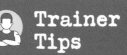
POWERWALKING

HOW DOES IT WORK?

This technique involves pulling a sled with a harness or attached to your training belt for several minutes. An optimal starting load should be 10 kg for women and 20 kg for men. Ideally, for very long distances, you should split your training into intervals. For example, a person training for 5 or 10 kilometers could walk the sled nonstop for 20-40 minutes. However, a person who completes a half-marathon in 90 minutes should complete three 30-minute intervals with a recovery time between intervals that allows the heart rate to drop below 75% of maximum heart rate (HRmax), then gradually increase the duration of effort to 45, 60, and even 90 minutes without stopping.

ADVANTAGES

→ This technique improves muscular endurance for long-distance running events.

DISADVANTAGES

→ It requires access to a turf area (indoor training) or flat lawn and a sled.

PRESCRIPTION TABLE

Load	Number of repetitions per set	Number of sets per exercise	Number of exercises per muscle group	Target heart rate
10-50 kg	1-6	1	N/A	<75% HRmax

Powerwalking can also be used by 60- to 800-meter sprinters. For sprints of less than 200 meters, run the same duration as your race, but with more weight on the sled (you can even use a load beyond 50 kg). For 400- and 800-meter sprints, try to complete half the distance with a load in the same amount of time as your planned event (e.g., run 400 meters with a 30 kg load in the same amount of time as 800 meters without a load). For powerwalking 200-800 meters, women should use a 20 kg sled and men should use 30-50 kg.

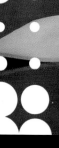

CHAPTER 9

FLEXIBILITY TRAINING

TRAINING PROGRAM

+ Intensity: **None or partner pressure only**

+ Duration of repetition: **<2-60 seconds**

+ Number of repetitions: **8-15**

+ Rest between reps: **0-30 seconds**

+ Sets per exercise: **1-5**

+ Rest between sets: **1-3 minutes**

+ Rest between workouts: **No restriction**

#9

FLEXIBILITY TRAINING

The development of flexibility is essential to obtain an adequate range of motion, both for the athlete (according to the needs of his sport) and for the individual who wishes to maintain ease of activities of daily life. In general, we will need to stretch in different ways in order to improve range of motion, reduce muscle tension, and increase the extensibility of connective tissues in muscles and joints. However, several factors can influence flexibility, including the following:

→ Muscle tension
→ Hormones
→ Pelvic structure
→ Obesity
→ Joint limitations
→ Postural misalignment (e.g., scoliosis)
→ Elasticity of connective tissues (or lack thereof)
→ Length of tendons and ligaments
→ Inflammation
→ Muscle mass
→ Temperature
→ Age
→ Fear
→ Pain tolerance
→ Training level

There are many benefits to stretching. It reduces muscle tension, stretches shortened muscles, and can be easily individualized and practiced anywhere. Ideally, you should stretch after 5 minutes of warming up to help the muscle components (e.g., actin and myosin) move more smoothly. Consider hot honey versus cold honey in a syringe: Which will move more easily? It's a similar concept to your muscles; warm them up before starting a muscular effort or stretching. Thereafter, increase the intensity of the stretch gradually without jerking and hold the position for at least 10 seconds (otherwise the myotatic stretch reflex will not be inhibited). Stretching should be done with regular, deep, and calm breathing.

The Impact of the Nervous System on Flexibility

The nervous system plays a protective role through three main mechanisms: the myotatic reflex, the reverse myotatic reflex, and reciprocal inhibition. First, the **myotatic reflex** is a mechanism that protects the joints by sending a muscle contraction in the muscle subjected to a rapid stretch. The knee jerk test (when the doctor taps your knee with a hammer and you extend it) reflects this mode of action. Inside a muscle, there are specialized fibers called **muscle spindles** that govern this mechanism. During a sudden stretch, they contract to protect the joint from potential injury. This is the contraction you feel when you begin your static stretch. After a few seconds, the nervous system will relax and disengage the contraction of muscle spindles, suddenly giving you more range of motion.

Second, the **reverse myotatic reflex** involves elements within the tendon called Golgi tendon organs. These mechanoreceptors analyze the tension in the tendon and, when it becomes too great, send a signal to the spinal cord to stop the muscle contraction, thus avoiding excessive tension and potential tearing of the tendon. We will try to activate this reflex in order to obtain greater amplitude of movement using various proprioceptive neuromuscular facilitation (PNF) techniques in this chapter.

The third mechanism, **reciprocal inhibition**, is very simple. When a muscle contracts, your brain decreases the contraction of the opposing muscle to facilitate the movement. For example, when you contract your biceps, your brain will inhibit your triceps to promote elbow movement. Therefore, if you are attempting to stretch your hamstrings, contracting your quadriceps will help you achieve a greater range of motion by decreasing the contraction in your hamstrings.

Improving flexibility takes time. You will be asking your body to both reduce the intensity of your nervous system's protective mechanisms and to increase the number of sarcomeres (small muscle units) in series to increase the length of your muscle fibers. And unfortunately, if you stop stretching for a few weeks, you will lose some of these achievements. Rigor and consistency are therefore essential in order to continue improving your flexibility. To achieve this, do not tell yourself that you will do your stretches at home, because very few of us actually do it. Also, do not do your stretches (apart from joint mobilization) at the start of your workout, which may affect your performance in terms of strength and power. Therefore, the best times to stretch are at the end of the workout (once the body is warm) or during rest periods between sets. Personally, I prefer the latter option because it doesn't lengthen my workouts; however, it may be difficult to find adequate space to stretch near your weight training equipment.

In the beginning, you will see substantial gains with 2-3 stretching sessions a week. However, the more time goes by, the smaller the change in your range of motion will be. To see further progress, you will have to increase the frequency of your flexibility sessions per week (e.g., stretching

5 days a week instead of 3) and per day (e.g., stretching in the morning and evening instead of morning only). The techniques in this chapter will help you design each of your sessions. Vary the techniques with each session to find the ones that work best for you. In general, and as you will see in the following prescription tables, training your flexibility requires 3-5 sets of 10-15 repetitions, with each repetition lasting between 10 and 60 seconds. One of the reasons many people quickly become demotivated from doing flexibility exercises is that we don't see results from stretching just 30 seconds per muscle after our workouts. The volume is actually too low. Instead, complete, for example, 3 sets of 15 reps (10 seconds) for each leg. This will then total a session of 900 seconds, or 15 minutes. You must take the time to stretch like you take the time to train. You will get many benefits from it!

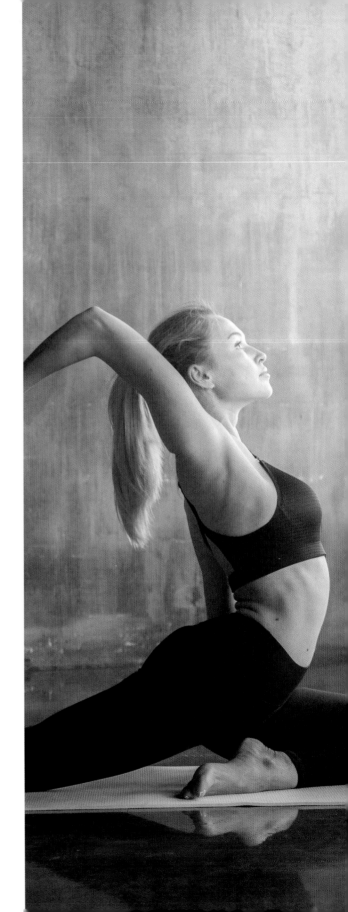

Technique #223

Perceived effort

Effect on passive flexibility

Effect on active flexibility

Effect on muscular endurance

Experience required

✓ With partner

✓ Without partner

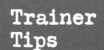
PASSIVE STATIC STRETCHING

Ⓢ

HOW DOES IT WORK?

This technique consists of performing a stretch while maintaining an isometric position at the end of the movement for an extended period. The desired position can be achieved with a partner, a device, the contraction of muscles surrounding the mobilized joint, or gravity. Because it uses slow movement, the stretch reflex will not be involved—unlike, for example, ballistic stretching (technique #227).

ADVANTAGES

→ It is ideal to integrate at the end of training for a return to calm or during rest periods during the training session.
→ It increases flexibility with maximum control over movement and minimal or no joint velocity.

DISADVANTAGES

→ It does not strengthen the agonist muscles so that the joint can actively reach the new range of motion.

PRESCRIPTION TABLE

Load	Duration of each repetition	Number of repetitions per set	Rest between repetitions	Number of sets per exercise
None	10-60 seconds	10-15	10-30 seconds	3-5

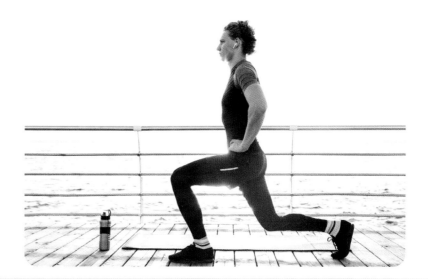

Technique #224

Perceived effort

▮▮▯▯▯

Effect on passive flexibility

▮▮▯▯▯

Effect on active flexibility

▮▮▮▮▯

Effect on muscular endurance

▮▮▯▯▯

Experience required

▮▮▮

✓ With partner

✓ Without partner

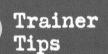
ACTIVE STATIC STRETCHING (S)

HOW DOES IT WORK?

This method consists of performing a stretch with only the use of your agonist muscles without assistance or ballistic movement. For example, if you want to stretch your hamstrings, you lie on the floor and contract your quadriceps (agonist muscle for the movement you will do, a hip flexion). You then hold the position for several seconds.

ADVANTAGES

→ It strengthens the weak agonist muscles that oppose the tense muscles to be stretched.
→ It is useful for sports such as ballet or dance for which positions in large ranges of motion must be maintained for several seconds.

DISADVANTAGES

→ It does not continually improve passive flexibility and therefore does not contribute to improving range of motion.

PRESCRIPTION TABLE

Load	Duration of each repetition	Number of repetitions per set	Rest between repetitions	Number of sets per exercise
None	10-60 seconds	10-15	10-30 seconds	3-5

Hold the position with your muscles

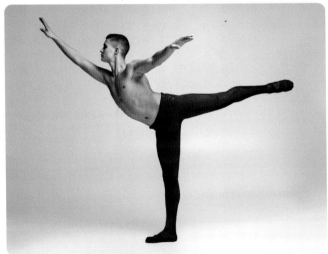

Technique #225

Perceived effort

▮▮▯▯▯

Effect on passive flexibility

▮▮▮▮▯

Effect on active flexibility

▮▮▮▮▯

Effect on muscular endurance

▮▮▯▯▯

Experience required

▮▮▯

☑ With partner

☐ Without partner

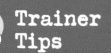

Trainer Tips

As with active static stretching (technique #224), you may need support, particularly because a partner will exert pressure on you in this technique, risking tipping you over. A wall or a weight machine will suffice.

ASSISTED ACTIVE STATIC STRETCHING

Ⓢ

HOW DOES IT WORK?

This method involves performing an active static stretch. When the limit of active flexibility is reached, the rest of passive flexibility is accomplished by a partner.

ADVANTAGES

→ It strengthens the weak agonist muscles that oppose the tense muscles to be stretched.

→ It is useful for sports such as ballet or dance for which positions in large ranges of motion must be maintained for several seconds.

DISADVANTAGES

→ It requires a partner.

PRESCRIPTION TABLE

Load	Duration of each repetition	Number of repetitions per set	Rest between repetitions	Number of sets per exercise
None	10-60 seconds	10-15	10-30 seconds	3-5

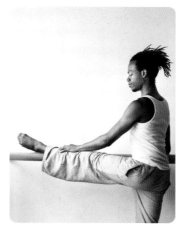

Reach your active flexibility

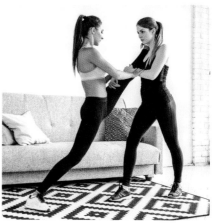

Use the help of a partner to complete the rest of the range of motion

Technique #226

Perceived effort

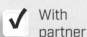

Effect on passive
flexibility

Effect on active
flexibility

Effect on muscular
endurance

Experience required

✓ With
partner

✓ Without
partner

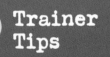

Trainer Tips

To get the most out of this
technique, try it with a partner.
At each repetition, your partner
will help you to gain 1-4 degrees
beyond the previous movement
by pushing or pulling a little bit.

ISOLATED ACTIVE STRETCHING

HOW DOES IT WORK?

This method, also called the Mattes method after its developer Aaron L. Mattes,[27] is believed to improve active and passive flexibility.[35] Other authors deem the Mattes method a good way to improve range of motion,[33] but don't consider it the most effective method for gaining flexibility. It consists of the following process:

1. Target one muscle at a time.
2. Contract the opposing muscle (agonist) to relax the muscle you are stretching.
3. Stretch the muscle quickly and hold the stretch for a maximum of 2 seconds.
4. Release the stretch before the muscle causes a protective contraction and return to the initial position.
5. Repeat the stretch 8-10 times, always going 1-4 degrees beyond the previous movement.

ADVANTAGES

→ It uses reciprocal inhibition to obtain gains in range of motion.

DISADVANTAGES

→ It is difficult to quantify the 1-4 degrees subjectively on certain exercises.

PRESCRIPTION TABLE

Load	Duration of each repetition	Number of repetitions per set	Rest between repetitions	Number of sets per exercise
None	<2 seconds	8-10	5-10 seconds	1

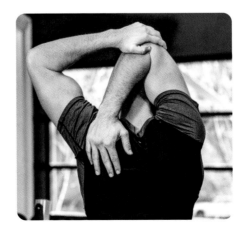

The following is an example of how to safely stretch the triceps using isolated active stretching:

→ Contract your biceps while stretching your triceps (promotes reciprocal inhibition).
→ Raise and lower your shoulder 8-10 times, going a little farther each time (decreases the intensity of the myotatic reflex).

Technique #227

Perceived effort

▮▯▯▯▯

Effect on passive flexibility

▮▮▮▮▯

Effect on active flexibility

▮▮▮▯▯

Effect on muscular endurance

▮▯▯▯▯

Experience required

▮▯▯

☐ With partner

☑ Without partner

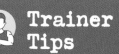

Trainer Tips

Zachazewski recommends ballistic stretching presented in a certain order within his progressive velocity flexibility program.[38] After a warm-up, you will do static stretches; then slow, low range-of-motion ballistic stretches; then slow, full range-of-motion ballistic stretches; then fast, low range-of-motion ballistic stretches; and finally fast ballistic stretches at full range of motion.

BALLISTIC STRETCHING

HOW DOES IT WORK?

This method involves performing a flexibility exercise using a swing or bounce in motion. In a ballistic stretch, there is no time when you should hold the position statically. Leg swings from front to back or from right to left are examples of ballistic stretches.

ADVANTAGES

→ It helps to develop active (dynamic) flexibility.

→ It increases the stretch reflex.[25]

→ Ballistic stretching is less monotonous than static stretching.

DISADVANTAGES

→ There is a risk of injury if you bounce or swing too far for your individual ability (see Trainer Tips for a safe progression).

PRESCRIPTION TABLE

Load	Duration of each repetition	Number of repetitions per set	Rest between repetitions	Number of sets per exercise
None	<2 seconds	8-10	<2 seconds	2-4

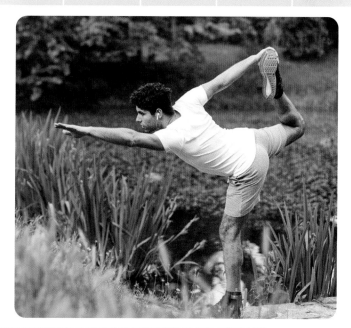

Technique #228

Perceived effort

■■■□□

Effect on passive
flexibility

■■■■■

Effect on active
flexibility

■■□□□

Effect on muscular
endurance

■■□□□

Experience required

■□□

✓ With
partner

☐ Without
partner

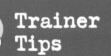

Trainer Tips

Be careful to not perform the Valsalva maneuver while using PNF techniques—that is, to hold your breath while bearing down, potentially causing a dangerous rise in blood pressure. Try to exhale while stretching in order to avoid this phenomenon.

PROPRIOCEPTIVE NEUROMUSCULAR FACILITATION (PNF)

HOW DOES IT WORK?

Proprioceptive neuromuscular facilitation (PNF) is a method that promotes or inhibits neuromuscular mechanisms by stimulating proprioceptors. It was developed in the late 1940s by neurologist Herman Kabat to treat his patients with neurological disorders. It involves the three mechanisms explained at the beginning of this chapter (the myotatic reflex, the reverse myotatic reflex, and reciprocal inhibition). This and the following 9 techniques exploit one or more of these mechanisms to potentiate gains in flexibility. You will contract either your agonist muscle or your antagonist muscle to create a lower contraction in the muscle that you want to stretch.

ADVANTAGES

→ It is one of the best ways to improve passive flexibility.
→ Muscle contractions increase intramuscular temperature and decrease muscle stiffness.

DISADVANTAGES

→ It usually requires a training partner to exert pressure, either to achieve a greater amplitude or against which we will have to resist with a voluntary contraction.

PRESCRIPTION TABLE

Load	Duration of each repetition	Number of repetitions per set	Rest between repetitions	Number of sets per exercise
None or produced by the partner	10-60 seconds	10-15	None	3-5

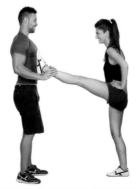

Technique #229

Perceived effort

▣ ▣ ▢ ▢ ▢

Effect on passive flexibility

▣ ▣ ▣ ▣ ▣

Effect on active flexibility

▣ ▣ ▣ ▣ ▢

Effect on muscular endurance

▣ ▣ ▣ ▢ ▢

Experience required

▣ ▢ ▢

✓ With partner

☐ Without partner

🏋 Trainer Tips

Passively stretch the targeted muscle for 20-30 seconds. Then perform a contraction of the opposite muscle for 3 seconds with the help of your partner, followed by 3 seconds without help, then 3 seconds with additional pressure. Repeat 10-15 times.

PNF, RHYTHMIC INITIATION

HOW DOES IT WORK?

This PNF method consists of the following steps:

1. Passively stretch the antagonist (e.g., hamstrings).
2. Contract the agonist (e.g., quadriceps) with a little help (e.g., the partner helps lift the leg).
3. Contract the agonist without help.
4. Contract the agonist with resistance (e.g., the partner pushes on the knee slightly).
5. Start the cycle again.

ADVANTAGES

→ It improves the ability to initiate movement.
→ It improves coordination and sense of movement.
→ It helps with relaxation.

DISADVANTAGES

→ It requires a partner.

PRESCRIPTION TABLE

Load	Duration of each repetition	Number of repetitions per set	Rest between repetitions	Number of sets per exercise
None or produced by the partner	20-60 seconds	10-15	None	3-5

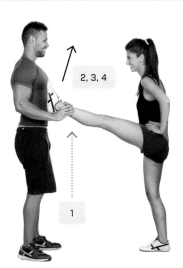

········> Dotted line: Passive flexibility

⟶ Black line: Isometric contraction

Technique #230

Perceived effort

■ ■ □ □ □

Effect on passive flexibility

■ ■ ■ ■ ■

Effect on active flexibility

■ ■ ■ □ □

Effect on muscular endurance

■ ■ ■ □ □

Experience required

■ □ □

☑ With partner

☐ Without partner

HOW DOES IT WORK?

This PNF method consists of the following steps:

1. Contract the antagonist (e.g., hamstrings) with a joint movement (e.g., hip extension).
2. Contract the agonist (e.g., quadriceps) with a joint movement (e.g., hip flexion).

ADVANTAGES

→ It develops strength of the agonist muscles in a better range of motion than PNF, rhythmic initiation (technique #229).

→ It facilitates the reciprocal inhibition of antagonistic muscles.

→ It develops the strength of antagonistic muscles.

DISADVANTAGES

→ It requires a partner.

PRESCRIPTION TABLE

Load	Duration of each repetition	Number of repetitions per set	Rest between repetitions	Number of sets per exercise
None	6-10 seconds	10-15	None	3-5

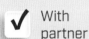

Trainer Tips

Contract the muscle you want to stretch for 3-5 seconds with a slight joint movement (resisted by a partner), then release to contract the opposite muscle for the same duration, but with slightly greater amplitude (not resisted by a partner). Alternate these two contractions 10-15 times, trying to bring the joint a little farther each time.

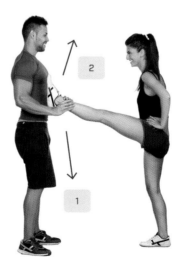

→
Red line:
Isotonic contraction

Technique #231

Perceived effort

▪▪▪▫▫

Effect on passive flexibility

▪▪▪▪▪

Effect on active flexibility

▪▪▪▪▪

Effect on muscular endurance

▪▪▪▫▫

Experience required

▪▪▫

☑ With partner

☐ Without partner

Trainer Tips

Contract the muscle you want to stretch for 3-5 seconds (resisted by a partner), hold the position in tension for 3-5 seconds, then release to contract its opposite muscle for the same duration with the isometric phase. Alternate these 4 contractions 10-15 times, trying to bring the joint a little farther each time. The partner increases the amplitude of the stretch when the opposite muscle is contracted.

PNF, SLOW REVERSAL–HOLD

HOW DOES IT WORK?

This PNF method consists of the following steps:

1. Contract the antagonist (e.g., hamstrings) with a joint movement (e.g., hip extension).
2. Hold the antagonist contraction isometrically.
3. Contract the agonist (e.g., quadriceps) with a joint movement (e.g., hip flexion).
4. Hold the agonist contraction isometrically.
5. Start the cycle again.

ADVANTAGES

→ It develops strength of the agonist muscles in a better range of motion than PNF, rhythmic initiation (technique #229).
→ It facilitates the reciprocal inhibition of antagonistic muscles.
→ It develops the strength of antagonistic muscles.

DISADVANTAGES

→ It requires a partner.

PRESCRIPTION TABLE

Load	Duration of each repetition	Number of repetitions per set	Rest between repetitions	Number of sets per exercise
None	12-20 seconds	10-15	None	3-5

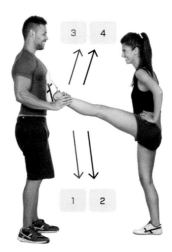

→ Black line: Isometric contraction

→ Red line: Isotonic contraction

Technique #232

Perceived effort

Effect on passive flexibility

Effect on active flexibility

Effect on muscular endurance

Experience required

✓ With partner

☐ Without partner

Trainer Tips

Contract the opposite muscle to the one you want to stretch for 3-5 seconds (resisted by a partner), then release and contract the muscle you want to stretch for the same duration. Alternate these contractions 10-15 times, trying to bring the joint a little farther each time.

PNF, RHYTHMIC STABILIZATION

HOW DOES IT WORK?

This PNF method consists of the following alternating isometric contractions of agonists and antagonists:

1. Contract the agonist (e.g., quadriceps) without joint movement.
2. Contract the antagonist (e.g., hamstrings) without joint movement.
3. Alternate these steps by gradually increasing the strength of your contractions while increasing the range of motion achieved.

ADVANTAGES

→ This technique improves passive and active flexibility.
→ It improves stability and balance.
→ It improves local circulation and helps relaxation.

DISADVANTAGES

→ It requires a partner.

PRESCRIPTION TABLE

Load	Duration of each repetition	Number of repetitions per set	Rest between repetitions	Number of sets per exercise
None	6-10 seconds	10-15	None	3-5

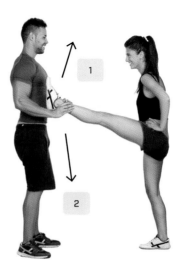

⟶
Black line:
Isometric contraction

Technique #233

Perceived effort

■ ■ ■ ▢ ▢

Effect on passive flexibility

■ ■ ■ ■ ■

Effect on active flexibility

■ ▢ ▢ ▢ ▢

Effect on muscular endurance

■ ■ ▢ ▢ ▢

Experience required

■ ■ ▢

✓ With partner

☐ Without partner

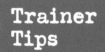

Trainer Tips

You can use a similar PNF technique called CRAC (contract, relax, agonist contraction), which consists of performing the same sequence. However, during the final stretching phase, the agonist muscle (e.g., quadriceps) is contracted for 3-5 seconds.

PNF, CONTRACT-RELAX

HOW DOES IT WORK?

This PNF method consists of executing a maximum contraction of the antagonist muscle (e.g., hamstrings) against resistance (produced by a partner) at the limit of your range of motion, followed by a period of rest. Subsequently, your partner then brings the limb (e.g., the leg) passively through a greater range of motion until a new limit is reached.

1. Contract the antagonist (e.g., hamstrings) with a joint movement (e.g., hip extension) for 3-5 seconds.
2. Relax the muscle.
3. Passively stretch the antagonist muscle (e.g., hamstrings) for 15-30 seconds.

ADVANTAGES

→ This technique improves passive range of motion.

DISADVANTAGES

→ It requires a partner.
→ It carries a greater risk of injury than static stretching due to increased tension in the muscle (maximum contraction).

PRESCRIPTION TABLE

Load	Duration of each repetition	Number of repetitions per set	Rest between repetitions	Number of sets per exercise
None	18-35 seconds	10-15	None	3-5

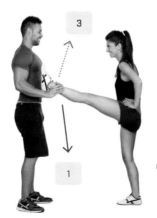

Dotted line: Passive flexibility

Red line: Isotonic contraction

Passive relaxation

Perceived effort

Effect on passive flexibility

Effect on active flexibility

Effect on muscular endurance

Experience required

✓ With partner

☐ Without partner

Trainer Tips

This technique is similar to the CRAC (contract, relax, agonist contraction) technique, which is a variant of PNF, contract–relax (technique #233), except that the first step is an isotonic contraction instead of isometric.

PNF, HOLD-RELAX

HOW DOES IT WORK?

This PNF method consists of executing an isometric contraction of the antagonist muscle (e.g., hamstrings) against resistance (produced by a partner) at the limit of your range of motion, followed by a period of rest. Next, you contract the agonist muscle (e.g., quadriceps) against a weak resistance (produced by the partner) with greater amplitude until the new limit is reached.

1. Contract the antagonist (e.g., hamstrings) with a joint movement (e.g., hip extension) for 3-5 seconds.
2. Relax the muscle.
3. Contract the agonist (e.g., quadriceps) with a joint movement (e.g., hip flexion) for 3-5 seconds.

ADVANTAGES

→ This technique is effective when the range of motion is decreased because one of the muscles on either side of a joint is tight.

DISADVANTAGES

→ It requires a partner.

PRESCRIPTION TABLE

Load	Duration of each repetition	Number of repetitions per set	Rest between repetitions	Number of sets per exercise
None	6-10 seconds	10-15	None	3-5

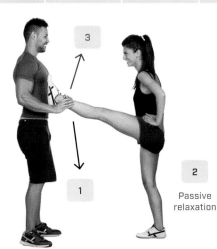

Black line: Isometric contraction

Red line: Isotonic contraction

Passive relaxation

Technique #235

Perceived effort

■■■□□

Effect on passive
flexibility

■■■■■

Effect on active
flexibility

■■□□□

Effect on muscular
endurance

■■□□□

Experience required

■□□

✓ With
partner

☐ Without
partner

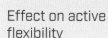

Trainer Tips

As in all PNF techniques, the isometric contraction, relaxation, and isotonic contraction phases should last 3-5 seconds each. Count out loud to make sure you are keeping correct time.

PNF, SLOW REVERSAL–HOLD–RELAX

Ⓢ

HOW DOES IT WORK?

This PNF method consists of the following steps:

1. Contract the antagonist (e.g., hamstrings) with a joint movement (e.g., hip extension).
2. Hold the antagonist contraction isometrically.
3. Relax the muscle.
4. Contract the agonist (e.g., quadriceps) with a joint movement (e.g., hip flexion).
5. Start the cycle again.

ADVANTAGES

→ This technique develops strength in antagonistic muscles.

DISADVANTAGES

→ It requires a partner.

PRESCRIPTION TABLE

Load	Duration of each repetition	Number of repetitions per set	Rest between repetitions	Number of sets per exercise
None	12-20 seconds	10-15	None	3-5

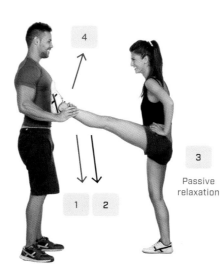

→ Black line:
Isometric contraction

→ Red line:
Isotonic contraction

Technique #236

Perceived effort

Effect on passive flexibility

Effect on active flexibility

Effect on muscular endurance

Experience required

✓ With partner

☐ Without partner

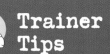

Trainer Tips

This technique involves eccentric contractions. You can start by moving your joint in the opposite direction to improve the strength and endurance of your agonist muscles in this range. Thereafter, you can ask your partner to apply slight resistance.

PNF, AGONISTIC REVERSAL

HOW DOES IT WORK?

This PNF method consists of the following steps:

1. Contract the agonist (e.g., quadriceps) with a joint movement (e.g., hip flexion) until the end of the concentric range.
2. Execute a slow and controlled eccentric contraction (e.g., without or with pressure from the partner in hip extension).
3. Relax the muscle halfway (e.g., place the foot on the partner, but do not have the partner stretch the hamstrings at this point).
4. Execute another slow and controlled eccentric contraction.
5. Start the cycle again.

ADVANTAGES

→ This technique improves the muscle strength of the agonist at the end of the concentric movement, which is beneficial for active flexibility.

DISADVANTAGES

→ It requires a partner.

PRESCRIPTION TABLE

Load	Duration of each repetition	Number of repetitions per set	Rest between repetitions	Number of sets per exercise
None	12-20 seconds	10-15	None	3-5

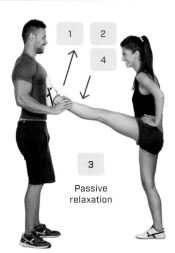

→ Red line: Isotonic contraction

Technique #237

Perceived effort

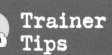

Effect on passive flexibility

Effect on active flexibility

Effect on muscular endurance

Experience required

✓ With partner

☐ Without partner

PNF, REPEATED CONTRACTIONS

HOW DOES IT WORK?

This PNF method consists of the following steps:

1. Contract the antagonist (e.g., hamstrings) with a joint movement (e.g., hip extension) for 3-5 seconds while your partner provides resistance for this concentric phase.
2. Contract the agonist (e.g., quadriceps) with a joint movement (e.g., hip flexion) until the end range for 3-5 seconds (without partner).
3. Hold the position isometrically for 3-5 seconds.
4. Start the cycle again.

ADVANTAGES

→ This technique helps develop muscle strength and endurance with concentric and isometric contractions.

DISADVANTAGES

→ It requires a partner.

PRESCRIPTION TABLE

Load	Duration of each repetition	Number of repetitions per set	Rest between repetitions	Number of sets per exercise
None	9-15 seconds	10-15	None	3-5

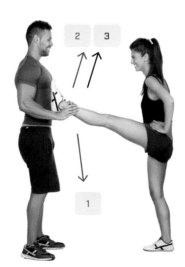

→ Black line: Isometric contraction

→ Red line: Isotonic contraction

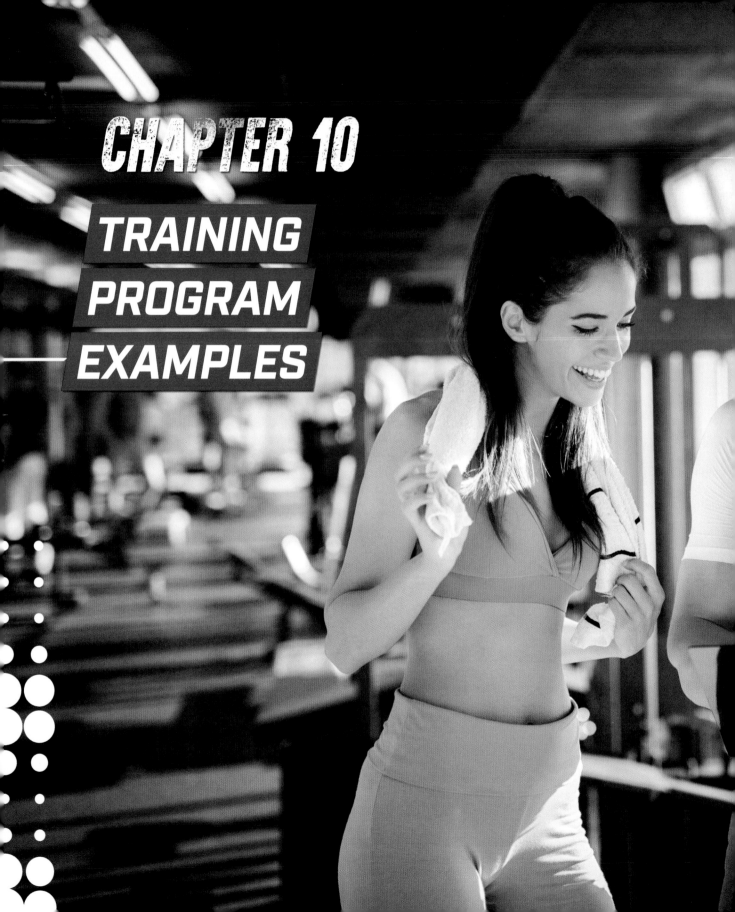

CHAPTER 10

TRAINING PROGRAM EXAMPLES

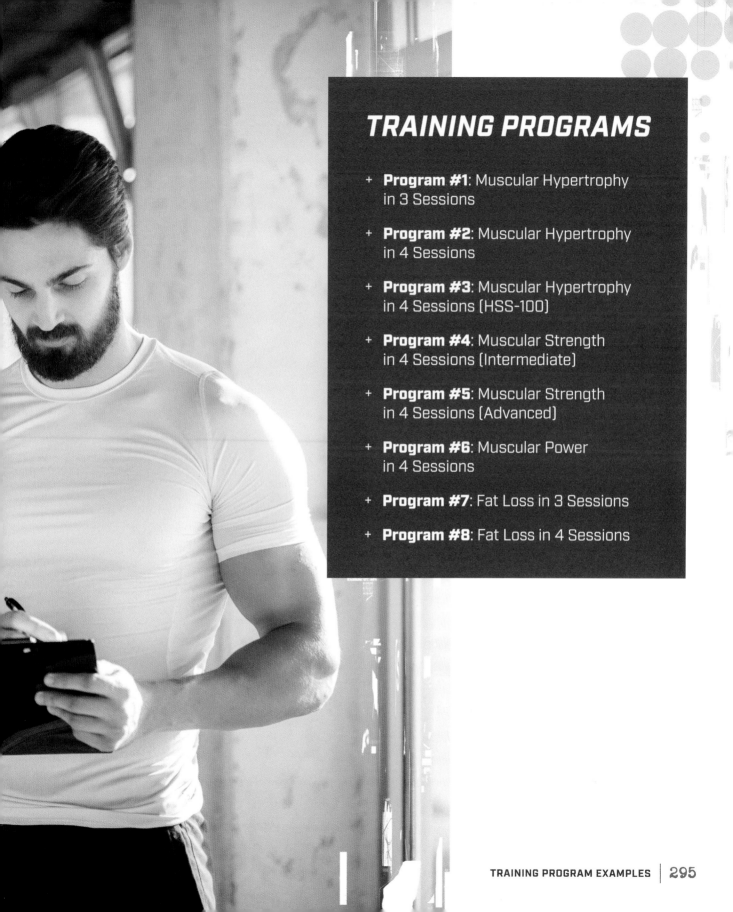

TRAINING PROGRAMS

+ **Program #1**: Muscular Hypertrophy in 3 Sessions

+ **Program #2**: Muscular Hypertrophy in 4 Sessions

+ **Program #3**: Muscular Hypertrophy in 4 Sessions (HSS-100)

+ **Program #4**: Muscular Strength in 4 Sessions (Intermediate)

+ **Program #5**: Muscular Strength in 4 Sessions (Advanced)

+ **Program #6**: Muscular Power in 4 Sessions

+ **Program #7**: Fat Loss in 3 Sessions

+ **Program #8**: Fat Loss in 4 Sessions

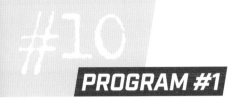

PROGRAM #1

MUSCULAR HYPERTROPHY IN 3 SESSIONS

The techniques used in this program are the 4 × 10 per minute (#110), double contraction (#108), agonist superset (#71), and dropset (#74). If an exercise doesn't have a number in parentheses, do it with the classic tempo of 3-0-1-0. Perform exercises labeled with the same letter as supersets.

	DAY 1: Chest, shoulders, triceps	Sets	Reps	Rest
A	Barbell bench press (#110)	4	10	1 min
B1	Dumbbell bench press (#108)	3	8-10	0 min
B2	Standing pulley cross-over	3	8-10	2 min
C	Chest press (#74)	3	8-10 + 8-10	2 min
D1	Dumbbell lateral raise (#108)	4	8-10	0 min
D2	Seated dumbbell shoulder press	4	8-10	2 min
E1	Overhead dumbbell triceps extension (#108)	4	8-10	0 min
E2	Triceps push-down (#71)	4	8-10	2 min

	DAY 2: Quadriceps, hamstrings, adductors	Sets	Reps	Rest
A	Hack squat (#110)	4	10	1 min
B1	Leg extension (#108)	3	8-10	0 min
B2	Dumbbell walking lunge	3	8-10 per leg	2 min
C	Leg press (#74)	3	8-10 + 8-10	2 min
D	Seated leg curl (#110)	4	10	1 min
E1	Lying leg curl (#108)	4	8-10	0 min
E2	Dumbbell Romanian deadlift	4	8-10	2 min
F	Hip adductor machine (#74)	4	8-10 + 8-10	2 min

	DAY 3: Back, upper back, biceps	Sets	Reps	Rest
A	Assisted pull-up machine (#110)	4	10	1 min
B1	Seated cable row (#108)	3	8-10	0 min
B2	Bent-over dumbbell row	3	8-10	2 min
C	T-bar row machine, neutral grip (#74)	3	8-10 + 8-10	2 min
D1	Seated cable row to chest (#108)	4	8-10	0 min
D2	Dumbbell rear delt fly	4	8-10	2 min
E1	Standing barbell curl (#108)	4	8-10	0 min
E2	Dumbbell hammer curl	4	8-10	2 min

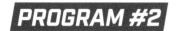

MUSCULAR HYPERTROPHY IN 4 SESSIONS

The techniques used in this program are the maximal duration isometric (#164), plyometrics with or without load (#184), agonist superset (#71), and super slow reps 10-4 (#103). If an exercise doesn't have a number in parentheses, do it with the classic tempo of 3-0-1-0. Perform exercises labeled with the same letter as supersets. If a fifth session is desired, add a day that includes work on the glutes and latissimus dorsi.

DAY 1: Chest, biceps				
	Exercises	Sets	Reps	Rest
A1	Barbell bench press (#164)	4	2-10 s per position*	1 min
A2	Dumbbell bench press	4	6-8	2 min
B1	Clap push-ups (#184)	3	8-10 (fast)	0 min
B2	Pec deck machine (#103)	3	4-5	2 min
C1	Standing barbell curl (#164)	4	2-10 s per position*	1 min
C2	Dumbbell hammer curl	4	6-8	2 min
D1	Explosive standing curl with band (moderate tension) (#184)	3	8-10 (fast)	0 min
D2	Barbell pronated Scott curl (#103)	3	4-5	2 min

DAY 2: Quadriceps, hamstrings				
	Exercises	Sets	Reps	Rest
A1	Leg press (#164)	4	2-10 s per position*	1 min
A2	Back squat	4	6-8	2 min
B1	Depth jump between boxes (#184)	3	8-10 (fast)	0 min
B2	Front squat (#103)	3	4-5	2 min
C1	Lying leg curl (#164)	4	2-10 s per position*	1 min
C2	Barbell Romanian deadlift	4	6-8	2 min
D1	Explosive alternating lying single-leg curl (#184)	3	8-10 per leg (fast)	0 min
D2	Good morning (#103)	3	4-5	2 min

DAY 3: Shoulders, triceps				
	Exercises	Sets	Reps	Rest
A1	30-degree incline dumbbell bench press (#164)	4	2-10 s per position*	1 min
A2	Dumbbell lateral raise	4	6-8	2 min
B1	One-arm dumbbell shoulder press (#184)	3	8-10 per arm (fast)	0 min
B2	Upright barbell row (#103)	3	4-5	2 min
C1	Triceps push-down (#164)	4	2-10 s per position*	1 min
C2	Lying barbell triceps extension	4	6-8	2 min
D1	Explosive push-up, alternating close and wide grip (#184)	3	8-10 (fast) total	0 min
D2	Rope triceps push-down (#103)	3	4-5	2 min

DAY 4: Upper back, back, abdominals				
	Exercises	Sets	Reps	Rest
A1	Chest-supported T-bar row to chest (#164)	4	2-10 s per position*	1 min
A2	Dumbbell rear delt fly	4	6-8	2 min
B1	Explosive pronated inverted row, alternating wide and close grip (#184)	3	8-10 (fast) total	0 min
B2	Seated cable row to chest (#103)	3	4-5	2 min
C1	Kneeling cable crunch (#164)	4	2-10 s per position*	1 min
C2	Reverse crunch	4	6-8	2 min
D1	V sit-up (#184)	3	8-10 (fast)	0 min
D2	Roman chair leg raise (#103)	3	4-5	2 min

*The 2 positions for the maximal duration isometric are generally at the beginning and halfway through the movement.

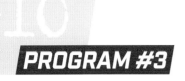

#10

PROGRAM #3

MUSCULAR HYPERTROPHY IN 4 SESSIONS (HSS-100)

The technique used in this program is the HSS-100 (#161). The heavy technique (H) used is grouping (#33) and the special technique used is uniangular triset (#89). If an exercise doesn't have a number in parentheses, do it with the classic tempo of 3-0-1-0. Perform exercises labeled with the same letter as supersets.

	DAY 1: Chest, biceps			
	Exercises	Sets	Reps	Rest
A	Chest press (#33)	3	4 + 1 + 1*	3 min
B1	30-degree incline dumbbell bench press	3	8-10	0 min
B2	Pec deck machine	3	8-10	2 min
C	Barbell bench press (close, medium, wide grip) (#89)	3	5 + 5 + 5	2 min
D	Push-up with hands on bench (#214)	1	100	2 min
E	Standing barbell curl (#33)	3	4 + 1 + 1*	3 min
F1	Chin-up	3	8-10	0 min
F2	Dumbbell hammer curl	3	8-10	2 min
G	Standing barbell curl (close, medium, wide grip) (#89)	3	5 + 5 + 5	2 min
H	Curl machine (#214)	1	100	2 min

	DAY 2: Quadriceps, hamstrings			
	Exercises	Sets	Reps	Rest
A	Back squat (#33)	3	4 + 1 + 1*	3 min
B1	One-leg squat, back on Swiss ball	3	8-10 per leg	0 min
B2	Single-leg extension (superset on each leg)	3	8-10 per leg	2 min
C	Hack squat (low-half, complete, high-half) (#89)	3	5 + 5 + 5	2 min
D	Leg press (#214)	1	100	2 min
E	Standing one-leg curl on machine (#33)	3	4 + 1 + 1* per leg	3 min
F1	Seated leg curl	3	8-10	0 min
F2	Back extension	3	8-10	2 min
G	Lying leg curl (internal rotation, external rotation, neutral) (#89)	3	5 + 5 + 5	2 min
H	Standing calf with machine (#214)	1	100	2 min

	DAY 3: Shoulders, triceps			
	Exercises	Sets	Reps	Rest
A	One-arm lateral raise on low pulley (#33)	3	4 + 1 + 1* per arm	3 min
B1	Lateral machine raise	3	8-10	0 min
B2	Standing barbell military press	3	8-10	2 min
C	Upright barbell row (close, medium, wide grip) (#89)	3	5 + 5 + 5	2 min
D	Dumbbell lateral raise (#214)	1	100	2 min
E	Barbell close-grip bench press (#33)	3	4 + 1 + 1*	3 min
F1	Supinated triceps push-down	3	8-10	0 min
F2	Lying supinated EZ-bar extension	3	8-10	2 min
G	Dumbbell triceps extension (overhead, incline, flat) (#89)	3	5 + 5 + 5	2 min
H	Pronated triceps push-down, V bar (#214)	1	100	2 min

	DAY 4: Back, abdominals			
	Exercises	Sets	Reps	Rest
A	Bent-over barbell row	3	4 + 1 + 1*	3 min
B1	Pull-up neutral grip	3	8-10	0 min
B2	Dumbbell chest-supported row	3	8-10	2 min
C	Lat pull-down (close, medium, wide grip) (#89)	3	5 + 5 + 5	2 min
D	Seated cable row (#214)	1	100	2 min
E	Kneeling cable crunch (#33)	3	4 + 1 + 1*	3 min
F1	Ab slide	3	8-10	0 min
F2	Bicycle crunch	3	8-10 per side	2 min
G	Roman chair leg raise (low-half, complete, high-half) (#89)	3	5 + 5 + 5	2 min
H	Crunch (touch knees with fingers) (#214)	1	100	2 min

*Rest for 10 seconds between each group of reps.

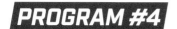

PROGRAM #4

MUSCULAR STRENGTH IN 4 SESSIONS (INTERMEDIATE)

The techniques used in this program are the overload in big waves (#111) adapted for muscle strength and progression over the weeks, general standards 1RM-5RM (#22), and pure concentric (#117). If an exercise doesn't have a number in parentheses, do it with the classic tempo of 3-0-1-0. Perform exercises labeled with the same letter as supersets.

DAY 1: Upper-body strength 1		Sets	Reps	Rest
	Exercises	Sets	Reps	Rest
A	Barbell bench press (#111)	6	8 + 6 + 4 + 8 + 6 + 4*	3 min
B	Dumbbell bench press (#22)	3	3-5	2 min
C	Seated cable row to chest (#111)	6	8 + 6 + 4 + 8 + 6 + 4*	3 min
D	Dumbbell chest-supported row to chest (#22)	3	3-5	2 min
E1	Rear delt fly machine	5	4-6	0 min
E2	Dumbbell lateral raise deadstart on bench (#117)	5	4-6	2 min

DAY 2: Lower-body strength 1		Sets	Reps	Rest
	Exercises	Sets	Reps	Rest
A	Back squat (#111)	6	8 + 6 + 4 + 8 + 6 + 4*	3 min
B	Leg press (#22)	3	3-5	2 min
C	Lying leg curl (#111)	6	8 + 6 + 4 + 8 + 6 + 4*	3 min
D	Barbell hip thrust (#22)	3	3-5	2 min
E1	Good morning	5	4-6	0 min
E2	Standing calf with machine	5	4-6	2 min

DAY 3: Upper-body strength 2		Sets	Reps	Rest
	Exercises	Sets	Reps	Rest
A1	Barbell bench press (#22)	4	5**	1 min
A2	Barbell bench press at 50%, lay on chest (#117)	4	6	2 min
B	Dumbbell fly	3	4-6	2 min
C	Lying barbell triceps extension (#22)	3	5**	3 min
D1	Lat pull-down, neutral grip (#22)	4	5**	1 min
D2	Lat pull-down, neutral grip at 50% (#117)	4	6	2 min
E	Seated cable row, supinated grip	3	4-6	2 min
F	Standing barbell curl (#22)	4	5**	2 min

DAY 4: Lower-body strength 2		Sets	Reps	Rest
	Exercises	Sets	Reps	Rest
A1	Back squat (#22)	4	5**	1 min
A2	Box squat at 50%, sit down 3 seconds on box (#117)	4	6	2 min
B1	Leg extension	4	4-6	1 min
B2	Hip adductor machine	4	4-6	2 min
C1	Barbell Romanian deadlift (#22)	4	5**	1 min
C2	Lying leg curl, pause for 3 seconds (#117)	4	6	2 min
D1	Back extension	3	4-6	1 min
D2	Hip abductor machine (#22)	3	5**	2 min

*Change your repetitions each week. For example, in week 1, you will do 8 + 6 + 4 + 8 + 6 + 4; in week 2, you will do 7 + 5 + 3 + 7 + 5 + 3; in week 3, you will do 6 + 4 + 2 + 6 + 4 + 2; in week 4, you will do 5 + 3 + 1 + 5 + 3 + 1; and in week 5, you will go back to 8 + 6 + 4 + 8 + 6 + 4 to compare your strength gains.

**Change your repetitions each week. For example, in week 1, you will do 5 repetitions; in week 2, you will do 4 repetitions; in week 3, you will do 3 repetitions; in week 4, you will do 2 repetitions; and in week 5, you will go back to 5 repetitions to compare your strength gains.

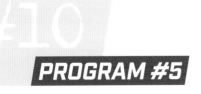

MUSCULAR STRENGTH IN 4 SESSIONS (ADVANCED)

The techniques used in this program are the functional isometric cluster (#55), super-Pletnev (#36), and pre-post-fatigue (#87). If an exercise doesn't have a number in parentheses, do it with the classic tempo of 3-0-1-0. Perform exercises labeled with the same letter as supersets.

DAY 1: Chest and biceps		Sets	Reps	Rest
A	Barbell bench press (#55)	3	2 per position*	3 min
B1	Eccentric chest press in 3-5 seconds (with assistance in concentric phase) (#36)	3	4	0 min
B2	Clap push-up (#36)	3	6	0 min
B3	Isometric push-up with elbows at 90 degrees (#36)	3	30 s	0 min
B4	Dumbbell bench press (#36)	3	4-6	3 min
C	Standing barbell curl (#55)	3	2 per position*	2 min
D1	Barbell Scott curl (#87)	4	4-6	0 min
D2	Chin-up (#87)	4	4-6	0 min
D3	Dumbbell hammer curl (#87)	4	4-6	3 min

DAY 2: Quadriceps and hamstrings		Sets	Reps	Rest
A	Leg press (#55)	3	2 per position*	3 min
B1	Eccentric single-leg press in 3-5 seconds (with assistance in concentric phase) (#36)	3	4	0 min
B2	Dumbbell jump squat (#36)	3	6	0 min
B3	Isometric leg extension (full extension) (#36)	3	30 s	0 min
B4	Walking dumbbell lunge (#36)	3	4-6	3 min
C	Lying leg curl (#55)	3	2 per position*	2 min
D1	Seated leg curl (#87)	4	4-6	0 min
D2	Barbell Romanian deadlift (#87)	4	4-6	0 min
D3	Back extension (#87)	4	4-6	3 min

DAY 3: Shoulders and abdominals		Sets	Reps	Rest
A	Seated shoulder press on Smith machine (#55)	3	2 per position*	3 min
B1	Eccentric low-pulley lateral raise in 3-5 seconds (with assistance in concentric phase) (#36)	3	4	0 min
B2	Explosive barbell military press (#36)	3	6	0 min
B3	Isometric barbell upright row (above navel) (#36)	3	30 s	0 min
B4	Dumbbell lateral raise (#36)	3	4-6	3 min
C	Kneeling cable crunch (#55)	3	2 per position*	2 min
D1	Reverse crunch (#87)	4	4-6	0 min
D2	Ab slide (#87)	4	4-6	0 min
D3	Weighted crunch on floor (#87)	4	4-6	3 min

DAY 4: Back and triceps		Sets	Reps	Rest
A	Lat pull-down (#55)	3	2 per position*	3 min
B1	Eccentric pull-up in 3-5 seconds (#36)	3	4	0 min
B2	Bent-over explosive dumbbell row (#36)	3	6	0 min
B3	Seated isometric cable row (hold at stomach) (#36)	3	30 s	0 min
B4	Dumbbell chest-supported row (#36)	3	4-6	3 min
C	Triceps push-down (#55)	3	2 per position*	2 min
D1	Lying barbell triceps extension (#87)	4	4-6	0 min
D2	Dip (elbows out) (#87)	4	4-6	0 min
D3	Dumbbell overhead triceps extension (#87)	4	4-6	3 min

*The three positions for the functional isometric cluster are at 1/4, 1/2, and 3/4 of the movements. Hold each position for 5 seconds and rest for 10 seconds before moving to the next position.

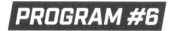

MUSCULAR POWER IN 4 SESSIONS

The techniques used in this program are the big Kahuna (#198), variable resistance with bands (#187), explosive static-dynamic (#182), plyometrics with or without load (#184), and ballistic exercises (#188). If an exercise doesn't have a number in parentheses, do it with the classic tempo of 3-0-1-0. Perform exercises labeled with the same letter as supersets.

DAY 1: Upper-body power 1 (emphasis on strength)

	Exercises	Sets	Reps	Rest
A	Barbell bench press (#198)	3	2 + 3 + max*	3 min
B	Dumbbell bench press (#182)	3	6-8	2 min
C	Lat pull-down (#198)	3	2 + 3 + max*	3 min
D	Bent-over dumbbell row (hold at mid-thigh) (#182)	3	6-8	2 min
E1	Lying barbell triceps extension	3	6-8	0 min
E2	Standing barbell curl (#182)	3	6-8	2 min
F	Kneeling cable crunch (#198)	4	2 + 3 + max*	2 min

DAY 2: Lower-body power 1 (emphasis on strength)

	Exercises	Sets	Reps	Rest
A	Hack squat (#198)	3	2 + 3 + max*	3 min
B	Back squat + jump after 3-second pause (#182)	3	6-8	2 min
C	Lying leg curl (#198)	3	2 + 3 + max*	3 min
D	Barbell Romanian deadlift (pause at knee level) (#182)	3	6-8	2 min
E	Hip abductor machine (#198)	3	2 + 3 + max*	2 min
F	Reverse hyper machine (#182)	3	6-8	2 min
G	Seated calf machine	3	4-6	1 min
H1	Barbell Romanian deadlift	4	4-6	0 min
H2	Back extension	4	4-6	3 min

DAY 3: Upper-body power 2 (emphasis on speed)

	Exercises	Sets	Reps	Rest
A	Barbell bench press with superbands at 50% (#187)	8	3	1 min
B	Barbell bench press throw on Smith machine at 30% (#188)	5	8	1 min
C	Bent-over barbell row at 50% (feet on the middle of the superbands at the ends of the bar) (#187)	8	3	1 min
D	Explosive inverted row alternating close and wide grip (#184)	5	8 total	1 min
E1	Standing landmine trunk rotation	3	6-8 per side	0 min
E2	V sit-up	3	6-8	1 min

DAY 4: Lower-body power 2 (emphasis on speed)

	Exercises	Sets	Reps	Rest
A	Hang power clean at 50%	8	2	1 min
B	Box squat with superbands at 50% (#187)	8	2	1 min
C	Box jump (#184)	5	8	1 min
D	Deadlift at 50% with superbands (#187)	8	1	1 min
E1	Hip adductor machine	3	6-8	0 min
E2	Standing calf with machine	3	6-8	1 min

*Maximum reps should be performed slowly (3-1-3-0 tempo) at 60%.

#10
PROGRAM #7

FAT LOSS IN 3 SESSIONS

The techniques used in this program are the antagonist superset (#72), Tabata method (#221), and metabolic training (#207). Perform exercises labeled with the same letter as supersets.

DAY 1: Antagonist superset and cardiovascular				
	Exercises	Sets	Reps	Rest
A1	Back squat [#72]	4	12-15	0 min
A2	Lying leg curl [#72]	4	12-15	1 min
B	Cardiovascular exercise in intervals	2	8*	2 min
C1	Barbell bench press [#72]	4	12-15	0 min
C2	Bent-over barbell row [#72]	4	12-15	1 min
D	Cardiovascular exercise in intervals	2	8*	2 min
E1	Lat pull-down [#72]	4	12-15	0 min
E2	Standing dumbbell military press [#72]	4	12-15	1 min
F	Cardiovascular exercise in intervals	2	8*	2 min

DAY 2: Tabata method with strength exercises				
	Exercises	Sets	Reps	Rest
A	Barbell hang clean [#221]	1	8**	2 min
B	Dumbbell Romanian deadlift [#221]	1	8**	2 min
C	Air squat [#221]	1	8**	2 min
D	Walking dumbbell lunge [#221]	1	8**	2 min
E	Dumbbell bench press [#221]	1	8**	2 min
F	Seated cable row [#221]	1	8**	2 min
G	Dumbbell lateral raise [#221]	1	8**	2 min
H	Dumbbell curl and press [#221]	1	8**	2 min
I	Crunch on floor [#221]	1	8**	N/A

DAY 3: Metabolic training				
	Exercises	Sets	Reps	Rest
A1	Push-up [#207]	10	10	0 min
A2	Knees to elbows [#207]	10	10	0 min
A3	Barbell deadlift [#207]	10	10	0 min
A4	Burpee [#207]	10	10	0 min
A5	V sit-up [#207]	10	10	0 min
A6	Dumbbell thruster [#207]	10	10	0 min
A7	Jumping pull-up [#207]	10	10	0 min

*1 rep = 15 seconds of effort (run, elliptical, bike, rower) and 15 seconds of rest.

**1 rep = 20 seconds of effort and 10 seconds of rest.

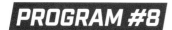

FAT LOSS IN 4 SESSIONS

The techniques used in this program are strength intervals (cardioacceleration) (#216) and triset (#86). Perform exercises labeled with the same letter as supersets.

DAY 1: Lower-body training 1				
	Exercises	Sets	Reps	Rest
A	Cardiovascular exercise in intervals	2	10*	2 min
B1	Bench step-up and over	3	12-15 per side	0 min
B2	Bulgarian split squat (#216)	3	12-15 per side	2 min**
C1	Jump over bench	3	12-15 per side	0 min
C2	Walking dumbbell lunge (#216)	3	12-15 per side	2 min**
D1	One-leg hip thrust on floor	3	12-15 per side	0 min
D2	Air squat (#216)	3	12-15	2 min**

DAY 2: Upper-body training 1				
	Exercises	Sets	Reps	Rest
A	Cardiovascular exercise in intervals	2	10*	2 min
B1	Push-up with hands on bench (#86)	5	12-15	0 min
B2	One-arm dumbbell row, knee on bench (#86)	5	12-15 per side	0 min
B3	Dumbbell bench press (#86)	5	12-15	1 min
C1	Chest press	5	12-15	0 min
C2	Vertical press with dumbbells	5	12-15	0 min
C3	Bent-over barbell row to chest	5	12-15	1 min

DAY 3: Lower-body training 2				
	Exercises	Sets	Reps	Rest
A	Cardiovascular exercise in intervals	2	10*	2 min
B1	Swiss ball squat (#86)	5	12-15	0 min
B2	Hip thrust + knee flexion with feet on Swiss ball (#86)	5	12-15	0 min
B3	Crunch on Swiss ball (#86)	5	12-15	1 min
C1	Jump squat	5	12-15	0 min
C2	Back extension	5	12-15	0 min
C3	Wall sit + raise a foot	5	12-15 per side	1 min

DAY 4: Upper-body training 2				
	Exercises	Sets	Reps	Rest
A	Cardiovascular exercise in intervals	2	10*	2 min
B1	Incline dumbbell bench press	3	12-15	0 min
B2	Dumbbell chest-supported row (#216)	3	12-15	2 min**
C1	Lat pull-down	3	12-15	0 min
C2	Barbell curl and press (#216)	3	12-15	2 min**
D1	Crunch on floor	3	12-15	0 min
D2	Plank + touch the wall with your hand (3 support points) (#216)	3	12-15 per side	2 min**

*1 rep = 30 seconds of effort (run, elliptical, bike, rower) and 30 seconds of rest.

**Because this superset is part of strength intervals (cardioacceleration) (#216), you should work on a cardio machine during the 2-minute break. After about 40-60 seconds, increase the intensity for 15-20 seconds. Once all 3 sets have been completed, take a 3-minute break before moving on to the next superset.

#10

EXAMPLE OF EVOLUTION OF HYPERTROPHY TRAINING TECHNIQUES OVER 5 YEARS

P	YEAR 1	YEAR 2	YEAR 3	YEAR 4	YEAR 5
	Beginner	Intermediate	Advanced I	Advanced II	Elite
1	Failure set	General standards 1RM-5RM; overload in small waves	Russian complex training; maximum weight 1; pure concentric	Extended 5's cluster; Bulgarian method	Mentzer cluster; stage 5RM-3RM
2	Antagonist superset	4 × 10 per minute; metabolic postfatigue	German volume phase 1; Nubret pro-set	German volume phase 2; speed-set training	German volume phase 3; tempo contrast
3	Agonist superset; hypertrophy 12RM-10RM-8RM-6RM	Concentric static-dynamic; negative reps	Maximum contraction; postpotentiation	Breathing squat; 1-minute intervals at 85%; big Kahuna	Giant organic set 4; the 21
	WEEK OFF				
4	Squat–bench–deadlift split; double contraction	Stage 10RM-6RM; postactivation	HSS-100 [S: uniangular triset]	The layer system	Descending sets 2; giant organic set 5
5	Dropset; super slow reps 5-5	Overload in big waves; plyometrics with or without load	Kulesza method; grouping dropset	Olympic weightlifting variations; classic cluster; ballistic isometric	Dropset cluster; depth landing
6	Constant tension; burn set	Super-pump set short version; isometric with perturbations	Maximum duration isometric; super slow reps 10-4	Descending sets 1; posing	Extended 7's; variable resistance training; bookend training
	WEEK OFF				

Each program (P in the table) is for a suggested duration of 4 weeks.

P	YEAR 1	YEAR 2	YEAR 3	YEAR 4	YEAR 5
	Beginner	Intermediate	Advanced I	Advanced II	Elite
7	Prefatigue; forced set	Eccentric–isometric contrast 1; continuous work at 40%	Potentiation + metabolic; eccentric–concentric contrast	Big Kahuna progression; holistic set; postfatigue	Antagonist cluster; super negative reps
8	Double dropset; 5 × 5	Stage 6RM-10RM; dropset with progressive reps	5 × 10; giant organic set 1	Grouping; giant organic set 2	Full giant organic set
9	Internal pyramid method; preactivation; short intervals at 60%	5 × 5 higher strength; traditional exercises with max power	Grouping; Wendler method	Antagonist cluster; depth jump; 2/1 technique	Pure eccentric (maximal and supramaximal); maximum intensity isometric; drop, catch, and lift
	WEEK OFF				
10	Triset; metabolic training	Rest-pause; metabolic postfatigue	Hypertrophy circuit; failure set; double contraction; maximal fatigue	Giant organic set 3; explosive static-dynamic; strength intervals (2 exercises)	Muscular chaos (for the last 4 workouts)
11	Maximal fatigue; 5 × 6	Partial reps with max effort; super-pump set regressive version; super slow eccentric reps	Iso-max eccentric; strength intervals (1 exercise)	1-minute intervals at 90%; dropset with progressive reps	Alternating rest-pause; 4-minute muscle
12	Double progression method; small-angle training; long intervals at 60%	Heavy lifting and manual isometrics	Interset decreasing loads; 2-movements technique	Metabolic training; mechanical dropset; unilateral exercises	Functional isometric cluster; super-Pletnev; pre-post-fatigue
	WEEK OFF				

Each program (P in the table) is for a suggested duration of 4 weeks.

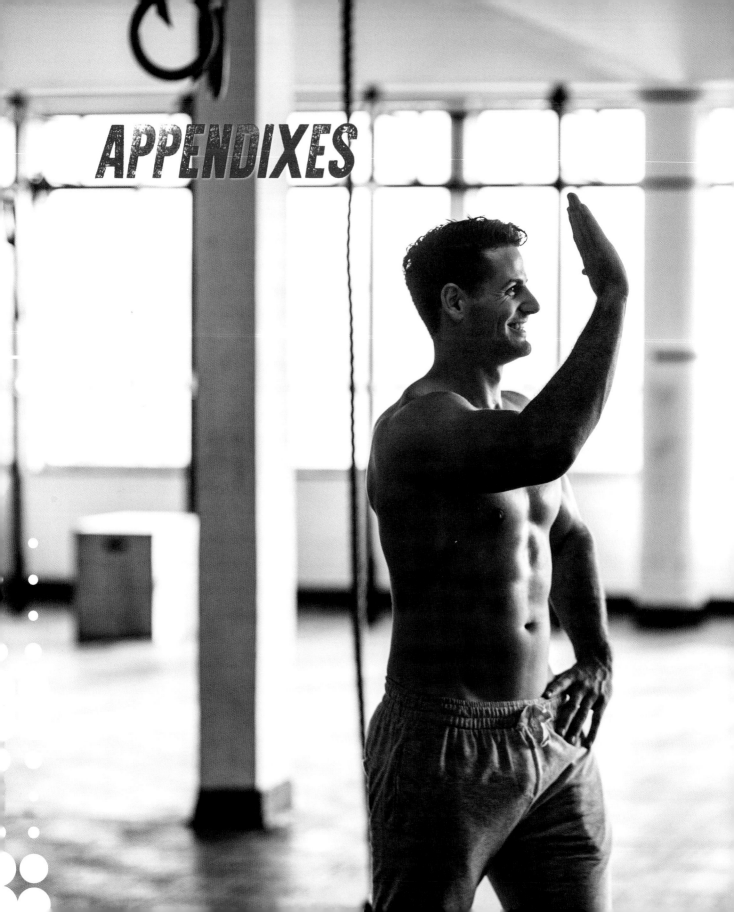

APPENDIXES

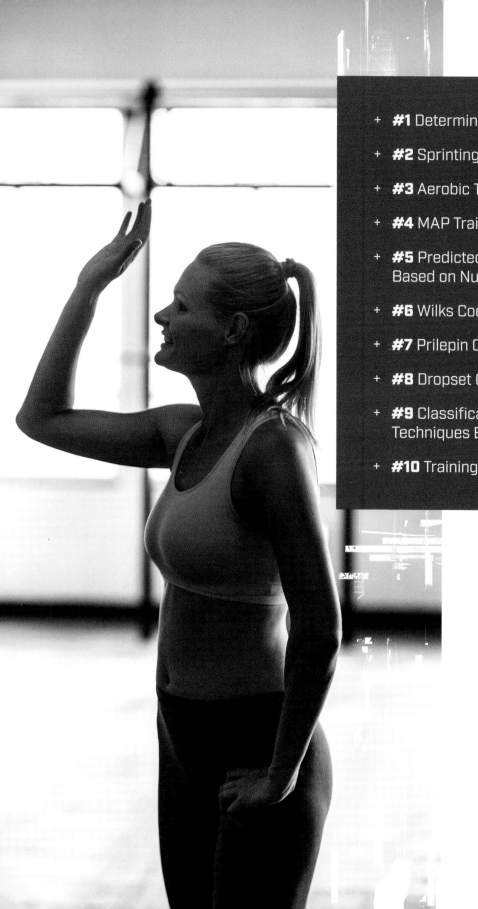

In this section, you will find many useful tools to help you with your workouts and with the application of the training techniques found in this book. Here is a brief description of each of these tools to help you make the most of them.

Appendix #1
Determining Needs

This two-page document allows you to concretely establish the needs of your client or your personal sport goals. You may need to do research in order to properly answer all of the questions—this is completely normal. The objective is to establish a good working basis to ensure the development of good physical qualities for the goal in question. Once these components have been determined, you can then design training programs around these components using techniques from this book.

Appendix #2
Sprinting Warm-Up

The sprinting warm-up is a planned warm-up sequence designed to enhance the performance of very high-intensity acceleration or running sessions while minimizing the risk of injury or strain. The warm-up can last on average between 10 and 20 minutes before the sprint session begins. It consists of the following, in order:

→ A global body warm-up such as a run
→ A global mobilization of the body back and forth over 4 meters
→ More precise joint mobilization in a greater range of motion, always back and forth over 4 meters
→ Running drills promoting coordination and agility
→ Strength exercises (usually on the floor) combined with straight-leg runs (for greater hamstring recruitment)

→ Progressive accelerations (70%, 80%, 90%, and 100% of your maximum speed) to prepare your body to run at its maximum speed during the training session

Appendix #3
Aerobic Treadmill Test

When the shuttle test is not an option, a cardiovascular test on a treadmill can be a good alternative to determine more personalized guidelines for your running. In fact, by determining your maximum aerobic speed (MAS), this test will allow you to determine the running speeds to use during your training according to your cardiovascular capacity (e.g., MAP training, endurance aerobic limit, long-term aerobic endurance). You will then work according to your maximum aerobic capacity rather than random speeds.

Each stage of the test consists of 3 minutes of effort and 3 minutes of rest at an incline of 0%. You must complete at least 4 stages for the test to be valid. If you are an experienced runner, you do not have to start at stage 1. As a reference, the majority of runners will start the test at stage 4 or 5. The test chart shows speed in miles per hour and in kilometers per hour for each stage, and you can enter your heart rate at the end of each stage for follow-up. If you have previously determined your estimated maximum heart rate (e.g., 207 − [70% × age]), you will be able to estimate the approach of your final stage.

For example, if you are a good runner, you may start the test at stage 5 (i.e., at 10.3 km/h). You will run for 3 minutes, then take 3 minutes of rest while walking slowly. At 6 minutes you will start stage 6 (11.9 km/h) for another 3 minutes followed by 3 minutes of rest, and so on until you are no longer able to keep up. If you only complete 2 minutes and 3 seconds of level 10, this would mean that your MAS is 15.8 METS (see the 2:00 column of stage 10). A MET is a metabolic equivalent corresponding to your oxygen consumption (1 MET = 3.5 ml O_2/min/kg body weight), so 15.8 METS means that your MAS (100%) is 15.8 km/h. Thus, if you are subsequently asked to run at 90% of your MAS, the speed to be used on the treadmill would therefore be 14.2 km/h (15.8 × 0.9). Don't forget to reassess your cardiovascular condition after 3 months in order to adjust the values as necessary because aerobic training should normally improve it.

Appendix #4
MAP Training
These tables allow you to quickly identify the speeds or distances to use to complete intervals of medium, short, or very short runs based on your beep test (Léger-Boucher), 20 m shuttle run test (Léger-Lambert), or MAS results. The tables provide speeds in kilometers per hour as well as distances in meters.

Appendix #5
Predicted Absolute Maximum Based on Number of Repetitions
This table will help you quickly locate a number of max reps based on another (e.g., if you do 6 max reps with 50 kg, you may have to use 35 kg to do 12 max reps). This table uses statistical data from a number of trainers and the modified Berger table. The number of reps may vary from muscle to muscle, however, because they depend primarily on the muscle type and training frequency.

Appendix #6
Wilks Coefficient
These tables show the strength coefficients based on body weight in kilograms to help you compare your level of strength to others. It is often used in strength competitions, including the powerlifting competitions of the CPA (Canadian Powerlifting Association), by accounting for the world records of the squat, bench press, and deadlift. This then avoids the biases that relative strength can present. Tables for both men and women are presented for cross-gender comparisons.

Take, for example, two male individuals weighing 80.4 kg and 100.1 kg, who can deadlift 200 kg and 220 kg, respectively. If we only look at brute strength, the individual weighing 100.1 kg wins. However, if we use the Wilks coefficient, is he still the winner? Let's use the tables in appendix #6.
→ Individual weighing 80.4 kg: Strength coefficient found in the table = 0.6806. If we multiply the coefficient by the load lifted, we get 136.12 (0.6806 × 200).
→ Individual weighing 100.1 kg: Strength coefficient found in the table = 0.6083. If we multiply the coefficient by the load lifted, we get 133.826 (0.6083 × 220).

Using the Wilks coefficient, we see that, in terms of relative strength, the 80.4 kg individual is stronger than the 100.1 kg individual. Take note, however, that there is no perfect formula for actually comparing the relative strength between two individuals. Even the Wilks coefficient favors certain competitors and has not been updated since 1994.

Appendix #7
Prilepin Chart
Alexander Prilepin created his chart after he analyzed the training books of more than a thousand national

and international weightlifting champions to determine the intensity with which an athlete should train and the number of repetitions and sets to complete per workout without placing too much stress on the nervous system. The Prilepin chart will allow you to optimize the volume of your training sessions or those of your clients.

Appendix #8
Dropset Cluster Chart

These tables will help you apply the dropset cluster technique found in chapter 2. The version shown here is for traditional barbell exercises (e.g., bench press, bent-over barbell row). To use these tables for the squat, you must include your body weight in the calculation.

Load used to squat = ([Body weight + load lifted] × desired percentage) – body weight

To give you an example, an 80 kg individual who can lift 150 kg in the squat actually lifts 230 kg (rather, a little less, because he does not lift his calves). In order to calculate the percentage to use, he will have to consider his body weight in the equation. Using a load of 90% without this consideration would be equivalent to using 135 kg, whereas the more sensible load to use (taking into account the individual's body weight of 80 kg) would be 127 kg ([80 + 150] × 90%) – 80.

Appendix #9
Classification of Training Techniques Based on Experience
These tables provide a directory of training techniques based on the level of experience required.

Appendix #10
Training Technique Template
This blank template can be used to create your own training techniques.

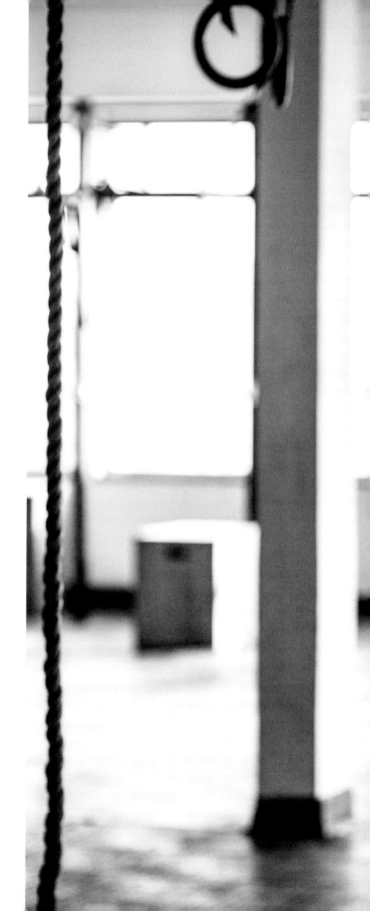

APPENDIX #1: DETERMINING NEEDS

Task analysis

Sport: _____   Level: ☐ Amateur ☐ Elite ☐ Pro ☐ All

External load
(identify the mechanical constraints of the main motor actions)

Breakdown of active time and downtime	
→ Duration of discipline	....
→ % high-intensity actions	....
→ % moderate-intensity actions	....
→ % low-intensity actions	....
→ Duration of rest between actions	....

Internal load
(identify physiological and biological reactions)

Breakdown of active time and downtime	
→ % heart rate	....
→ Lactatemia	....
→ % of VO$_2$	....

Additional features of the sport

_____

_____

_____

Physical qualities required

Determine the relative importance and contribution of each of these physical qualities to the achievement of the performance.

1 = important; 2 = secondary; 3 = complementary; N/A = not applicable

Anaerobic alactic system (AAS), running (chapter 1)				
→ Acceleration *(e.g., football, soccer)*	1	2	3	N/A
→ Maximum speed (cyclic) *(e.g., 50 m sprint)*	1	2	3	N/A
→ Maximum speed (acyclic) *(e.g., boxing, baseball, judo)*	1	2	3	N/A
→ Speed endurance *(e.g., 100 m and 20 m sprint)*	1	2	3	N/A
→ Acceleration with changes of direction *(e.g., football)*	1	2	3	N/A

Anaerobic alactic system (AAS), jumping + throwing + impulses (chapters 6 and 7)				
→ Impulses *(e.g., volleyball)*	1	2	3	N/A
→ Starting strength *(e.g., badminton, volleyball, judo)*	1	2	3	N/A
→ Ability to repeat jumps *(e.g., basketball, volleyball)*	1	2	3	N/A
→ Ability to repeat throws, strikes *(e.g., baseball, golf, tennis)*	1	2	3	N/A
→ Ability to repeat impulses (upper body) *(e.g., swimming, kayaking, boxing)*	1	2	3	N/A

Physical qualities required *(continued)*

Determine the relative importance and contribution of each of these physical qualities to the achievement of the performance.

1 = important; 2 = secondary; 3 = complementary; N/A = not applicable

Anaerobic lactic system (ALS) (chapter 1)				
→ Anaerobic lactic power (cyclic activity of 50-120 seconds) *(e.g., 400 m sprint, athletics)*	1	2	3	N/A
→ Anaerobic lactic power (intermittent sport) *(e.g., hockey)*	1	2	3	N/A
→ Anaerobic lactic capacity (cyclic activity of 50-120 seconds) *(e.g., alpine skiing, FireFit)*	1	2	3	N/A
→ Ability to repeat lower-body *(e.g., alpine skiing, snowboarding)* and upper-body *(e.g., swimming, rowing)* impulses continuously	1	2	3	N/A

Aerobic system (AS) (chapter 1)				
→ Maximum aerobic power (MAP), maximum aerobic speed (MAS) (cyclic activity of 2-8 minutes)	1	2	3	N/A
→ Maximum aerobic power (MAP), very short intermittent (intermittent sport recovery, oxidative power)	1	2	3	N/A
→ Limited aerobic endurance (cyclic activity of 30-60 minutes)	1	2	3	N/A
→ Aerobic endurance	1	2	3	N/A

Muscular qualities				
→ Maximal strength 1RM-5RM (absolute strength) (chapters 2, 4, and 5)	1	2	3	N/A
→ Maximal strength 6RM-12RM (hypertrophy) (chapters 3, 4, and 5)	1	2	3	N/A
→ Power-strength (chapter 6)	1	2	3	N/A
→ Power-speed (chapter 6)	1	2	3	N/A
→ Power endurance (chapter 7)	1	2	3	N/A
→ Strength endurance (chapter 8)	1	2	3	N/A
→ Range of motion (flexibility) (chapter 9)	1	2	3	N/A

Motor qualities (to be worked on by the trainer and/or by selecting exercises from the head coach)				
→ Reaction time (acceleration)	1	2	3	N/A
→ Movement speed (throws, impulses)	1	2	3	N/A
→ Coordination (low plyometric, power-speed)	1	2	3	N/A
→ Agility (low plyometric, power-speed)	1	2	3	N/A
→ Mobility *(e.g., cone-to-cone)*	1	2	3	N/A
→ Artistic rhythm (not cyclic), cyclic rate *(e.g., bike)*	1	2	3	N/A
→ Spatio-temporal orientation *(e.g., gymnastics, diving)*	1	2	3	N/A
→ Motor balance (proprioception)	1	2	3	N/A

From K. Arseneault, *The Complete Guide to Strength Training Methods* (Champaign, IL: Human Kinetics, 2024).

APPENDIX #2: SPRINTING WARM-UP

Use before acceleration, cone-to-cone, or anaerobic lactic system (ALS) training.

400-M JOGGING	
OVER 4 METERS	
BACK AND FORTH: GENERAL WARM-UP	
→ Walk on heels	→ Greek dance to the left
→ Walk on tiptoes	→ Greek dance to the right
→ Shuffle to the right with arm rotation	→ Jogging with feet in external rotation
→ Shuffle to the left with arm rotation	→ Backward jogging with arm rotation
→ Jogging with feet in internal rotation	

OVER 4 METERS	
BACK AND FORTH: JOINT MOBILIZATION (RANGE OF MOTION)	
→ Walk + hip flexion	→ Hip flexion + hip abduction
→ Walk + stretch hamstring	→ Left and right hip swing
→ Walk + stretch glute (knee at opposite shoulder)	→ Forward and backward hip swing
→ Hamstring stretch at each step (bent forward)	

OVER 4 METERS	
BACK AND FORTH: RUNNING DRILLS	
→ Heel-buttock, left leg only	→ High knees
→ Heel-buttock, right leg only	→ Heel-buttock in 3 parts (2 steps on floor + heel-buttock)
→ High knees, left leg only	
→ High knees, right leg only	→ High knees in 3 parts (2 steps on floor + high knees)
→ Heel-buttock	

OVER 4 METERS	
EXERCISE ON FLOOR + ACCELERATION WITH STRAIGHT LEGS	
→ Hamstring in concentric (6 each leg)	→ Hamstring in eccentric (6 each leg)
→ Stretch-stretch + hips-hips (6)	→ Fast stamping feet on floor (2 × 10 seconds)
→ One-leg hip thrust on floor (6 each leg)	→ Finnish compound (6)

OVER 15-45 METERS
PROGRESSIVE ACCELERATION AND RETURN TO WALKING
→ 70% for 15 meters
→ 80% for 25 meters
→ 90% for 35 meters
→ 100% for 45 meters

APPENDIX #3: AEROBIC TREADMILL TEST

MERCIER TEST

Date: _____   Name: _____

Stage	Speed (km/h)	Speed (mph)	Heart rate (bpm)	METS number								
				1:00	1:15	1:30	1:45	2:00	2:15	2:30	2:45	3:00
1	3.9	2.5		0.2	0.5	0.9	1.2	1.6	1.9	2.3	2.6	3.0
2	5.5	3.4		3.1	3.3	3.4	3.6	3.8	4.0	4.1	4.3	4.5
3	7.1	4.4		4.6	4.8	4.9	5.1	5.3	5.5	5.6	5.8	6.0
4	8.7	5.4		6.1	6.3	6.4	6.6	6.8	7.0	7.1	7.3	7.5
5	10.3	6.4		7.6	7.8	7.9	8.1	8.3	8.5	8.6	8.8	9.0
6	11.9	7.4		9.1	9.3	9.4	9.6	9.8	10.0	10.1	10.3	10.5
7	13.4	8.4		10.6	10.8	10.9	11.1	11.3	11.5	11.6	11.8	12.0
8	15.0	9.3		12.1	12.3	12.4	12.6	12.8	13.0	13.1	13.3	13.5
9	16.6	10.3		13.6	13.8	13.9	14.1	14.3	14.5	14.6	14.8	15.0
10	18.2	11.3		15.1	15.3	15.4	15.6	15.8	16.0	16.1	16.3	16.5
11	19.8	12.3		16.6	16.8	16.9	17.1	17.3	17.5	17.6	17.8	18.0
12	21.4	13.3		18.1	18.3	18.4	18.6	18.8	19.0	19.1	19.3	19.5
13	22.9	14.2		19.6	19.8	19.9	20.1	20.3	20.5	20.6	20.8	21.0
14	24.5	15.2		21.1	21.3	21.4	21.6	21.8	22.0	22.1	22.3	22.5
15	26.1	16.2		22.6	22.8	22.9	23.1	23.3	23.5	23.6	23.8	24.0

From K. Arseneault, *The Complete Guide to Strength Training Methods* (Champaign, IL: Human Kinetics, 2024).

MAP training compared to the result obtained with the 20 m shuttle test (Léger-Lambert, LL), the beep test (Léger-Boucher, LB), or the Mercier treadmill test

Stage LL	Speed LL [km/h]	MAS, METS, or LB speed [km/h]	VO₂MAX [1 MET = 3.5 ml O₂/kg/min]	Very short intermittent 10/10 (125%)		Very short intermittent 15/15 (120%)		Very short intermittent 20/20 (110%)		Very short intermittent 30/30 (100%)	
				km/h	meters	km/h	meters	km/h	meters	km/h	meters
1	8.5	8.5	29.8	10.6	30	10.2	43	9.4	52	8.5	71
2	9.0	9.0	31.5	11.3	31	10.8	45	9.9	55	9.0	75
3	9.5	9.5	33.3	11.9	33	11.4	48	10.5	58	9.5	79
4	10.0	10.0	35.0	12.5	35	12.0	50	11.0	61	10.0	83
5	10.5	10.5	36.8	13.1	36	12.6	53	11.6	64	10.5	88
6	11.0	11.0	38.5	13.8	38	13.2	55	12.1	67	11.0	92
		11.5	40.3	14.4	40	13.8	58	12.7	70	11.5	96
7	11.5	11.9	41.7	14.9	41	14.3	60	13.1	73	11.9	99
		12.0	42.0	15.0	42	14.4	60	13.2	73	12.0	100
		12.5	43.8	15.6	43	15.0	63	13.8	76	12.5	104
8	12.0	12.7	44.5	15.9	44	15.2	64	14.0	78	12.7	106
		13.0	45.5	16.3	45	15.6	65	14.3	79	13.0	108
		13.5	47.3	16.9	47	16.2	68	14.9	83	13.5	113
9	12.5	13.6	47.6	17.0	47	16.3	68	15.0	83	13.6	113
		14.0	49.0	17.5	49	16.8	70	15.4	86	14.0	117
10	13.0	14.5	50.8	18.1	50	17.4	73	16.0	89	14.5	121
		15.0	52.5	18.8	52	18.0	75	16.5	92	15.0	125
11	13.5	15.3	53.6	19.1	53	18.4	77	16.8	94	15.3	128
		15.5	54.3	19.4	54	18.6	78	17.1	95	15.5	129
		16.0	56.0	20.0	56	19.2	80	17.6	98	16.0	133
12	14.0	16.2	56.7	20.3	56	19.4	81	17.8	99	16.2	135
		16.5	57.8	20.6	57	19.8	83	18.2	101	16.5	138
13	14.5	17.0	59.5	21.3	59	20.4	85	18.7	104	17.0	142
		17.5	61.3	21.9	61	21.0	88	19.3	107	17.5	146
14	15.0	17.9	62.7	22.4	62	21.5	90	19.7	109	17.9	149
		18.0	63.0	22.5	63	21.6	90	19.8	110	18.0	150
		18.5	64.8	23.1	64	22.2	93	20.4	113	18.5	154
15	15.5	18.7	65.5	23.4	65	22.4	94	20.6	114	18.7	156
		19.0	66.5	23.8	66	22.8	95	20.9	116	19.0	158
		19.5	68.3	24.4	68	23.4	98	21.5	119	19.5	163
16	16.0	19.6	68.6	24.5	68	23.5	98	21.6	120	19.6	163
		20.0	70.0	25.0	69	24.0	100	22.0	122	20.0	167
17	16.5	20.5	71.8	25.6	71	24.6	103	22.6	125	20.5	171
		21.0	73.5	26.3	73	25.2	105	23.1	128	21.0	175
18	17.0	21.3	74.6	26.6	74	25.6	107	23.4	130	21.3	178
		21.5	75.3	26.9	75	25.8	108	23.7	131	21.5	179
		22.0	77.0	27.5	76	26.4	110	24.2	134	22.0	183
19	17.5	22.2	77.7	27.8	77	26.6	111	24.4	136	22.2	185
		22.5	78.8	28.1	78	27.0	113	24.8	138	22.5	188
20	18.0	23.0	80.5	28.8	80	27.6	115	25.3	141	23.0	192

MAP training compared to the result obtained with the 20 m shuttle test (Léger-Lambert, LL), the beep test (Léger-Boucher, LB), or the Mercier treadmill test

Stage LL	Speed LL (km/h)	MAS, METS, or LB speed (km/h)	VO_2MAX (1 MET = 3.5 ml O_2/kg/min)	Short intermittent (110%)		Short intermittent (105%)		Short intermittent (100%)	
				km/h	meters	km/h	meters	km/h	meters
1	8.5	8.5	29.8	9.4	156	8.9	149	8.5	142
2	9.0	9.0	31.5	9.9	165	9.5	158	9.0	150
3	9.5	9.5	33.3	10.5	174	10.0	166	9.5	158
4	10.0	10.0	35.0	11.0	183	10.5	175	10.0	167
5	10.5	10.5	36.8	11.6	193	11.0	184	10.5	175
6	11.0	11.0	38.5	12.1	202	11.6	193	11.0	183
		11.5	40.3	12.7	211	12.1	201	11.5	192
7	11.5	11.9	41.7	13.1	218	12.5	208	11.9	198
		12.0	42.0	13.2	220	12.6	210	12.0	200
		12.5	43.8	13.8	229	13.1	219	12.5	208
8	12.0	12.7	44.5	14.0	233	13.3	222	12.7	212
		13.0	45.5	14.3	238	13.7	228	13.0	217
		13.5	47.3	14.9	248	14.2	236	13.5	225
9	12.5	13.6	47.6	15.0	249	14.3	238	13.6	227
		14.0	49.0	15.4	257	14.7	245	14.0	233
10	13.0	14.5	50.8	16.0	266	15.2	254	14.5	242
		15.0	52.5	16.5	275	15.8	263	15.0	250
11	13.5	15.3	53.6	16.8	281	16.1	268	15.3	255
		15.5	54.3	17.1	284	16.3	271	15.5	258
		16.0	56.0	17.6	293	16.8	280	16.0	267
12	14.0	16.2	56.7	17.8	297	17.0	284	16.2	270
		16.5	57.8	18.2	303	17.3	289	16.5	275
13	14.5	17.0	59.5	18.7	312	17.9	298	17.0	283
		17.5	61.3	19.3	321	18.4	306	17.5	292
14	15.0	17.9	62.7	19.7	328	18.8	313	17.9	298
		18.0	63.0	19.8	330	18.9	315	18.0	300
		18.5	64.8	20.4	339	19.4	324	18.5	308
15	15.5	18.7	65.5	20.6	343	19.6	327	18.7	312
		19.0	66.5	20.9	348	20.0	333	19.0	317
		19.5	68.3	21.5	358	20.5	341	19.5	325
16	16.0	19.6	68.6	21.6	359	20.6	343	19.6	327
		20.0	70.0	22.0	367	21.0	350	20.0	333
17	16.5	20.5	71.8	22.6	376	21.5	359	20.5	342
		21.0	73.5	23.1	385	22.1	368	21.0	350
18	17.0	21.3	74.6	23.4	391	22.4	373	21.3	355
		21.5	75.3	23.7	394	22.6	376	21.5	358
		22.0	77.0	24.2	403	23.1	385	22.0	367
19	17.5	22.2	77.7	24.4	407	23.3	389	22.2	370
		22.5	78.8	24.8	413	23.6	394	22.5	375
20	18.0	23.0	80.5	25.3	422	24.2	403	23.0	383

(continued)

MAP training compared to the result obtained with the 20 m shuttle test (Léger-Lambert, LL), the beep test (Léger-Boucher, LB), or the Mercier treadmill test

Stage LL	Speed LL [km/h]	MAS, METS, or LB speed [km/h]	VO_2MAX (1 MET = 3.5 ml O_2/kg/min)	Medium intermittent (95%)		Medium intermittent (90%)		Medium intermittent (85%)	
				km/h	meters	km/h	meters	km/h	meters
1	8.5	8.5	29.8	8.1	135	7.7	128	7.2	120
2	9.0	9.0	31.5	8.6	143	8.1	135	7.7	128
3	9.5	9.5	33.3	9.0	150	8.6	143	8.1	135
4	10.0	10.0	35.0	9.5	158	9.0	150	8.5	142
5	10.5	10.5	36.8	10.0	166	9.5	158	8.9	149
6	11.0	11.0	38.5	10.5	174	9.9	165	9.4	156
		11.5	40.3	10.9	182	10.4	173	9.8	163
7	11.5	11.9	41.7	11.3	188	10.7	179	10.1	169
		12.0	42.0	11.4	190	10.8	180	10.2	170
		12.5	43.8	11.9	198	11.3	188	10.6	177
8	12.0	12.7	44.5	12.1	201	11.4	191	10.8	180
		13.0	45.5	12.4	206	11.7	195	11.1	184
		13.5	47.3	12.8	214	12.2	203	11.5	191
9	12.5	13.6	47.6	12.9	215	12.2	204	11.6	193
		14.0	49.0	13.3	222	12.6	210	11.9	198
10	13.0	14.5	50.8	13.8	230	13.1	218	12.3	205
		15.0	52.5	14.3	238	13.5	225	12.8	213
11	13.5	15.3	53.6	14.5	242	13.8	230	13.0	217
		15.5	54.3	14.7	245	14.0	233	13.2	220
		16.0	56.0	15.2	253	14.4	240	13.6	227
12	14.0	16.2	56.7	15.4	257	14.6	243	13.8	230
		16.5	57.8	15.7	261	14.9	248	14.0	234
13	14.5	17.0	59.5	16.2	269	15.3	255	14.5	241
		17.5	61.3	16.6	277	15.8	263	14.9	248
14	15.0	17.9	62.7	17.0	283	16.1	269	15.2	254
		18.0	63.0	17.1	285	16.2	270	15.3	255
		18.5	64.8	17.6	293	16.7	278	15.7	262
15	15.5	18.7	65.5	17.8	296	16.8	281	15.9	265
		19.0	66.5	18.1	301	17.1	285	16.2	269
		19.5	68.3	18.5	309	17.6	293	16.6	276
16	16.0	19.6	68.6	18.6	310	17.6	294	16.7	278
		20.0	70.0	19.0	317	18.0	300	17.0	283
17	16.5	20.5	71.8	19.5	325	18.5	308	17.4	290
		21.0	73.5	20.0	333	18.9	315	17.9	298
18	17.0	21.3	74.6	20.2	337	19.2	320	18.1	302
		21.5	75.3	20.4	340	19.4	323	18.3	305
		22.0	77.0	20.9	348	19.8	330	18.7	312
19	17.5	22.2	77.7	21.1	352	20.0	333	18.9	315
		22.5	78.8	21.4	356	20.3	338	19.1	319
20	18.0	23.0	80.5	21.9	364	20.7	345	19.6	326

APPENDIX #5: PREDICTED ABSOLUTE MAXIMUM BASED ON NUMBER OF REPETITIONS

100%	94.3%	90.6%	88.1%	85.6%	83.1%	80.7%	78.6%	76.5%	74.4%	72.3%	70.3%	68.8%	67.5%	66.2%	65.0%	63.8%	62.7%	61.6%	60.6%
30	28.3	27.2	26.4	25.7	24.9	24.2	23.6	23.0	22.3	21.7	21.1	20.6	20.3	19.9	19.5	19.1	18.8	18.5	18.2
40	37.7	36.2	35.2	34.2	33.2	32.3	31.4	30.6	29.8	28.9	28.1	27.5	27.0	26.5	26.0	25.5	25.1	24.6	24.2
50	47.2	45.3	44.1	42.8	41.6	40.4	39.3	38.3	37.2	36.2	35.2	34.4	33.8	33.1	32.5	31.9	31.4	30.8	30.3
60	56.6	54.4	52.9	51.4	49.9	48.4	47.2	45.9	44.6	43.4	42.2	41.3	40.5	39.7	39.0	38.3	37.6	37.0	36.4
70	66.0	63.4	61.7	59.9	58.2	56.5	55.0	53.6	52.1	50.6	49.2	48.2	47.3	46.3	45.5	44.7	43.9	43.1	42.4
80	75.4	72.5	70.5	68.5	66.5	64.6	62.9	61.2	59.5	57.8	56.2	55.0	54.0	53.0	52.0	51.0	50.2	49.3	48.5
90	84.9	81.5	79.3	77.0	74.8	72.6	70.7	68.9	67.0	65.1	63.3	61.9	60.8	59.6	58.5	57.4	56.4	55.4	54.5
100	94.3	90.6	88.1	85.6	83.1	80.7	78.6	76.5	74.4	72.3	70.3	68.8	67.5	66.2	65.0	63.8	62.7	61.6	60.6
110	103.7	99.7	96.9	94.2	91.4	88.8	86.5	84.2	81.8	79.5	77.3	75.7	74.3	72.8	71.5	70.2	69.0	67.8	66.7
120	113.2	108.7	105.7	102.7	99.7	96.8	94.3	91.8	89.3	86.8	84.4	82.6	81.0	79.4	78.0	76.6	75.2	73.9	72.7
130	122.6	117.8	114.5	111.3	108.0	104.9	102.2	99.5	96.7	94.0	91.4	89.4	87.8	86.1	84.5	82.9	81.5	80.1	78.8
140	132.0	126.8	123.3	119.8	116.3	113.0	110.0	107.1	104.2	101.2	98.4	96.3	94.5	92.7	91.0	89.3	87.8	86.2	84.8
150	141.5	135.9	132.2	128.4	124.7	121.1	117.9	114.8	111.6	108.5	105.5	103.2	101.3	99.3	97.5	95.7	94.1	92.4	90.9
160	150.9	145.0	141.0	137.0	133.0	129.1	125.8	122.4	119.0	115.7	112.5	110.1	108.0	105.9	104.0	102.1	100.3	98.6	97.0
170	160.3	154.0	149.8	145.5	141.3	137.2	133.6	130.1	126.5	122.9	119.5	117.0	114.8	112.5	110.5	108.5	106.6	104.7	103.0
180	169.7	163.1	158.6	154.1	149.6	145.3	141.5	137.7	133.9	130.1	126.5	123.8	121.5	119.2	117.0	114.8	112.9	110.9	109.1
190	179.2	172.1	167.4	162.6	157.9	153.3	149.3	145.4	141.4	137.4	133.6	130.7	128.3	125.8	123.5	121.2	119.1	117.0	115.1
200	188.6	181.2	176.2	171.2	166.2	161.4	157.2	153.0	148.8	144.6	140.6	137.6	135.0	132.4	130.0	127.6	125.4	123.2	121.2
210	198.0	190.3	185.0	179.8	174.5	169.5	165.1	160.7	156.2	151.8	147.6	144.5	141.8	139.0	136.5	134.0	131.7	129.4	127.3
220	207.5	199.3	193.8	188.3	182.8	177.5	172.9	168.3	163.7	159.1	154.7	151.4	148.5	145.6	143.0	140.4	137.9	135.5	133.3
230	216.9	208.4	202.6	196.9	191.1	185.6	180.8	176.0	171.1	166.3	161.7	158.2	155.3	152.3	149.5	146.7	144.2	141.7	139.4
1	2	3	4	5	6	7	8	9	10	11	12	13	14	15	16	17	18	19	20

(continued)

100%	94.3%	90.6%	88.1%	85.6%	83.1%	80.7%	78.6%	76.5%	74.4%	72.3%	70.3%	68.8%	67.5%	66.2%	65.0%	63.8%	62.7%	61.6%	60.6%
240	226.3	217.4	211.4	205.4	199.4	193.7	188.6	183.6	178.6	173.5	168.7	165.1	162.0	158.9	156.0	153.1	150.5	147.8	145.4
250	235.8	226.5	220.3	214.0	207.8	201.8	196.5	191.3	186.0	180.8	175.8	172.0	168.8	165.5	162.5	159.5	156.8	154.0	151.5
260	245.2	235.6	229.1	222.6	216.1	209.8	204.4	198.9	193.4	188.0	182.8	178.9	175.5	172.1	169.0	165.9	163.0	160.2	157.6
270	254.6	244.6	237.9	231.1	224.4	217.9	212.2	206.6	200.9	195.2	189.8	185.8	182.3	178.7	175.5	172.3	169.3	166.3	163.6
280	264.0	253.7	246.7	239.7	232.7	226.0	220.1	214.2	208.3	202.4	196.8	192.6	189.0	185.4	182.0	178.6	175.6	172.5	169.7
290	273.5	262.7	255.5	248.2	241.0	234.0	227.9	221.9	215.8	209.7	203.9	199.5	195.8	192.0	188.5	185.0	181.8	178.6	175.7
300	282.9	271.8	264.3	256.8	249.3	242.1	235.8	229.5	223.2	216.9	210.9	206.4	202.5	198.6	195.0	191.4	188.1	184.8	181.8
310	292.3	280.9	273.1	265.4	257.6	250.2	243.7	237.2	230.6	224.1	217.9	213.3	209.3	205.2	201.5	197.8	194.4	191.0	187.9
320	301.8	289.9	281.9	273.9	265.9	258.2	251.5	244.8	238.1	231.4	225.0	220.2	216.0	211.8	208.0	204.2	200.6	197.1	193.9
330	311.2	299.0	290.7	282.5	274.2	266.3	259.4	252.5	245.5	238.6	232.0	227.0	222.8	218.5	214.5	210.5	206.9	203.3	200.0
340	320.6	308.0	299.5	291.0	282.5	274.4	267.2	260.1	253.0	245.8	239.0	233.9	229.5	225.1	221.0	216.9	213.2	209.4	206.0
350	330.1	317.1	308.4	299.6	290.9	282.5	275.1	267.8	260.4	253.1	246.1	240.8	236.3	231.7	227.5	223.3	219.5	215.6	212.1
360	339.5	326.2	317.2	308.2	299.2	290.5	283.0	275.4	267.8	260.3	253.1	247.7	243.0	238.3	234.0	229.7	225.7	221.8	218.2
370	348.9	335.2	326.0	316.7	307.5	298.6	290.8	283.1	275.3	267.5	260.1	254.6	249.8	244.9	240.5	236.1	232.0	227.9	224.2
380	358.3	344.3	334.8	325.3	315.8	306.7	298.7	290.7	282.7	274.7	267.1	261.4	256.5	251.6	247.0	242.4	238.3	234.1	230.3
390	367.8	353.3	343.6	333.8	324.1	314.7	306.5	298.4	290.2	282.0	274.2	268.3	263.3	258.2	253.5	248.8	244.5	240.2	236.3
400	377.2	362.4	352.4	342.4	332.4	322.8	314.4	306.0	297.6	289.2	281.2	275.2	270.0	264.8	260.0	255.2	250.8	246.4	242.4
1	2	3	4	5	6	7	8	9	10	11	12	13	14	15	16	17	18	19	20

APPENDIX #6: WILKS COEFFICIENT

					Men (40-79 kg)					

Body weight (kg)	0	0.1	0.2	0.3	0.4	0.5	0.6	0.7	0.8	0.9
40	1.3354	1.3311	1.3268	1.3225	1.3182	1.3140	1.3098	1.3057	1.3016	1.2975
41	1.2934	1.2894	1.2854	1.2814	1.2775	1.2736	1.2697	1.2658	1.2620	1.2582
42	1.2545	1.2507	1.2470	1.2433	1.2397	1.2360	1.2324	1.2289	1.2253	1.2218
43	1.2183	1.2148	1.2113	1.2079	1.2045	1.2011	1.1978	1.1944	1.1911	1.1878
44	1.1846	1.1813	1.1781	1.1749	1.1717	1.1686	1.1654	1.1623	1.1592	1.1562
45	1.1531	1.1501	1.1471	1.1441	1.1411	1.1382	1.1352	1.1323	1.1294	1.1266
46	1.1237	1.1209	1.1181	1.1153	1.1125	1.1097	1.1070	1.1042	1.1015	1.0988
47	1.0962	1.0935	1.0909	1.0882	1.0856	1.0830	1.0805	1.0779	1.0754	1.0728
48	1.0703	1.0678	1.0653	1.0629	1.0604	1.0580	1.0556	1.0532	1.0508	1.0484
49	1.0460	1.0437	1.0413	1.0390	1.0367	1.0344	1.0321	1.0299	1.0276	1.0254
50	1.0232	1.0210	1.0188	1.0166	1.0144	1.0122	1.0101	1.0079	1.0058	1.0037
51	1.0016	0.9995	0.9975	0.9954	0.9933	0.9913	0.9893	0.9873	0.9853	0.9833
52	0.9813	0.9793	0.9773	0.9754	0.9735	0.9715	0.9696	0.9677	0.9658	0.9639
53	0.9621	0.9602	0.9583	0.9565	0.9547	0.9528	0.9510	0.9492	0.9474	0.9457
54	0.9439	0.9421	0.9404	0.9386	0.9369	0.9352	0.9334	0.9317	0.9300	0.9283
55	0.9267	0.9250	0.9233	0.9217	0.9200	0.9184	0.9168	0.9152	0.9135	0.9119
56	0.9103	0.9088	0.9072	0.9056	0.9041	0.9025	0.9010	0.8994	0.8979	0.8964
57	0.8949	0.8934	0.8919	0.8904	0.8889	0.8874	0.8859	0.8845	0.8830	0.8816
58	0.8802	0.8787	0.8773	0.8759	0.8745	0.8731	0.8717	0.8703	0.8689	0.8675
59	0.8662	0.8648	0.8635	0.8621	0.8608	0.8594	0.8581	0.8568	0.8555	0.8542
60	0.8529	0.8516	0.8503	0.8490	0.8477	0.8465	0.8452	0.8439	0.8427	0.8415
61	0.8402	0.8390	0.8378	0.8365	0.8353	0.8341	0.8329	0.8317	0.8305	0.8293
62	0.8281	0.8270	0.8258	0.8246	0.8235	0.8223	0.8212	0.8200	0.8189	0.8178
63	0.8166	0.8155	0.8144	0.8133	0.8122	0.8111	0.8100	0.8089	0.8078	0.8067
64	0.8057	0.8046	0.8035	0.8025	0.8014	0.8004	0.7993	0.7983	0.7973	0.7962
65	0.7952	0.7942	0.7932	0.7922	0.7911	0.7901	0.7891	0.7881	0.7872	0.7862
66	0.7852	0.7842	0.7832	0.7823	0.7813	0.7804	0.7794	0.7785	0.7775	0.7766
67	0.7756	0.7747	0.7738	0.7729	0.7719	0.7710	0.7701	0.7692	0.7683	0.7674
68	0.7665	0.7656	0.7647	0.7638	0.7630	0.7621	0.7612	0.7603	0.7595	0.7586
69	0.7578	0.7569	0.7561	0.7552	0.7544	0.7535	0.7527	0.7519	0.7510	0.7502
70	0.7494	0.7486	0.7478	0.7469	0.7461	0.7453	0.7445	0.7437	0.7430	0.7422
71	0.7414	0.7406	0.7398	0.7390	0.7383	0.7375	0.7367	0.7360	0.7352	0.7345
72	0.7337	0.7330	0.7322	0.7315	0.7307	0.7300	0.7293	0.7285	0.7278	0.7271
73	0.7264	0.7256	0.7249	0.7242	0.7235	0.7228	0.7221	0.7214	0.7207	0.7200
74	0.7193	0.7186	0.7179	0.7173	0.7166	0.7159	0.7152	0.7146	0.7139	0.7132
75	0.7126	0.7119	0.7112	0.7106	0.7099	0.7093	0.7086	0.7080	0.7074	0.7067
76	0.7061	0.7055	0.7048	0.7042	0.7036	0.7029	0.7023	0.7017	0.7011	0.7005
77	0.6999	0.6993	0.6987	0.6981	0.6975	0.6969	0.6963	0.6957	0.6951	0.6945
78	0.6939	0.6933	0.6927	0.6922	0.6916	0.6910	0.6905	0.6899	0.6893	0.6888
79	0.6882	0.6876	0.6871	0.6865	0.6860	0.6854	0.6849	0.6843	0.6838	0.6832

(continued)

Men (80-119 kg)

Body weight (kg)	0	0.1	0.2	0.3	0.4	0.5	0.6	0.7	0.8	0.9
80	0.6827	0.6822	0.6816	0.6811	0.6806	0.6800	0.6795	0.6790	0.6785	0.6779
81	0.6774	0.6769	0.6764	0.6759	0.6754	0.6749	0.6744	0.6739	0.6734	0.6729
82	0.6724	0.6719	0.6714	0.6709	0.6704	0.6699	0.6694	0.6689	0.6685	0.6680
83	0.6675	0.6670	0.6665	0.6661	0.6656	0.6651	0.6647	0.6642	0.6637	0.6633
84	0.6628	0.6624	0.6619	0.6615	0.6610	0.6606	0.6601	0.6597	0.6592	0.6588
85	0.6583	0.6579	0.6575	0.6570	0.6566	0.6562	0.6557	0.6553	0.6549	0.6545
86	0.6540	0.6536	0.6532	0.6528	0.6523	0.6519	0.6515	0.6511	0.6507	0.6503
87	0.6499	0.6495	0.6491	0.6487	0.6483	0.6479	0.6475	0.6471	0.6467	0.6463
88	0.6459	0.6455	0.6451	0.6447	0.6444	0.6440	0.6436	0.6432	0.6428	0.6424
89	0.6421	0.6417	0.6413	0.6410	0.6406	0.6402	0.6398	0.6395	0.6391	0.6388
90	0.6384	0.6380	0.6377	0.6373	0.6370	0.6366	0.6363	0.6359	0.6356	0.6352
91	0.6349	0.6345	0.6342	0.6338	0.6335	0.6331	0.6328	0.6325	0.6321	0.6318
92	0.6315	0.6311	0.6308	0.6305	0.6301	0.6298	0.6295	0.6292	0.6288	0.6285
93	0.6282	0.6279	0.6276	0.6272	0.6269	0.6266	0.6263	0.6260	0.6257	0.6254
94	0.6250	0.6247	0.6244	0.6241	0.6238	0.6235	0.6232	0.6229	0.6226	0.6223
95	0.6220	0.6217	0.6214	0.6211	0.6209	0.6206	0.6203	0.6200	0.6197	0.6194
96	0.6191	0.6188	0.6186	0.6183	0.6180	0.6177	0.6174	0.6172	0.6169	0.6166
97	0.6163	0.6161	0.6158	0.6155	0.6152	0.6150	0.6147	0.6144	0.6142	0.6139
98	0.6136	0.6134	0.6131	0.6129	0.6126	0.6123	0.6121	0.6118	0.6116	0.6113
99	0.6111	0.6108	0.6106	0.6103	0.6101	0.6098	0.6096	0.6093	0.6091	0.6088
100	0.6086	0.6083	0.6081	0.6079	0.6076	0.6074	0.6071	0.6069	0.6067	0.6064
101	0.6062	0.6060	0.6057	0.6055	0.6053	0.6050	0.6048	0.6046	0.6044	0.6041
102	0.6039	0.6037	0.6035	0.6032	0.6030	0.6028	0.6026	0.6024	0.6021	0.6019
103	0.6017	0.6015	0.6013	0.6011	0.6009	0.6006	0.6004	0.6002	0.6000	0.5998
104	0.5996	0.5994	0.5992	0.5990	0.5988	0.5986	0.5984	0.5982	0.5980	0.5978
105	0.5976	0.5974	0.5972	0.5970	0.5968	0.5966	0.5964	0.5962	0.5960	0.5958
106	0.5956	0.5954	0.5952	0.5950	0.5948	0.5946	0.5945	0.5943	0.5941	0.5939
107	0.5937	0.5935	0.5933	0.5932	0.5930	0.5928	0.5926	0.5924	0.5923	0.5921
108	0.5919	0.5917	0.5916	0.5914	0.5912	0.5910	0.5909	0.5907	0.5905	0.5903
109	0.5902	0.5900	0.5898	0.5897	0.5895	0.5893	0.5892	0.5890	0.5888	0.5887
110	0.5885	0.5883	0.5882	0.5880	0.5878	0.5877	0.5875	0.5874	0.5872	0.5870
111	0.5869	0.5867	0.5866	0.5864	0.5863	0.5861	0.5860	0.5858	0.5856	0.5855
112	0.5853	0.5852	0.5850	0.5849	0.5847	0.5846	0.5844	0.5843	0.5841	0.5840
113	0.5839	0.5837	0.5836	0.5834	0.5833	0.5831	0.5830	0.5828	0.5827	0.5826
114	0.5824	0.5823	0.5821	0.5820	0.5819	0.5817	0.5816	0.5815	0.5813	0.5812
115	0.5811	0.5809	0.5808	0.5806	0.5805	0.5804	0.5803	0.5801	0.5800	0.5799
116	0.5797	0.5796	0.5795	0.5793	0.5792	0.5791	0.5790	0.5788	0.5787	0.5786
117	0.5785	0.5783	0.5782	0.5781	0.5780	0.5778	0.5777	0.5776	0.5775	0.5774
118	0.5772	0.5771	0.5770	0.5769	0.5768	0.5766	0.5765	0.5764	0.5763	0.5762
119	0.5761	0.5759	0.5758	0.5757	0.5756	0.5755	0.5754	0.5753	0.5751	0.5750

Body weight (kg)	0	0.1	0.2	0.3	0.4	0.5	0.6	0.7	0.8	0.9
120	0.5749	0.5748	0.5747	0.5746	0.5745	0.5744	0.5743	0.5742	0.5740	0.5739
121	0.5738	0.5737	0.5736	0.5735	0.5734	0.5733	0.5732	0.5731	0.5730	0.5729
122	0.5728	0.5727	0.5726	0.5725	0.5724	0.5723	0.5722	0.5721	0.5720	0.5719
123	0.5718	0.5717	0.5716	0.5715	0.5714	0.5713	0.5712	0.5711	0.5710	0.5709
124	0.5708	0.5707	0.5706	0.5705	0.5704	0.5703	0.5702	0.5701	0.5700	0.5699
125	0.5698	0.5698	0.5697	0.5696	0.5695	0.5694	0.5693	0.5692	0.5691	0.5690
126	0.5689	0.5688	0.5688	0.5687	0.5686	0.5685	0.5684	0.5683	0.5682	0.5681
127	0.5681	0.5680	0.5679	0.5678	0.5677	0.5676	0.5675	0.5675	0.5674	0.5673
128	0.5672	0.5671	0.5670	0.5670	0.5669	0.5668	0.5667	0.5666	0.5665	0.5665
129	0.5664	0.5663	0.5662	0.5661	0.5661	0.5660	0.5659	0.5658	0.5658	0.5657
130	0.5656	0.5655	0.5654	0.5654	0.5653	0.5652	0.5651	0.5651	0.5650	0.5649
131	0.5648	0.5647	0.5647	0.5646	0.5645	0.5644	0.5644	0.5643	0.5642	0.5642
132	0.5641	0.5640	0.5639	0.5639	0.5638	0.5637	0.5636	0.5636	0.5635	0.5634
133	0.5634	0.5633	0.5632	0.5631	0.5631	0.5630	0.5629	0.5629	0.5628	0.5627
134	0.5627	0.5626	0.5625	0.5624	0.5624	0.5623	0.5622	0.5622	0.5621	0.5620
135	0.5620	0.5619	0.5618	0.5618	0.5617	0.5616	0.5616	0.5615	0.5614	0.5614
136	0.5613	0.5612	0.5612	0.5611	0.5610	0.5610	0.5609	0.5609	0.5608	0.5607
137	0.5607	0.5606	0.5605	0.5605	0.5604	0.5603	0.5603	0.5602	0.5602	0.5601
138	0.5600	0.5600	0.5599	0.5598	0.5598	0.5597	0.5597	0.5596	0.5595	0.5595
139	0.5594	0.5593	0.5593	0.5592	0.5592	0.5591	0.5590	0.5590	0.5589	0.5589
140	0.5588	0.5587	0.5587	0.5586	0.5586	0.5585	0.5584	0.5584	0.5583	0.5583
141	0.5582	0.5582	0.5581	0.5580	0.5580	0.5579	0.5579	0.5578	0.5578	0.5577
142	0.5576	0.5576	0.5575	0.5575	0.5574	0.5573	0.5573	0.5572	0.5572	0.5571
143	0.5571	0.5570	0.5570	0.5569	0.5568	0.5568	0.5567	0.5567	0.5566	0.5566
144	0.5565	0.5564	0.5564	0.5563	0.5563	0.5562	0.5562	0.5561	0.5561	0.5560
145	0.5560	0.5559	0.5558	0.5558	0.5557	0.5557	0.5556	0.5556	0.5555	0.5555
146	0.5554	0.5554	0.5553	0.5552	0.5552	0.5551	0.5551	0.5550	0.5550	0.5549
147	0.5549	0.5548	0.5548	0.5547	0.5547	0.5546	0.5546	0.5545	0.5544	0.5544
148	0.5543	0.5543	0.5542	0.5542	0.5541	0.5541	0.5540	0.5540	0.5539	0.5539
149	0.5538	0.5538	0.5537	0.5537	0.5536	0.5536	0.5535	0.5535	0.5534	0.5533
150	0.5533	0.5532	0.5532	0.5531	0.5531	0.5530	0.5530	0.5529	0.5529	0.5528
151	0.5528	0.5527	0.5527	0.5526	0.5526	0.5525	0.5525	0.5524	0.5524	0.5523
152	0.5523	0.5522	0.5522	0.5521	0.5521	0.5520	0.5520	0.5519	0.5519	0.5518
153	0.5518	0.5517	0.5516	0.5516	0.5515	0.5515	0.5514	0.5514	0.5513	0.5513
154	0.5512	0.5512	0.5511	0.5511	0.5510	0.5510	0.5509	0.5509	0.5508	0.5508
155	0.5507	0.5507	0.5506	0.5506	0.5505	0.5505	0.5504	0.5504	0.5503	0.5503
156	0.5502	0.5502	0.5501	0.5501	0.5500	0.5500	0.5499	0.5499	0.5498	0.5498
157	0.5497	0.5497	0.5496	0.5496	0.5495	0.5495	0.5494	0.5494	0.5493	0.5493
158	0.5492	0.5492	0.5491	0.5491	0.5490	0.5490	0.5489	0.5489	0.5488	0.5488
159	0.5487	0.5487	0.5486	0.5486	0.5485	0.5485	0.5484	0.5484	0.5483	0.5483

(continued)

Men (160-199 kg)

Body weight (kg)	0	0.1	0.2	0.3	0.4	0.5	0.6	0.7	0.8	0.9
160	0.5482	0.5482	0.5481	0.5481	0.5480	0.5480	0.5479	0.5479	0.5478	0.5478
161	0.5477	0.5477	0.5476	0.5476	0.5475	0.5475	0.5474	0.5474	0.5473	0.5472
162	0.5472	0.5471	0.5471	0.5470	0.5470	0.5469	0.5469	0.5468	0.5468	0.5467
163	0.5467	0.5466	0.5466	0.5465	0.5465	0.5464	0.5464	0.5463	0.5463	0.5462
164	0.5462	0.5461	0.5461	0.5460	0.5460	0.5459	0.5459	0.5458	0.5458	0.5457
165	0.5457	0.5456	0.5456	0.5455	0.5455	0.5454	0.5454	0.5453	0.5453	0.5452
166	0.5452	0.5451	0.5451	0.5450	0.5450	0.5449	0.5449	0.5448	0.5448	0.5447
167	0.5447	0.5446	0.5446	0.5445	0.5445	0.5444	0.5444	0.5443	0.5443	0.5442
168	0.5442	0.5441	0.5441	0.5440	0.5440	0.5439	0.5439	0.5438	0.5438	0.5437
169	0.5436	0.5436	0.5435	0.5435	0.5434	0.5434	0.5433	0.5433	0.5432	0.5432
170	0.5431	0.5431	0.5430	0.5430	0.5429	0.5429	0.5428	0.5428	0.5427	0.5427
171	0.5426	0.5426	0.5425	0.5425	0.5424	0.5424	0.5423	0.5423	0.5422	0.5422
172	0.5421	0.5421	0.5420	0.5420	0.5419	0.5419	0.5418	0.5418	0.5417	0.5417
173	0.5416	0.5416	0.5415	0.5415	0.5414	0.5414	0.5413	0.5413	0.5412	0.5412
174	0.5411	0.5411	0.5410	0.5410	0.5409	0.5409	0.5408	0.5408	0.5407	0.5407
175	0.5406	0.5406	0.5405	0.5405	0.5404	0.5404	0.5403	0.5403	0.5402	0.5402
176	0.5401	0.5401	0.5400	0.5400	0.5399	0.5399	0.5398	0.5398	0.5397	0.5397
177	0.5396	0.5396	0.5395	0.5395	0.5394	0.5394	0.5393	0.5393	0.5392	0.5392
178	0.5391	0.5391	0.5390	0.5390	0.5389	0.5389	0.5388	0.5388	0.5387	0.5387
179	0.5387	0.5386	0.5386	0.5385	0.5385	0.5384	0.5384	0.5383	0.5383	0.5382
180	0.5382	0.5381	0.5381	0.5380	0.5380	0.5379	0.5379	0.5378	0.5378	0.5377
181	0.5377	0.5377	0.5376	0.5376	0.5375	0.5375	0.5374	0.5374	0.5373	0.5373
182	0.5372	0.5372	0.5371	0.5371	0.5371	0.5370	0.5370	0.5369	0.5369	0.5368
183	0.5368	0.5367	0.5367	0.5366	0.5366	0.5366	0.5365	0.5365	0.5364	0.5364
184	0.5363	0.5363	0.5362	0.5362	0.5362	0.5361	0.5361	0.5360	0.5360	0.5359
185	0.5359	0.5359	0.5358	0.5358	0.5357	0.5357	0.5356	0.5356	0.5356	0.5355
186	0.5355	0.5354	0.5354	0.5353	0.5353	0.5353	0.5352	0.5352	0.5351	0.5351
187	0.5351	0.5350	0.5350	0.5349	0.5349	0.5349	0.5348	0.5348	0.5347	0.5347
188	0.5347	0.5346	0.5346	0.5345	0.5345	0.5345	0.5344	0.5344	0.5344	0.5343
189	0.5343	0.5342	0.5342	0.5342	0.5341	0.5341	0.5341	0.5340	0.5340	0.5340
190	0.5339	0.5339	0.5338	0.5338	0.5338	0.5337	0.5337	0.5337	0.5336	0.5336
191	0.5336	0.5335	0.5335	0.5335	0.5334	0.5334	0.5334	0.5333	0.5333	0.5333
192	0.5332	0.5332	0.5332	0.5332	0.5331	0.5331	0.5331	0.5330	0.5330	0.5330
193	0.5329	0.5329	0.5329	0.5329	0.5328	0.5328	0.5328	0.5327	0.5327	0.5327
194	0.5327	0.5326	0.5326	0.5326	0.5326	0.5325	0.5325	0.5325	0.5325	0.5324
195	0.5324	0.5324	0.5324	0.5323	0.5323	0.5323	0.5323	0.5322	0.5322	0.5322
196	0.5322	0.5322	0.5321	0.5321	0.5321	0.5321	0.5321	0.5320	0.5320	0.5320
197	0.5320	0.5320	0.5319	0.5319	0.5319	0.5319	0.5319	0.5319	0.5318	0.5318
198	0.5318	0.5318	0.5318	0.5318	0.5318	0.5317	0.5317	0.5317	0.5317	0.5317
199	0.5317	0.5317	0.5317	0.5317	0.5316	0.5316	0.5316	0.5316	0.5316	0.5316

Women (40-79 kg)

Body weight (kg)	0	0.1	0.2	0.3	0.4	0.5	0.6	0.7	0.8	0.9
40	1.4936	1.4915	1.4894	1.4872	1.4851	1.4830	1.4809	1.4788	1.4766	1.4745
41	1.4724	1.4702	1.4681	1.4660	1.4638	1.4617	1.4595	1.4574	1.4552	1.4531
42	1.4510	1.4488	1.4467	1.4445	1.4424	1.4402	1.4381	1.4359	1.4338	1.4316
43	1.4295	1.4273	1.4252	1.4231	1.4209	1.4188	1.4166	1.4145	1.4123	1.4102
44	1.4081	1.4059	1.4038	1.4017	1.3995	1.3974	1.3953	1.3932	1.3910	1.3889
45	1.3868	1.3847	1.3825	1.3804	1.3783	1.3762	1.3741	1.3720	1.3699	1.3678
46	1.3657	1.3636	1.3615	1.3594	1.3573	1.3553	1.3532	1.3511	1.3490	1.3470
47	1.3449	1.3428	1.3408	1.3387	1.3367	1.3346	1.3326	1.3305	1.3285	1.3265
48	1.3244	1.3224	1.3204	1.3183	1.3163	1.3143	1.3123	1.3103	1.3083	1.3063
49	1.3043	1.3023	1.3004	1.2984	1.2964	1.2944	1.2925	1.2905	1.2885	1.2866
50	1.2846	1.2827	1.2808	1.2788	1.2769	1.2750	1.2730	1.2711	1.2692	1.2673
51	1.2654	1.2635	1.2616	1.2597	1.2578	1.2560	1.2541	1.2522	1.2504	1.2485
52	1.2466	1.2448	1.2429	1.2411	1.2393	1.2374	1.2356	1.2338	1.2320	1.2302
53	1.2284	1.2266	1.2248	1.2230	1.2212	1.2194	1.2176	1.2159	1.2141	1.2123
54	1.2106	1.2088	1.2071	1.2054	1.2036	1.2019	1.2002	1.1985	1.1967	1.1950
55	1.1933	1.1916	1.1900	1.1883	1.1066	1.1049	1.1832	1.1818	1.1799	1.1783
56	1.1766	1.1750	1.1733	1.1717	1.1701	1.1684	1.1668	1.1652	1.1636	1.1620
57	1.1604	1.1588	1.1572	1.1556	1.1541	1.1525	1.1509	1.1494	1.1478	1.1463
58	1.1447	1.1432	1.1416	1.1401	1.1386	1.1371	1.1355	1.1340	1.1325	1.1310
59	1.1295	1.1281	1.1266	1.1251	1.1236	1.1221	1.1207	1.1192	1.1178	1.1163
60	1.1149	1.1134	1.1120	1.1106	1.1092	1.1078	1.1063	1.1049	1.1035	1.1021
61	1.1007	1.0994	1.0980	1.0966	1.0952	1.0939	1.0925	1.0911	1.0898	1.0884
62	1.0871	1.0858	1.0844	1.0831	1.0818	1.0805	1.0792	1.0779	1.0765	1.0753
63	1.0740	1.0727	1.0714	1.0701	1.0688	1.0676	1.0663	1.0650	1.0638	1.0625
64	1.0613	1.0601	1.0588	1.0576	1.0564	1.0551	1.0539	1.0527	1.0515	1.0503
65	1.0491	1.0479	1.0467	1.0455	1.0444	1.0432	1.0420	1.0408	1.0397	1.0385
66	1.0374	1.0362	1.0351	1.0339	1.0328	1.0317	1.0306	1.0294	1.0283	1.0272
67	1.0261	1.0250	1.0239	1.0228	1.0217	1.0206	1.0195	1.0185	1.0174	1.0163
68	1.0153	1.0142	1.0131	1.0121	1.0110	1.0100	1.0090	1.0079	1.0069	1.0059
69	1.0048	1.0038	1.0028	1.0018	1.0008	0.9998	0.9988	0.9978	0.9968	0.9958
70	0.9948	0.9939	0.9929	0.9919	0.9910	0.9900	0.9890	0.9881	0.9871	0.9862
71	0.9852	0.9843	0.9834	0.9824	0.9815	0.9806	0.9797	0.9788	0.9779	0.9769
72	0.9760	0.9751	0.9742	0.9734	0.9725	0.9716	0.9707	0.9698	0.9689	0.9681
73	0.9672	0.9663	0.9655	0.9646	0.9638	0.9629	0.9621	0.9613	0.9604	0.9596
74	0.9587	0.9579	0.9571	0.9563	0.9555	0.9547	0.9538	0.9530	0.9522	0.9514
75	0.9506	0.9498	0.9491	0.9483	0.9475	0.9467	0.9459	0.9452	0.9444	0.9436
76	0.9429	0.9421	0.9414	0.9406	0.9399	0.9391	0.9384	0.9376	0.9369	0.9362
77	0.9354	0.9347	0.9340	0.9333	0.9326	0.9318	0.9311	0.9304	0.9297	0.9290
78	0.9283	0.9276	0.9269	0.9263	0.9256	0.9249	0.9242	0.9235	0.9229	0.9222
79	0.9215	0.9209	0.9202	0.9195	0.9189	0.9182	0.9176	0.9169	0.9163	0.9156

(continued)

Women (80-119 kg)

Body weight (kg)	0	0.1	0.2	0.3	0.4	0.5	0.6	0.7	0.8	0.9
80	0.9150	0.9144	0.9137	0.9131	0.9125	0.9119	0.9112	0.9106	0.9100	0.9094
81	0.9088	0.9082	0.9076	0.9070	0.9064	0.9058	0.9052	0.9046	0.9040	0.9034
82	0.9028	0.9023	0.9017	0.9011	0.9005	0.9000	0.8994	0.8988	0.8983	0.8977
83	0.8972	0.8966	0.8961	0.8955	0.8950	0.8944	0.8939	0.8933	0.8928	0.8923
84	0.8917	0.8912	0.8907	0.8902	0.8896	0.8891	0.8886	0.8881	0.8876	0.8871
85	0.8866	0.8861	0.8856	0.8851	0.8846	0.8841	0.8836	0.8831	0.8826	0.8821
86	0.8816	0.8811	0.8807	0.8802	0.8797	0.8792	0.8788	0.8783	0.8778	0.8774
87	0.8769	0.8765	0.8760	0.8755	0.8751	0.8746	0.8742	0.8737	0.8733	0.8729
88	0.8724	0.8720	0.8716	0.8711	0.8707	0.8703	0.8698	0.8694	0.8690	0.8686
89	0.8681	0.8677	0.8673	0.8669	0.8665	0.8661	0.8657	0.8653	0.8649	0.8645
90	0.8641	0.8637	0.8633	0.8629	0.8625	0.8621	0.8617	0.8613	0.8609	0.8606
91	0.8602	0.8598	0.8594	0.8590	0.8587	0.8583	0.8579	0.8576	0.8572	0.8568
92	0.8565	0.8561	0.8558	0.8554	0.8550	0.8547	0.8543	0.8540	0.8536	0.8533
93	0.8530	0.8526	0.8523	0.8519	0.8516	0.8513	0.8509	0.8506	0.8503	0.8499
94	0.8496	0.8493	0.8489	0.8486	0.8483	0.8480	0.8477	0.8473	0.8470	0.8467
95	0.8464	0.8461	0.8458	0.8455	0.8452	0.8449	0.8446	0.8443	0.8440	0.8437
96	0.8434	0.8431	0.8428	0.8425	0.8422	0.8419	0.8416	0.8413	0.8410	0.8407
97	0.8405	0.8402	0.8399	0.8396	0.8393	0.8391	0.8388	0.8385	0.8382	0.8380
98	0.8377	0.8374	0.8372	0.8369	0.8366	0.8364	0.8361	0.8359	0.8356	0.8353
99	0.8351	0.8348	0.8346	0.8343	0.8341	0.8338	0.8336	0.8333	0.8331	0.8328
100	0.8326	0.8323	0.8321	0.8319	0.8316	0.8314	0.8311	0.8309	0.8307	0.8304
101	0.8302	0.8300	0.8297	0.8295	0.8293	0.8291	0.8288	0.8286	0.8284	0.8282
102	0.8279	0.8277	0.8275	0.8273	0.8271	0.8268	0.8266	0.8264	0.8262	0.8260
103	0.8258	0.8256	0.8253	0.8251	0.8249	0.8247	0.8245	0.8243	0.8241	0.8239
104	0.8237	0.8235	0.8233	0.8231	0.8229	0.8227	0.8225	0.8223	0.8221	0.8219
105	0.8217	0.8215	0.8214	0.8212	0.8210	0.8208	0.8206	0.8204	0.8202	0.8200
106	0.8198	0.8197	0.8195	0.8193	0.8191	0.8189	0.8188	0.8186	0.8184	0.8182
107	0.8180	0.8179	0.8177	0.8175	0.8173	0.8172	0.8170	0.8168	0.8167	0.8165
108	0.8163	0.8161	0.8160	0.8158	0.8156	0.8155	0.8153	0.8152	0.8150	0.8148
109	0.8147	0.8145	0.8143	0.8142	0.8140	0.8139	0.8137	0.8135	0.8134	0.8132
110	0.8131	0.8129	0.8128	0.8126	0.8124	0.8123	0.8121	0.8120	0.8118	0.8117
111	0.8115	0.8114	0.8112	0.8111	0.8109	0.8108	0.8106	0.8105	0.8103	0.8102
112	0.8101	0.8099	0.8098	0.8096	0.8095	0.8093	0.8092	0.8090	0.8089	0.8088
113	0.8086	0.8085	0.8083	0.8082	0.8081	0.8079	0.8078	0.8077	0.8075	0.8074
114	0.8072	0.8071	0.8070	0.8068	0.8067	0.8066	0.8064	0.8063	0.8062	0.8060
115	0.8059	0.8058	0.8056	0.8055	0.8054	0.8052	0.8051	0.8050	0.8049	0.8047
116	0.8046	0.8045	0.8043	0.8042	0.8041	0.8040	0.8038	0.8037	0.8036	0.8034
117	0.8033	0.8032	0.8031	0.8029	0.8028	0.8027	0.8026	0.8024	0.8023	0.8022
118	0.8021	0.8020	0.8018	0.8017	0.8016	0.8015	0.8013	0.8012	0.8011	0.8010
119	0.8009	0.8007	0.8006	0.8005	0.8004	0.8003	0.8001	0.8000	0.7999	0.7998

Women (120-150 kg)

Body weight (kg)	0	0.1	0.2	0.3	0.4	0.5	0.6	0.7	0.8	0.9
120	0.7997	0.7995	0.7994	0.7993	0.7992	0.7991	0.7989	0.7988	0.7987	0.7986
121	0.7985	0.7984	0.7982	0.7981	0.7980	0.7979	0.7978	0.7977	0.7975	0.7974
122	0.7973	0.7972	0.7971	0.7970	0.7969	0.7967	0.7966	0.7965	0.7964	0.7963
123	0.7962	0.7960	0.7959	0.7958	0.7957	0.7956	0.7955	0.7954	0.7953	0.7951
124	0.7950	0.7949	0.7948	0.7947	0.7946	0.7945	0.7943	0.7942	0.7941	0.7940
125	0.7939	0.7938	0.7937	0.7936	0.7934	0.7933	0.7932	0.7931	0.7930	0.7929
126	0.7928	0.7927	0.7926	0.7924	0.7923	0.7922	0.7921	0.7920	0.7919	0.7918
127	0.7917	0.7915	0.7914	0.7913	0.7912	0.7911	0.7910	0.7909	0.7908	0.7907
128	0.7905	0.7904	0.7903	0.7902	0.7901	0.7900	0.7899	0.7898	0.7897	0.7895
129	0.7894	0.7893	0.7892	0.7891	0.7890	0.7889	0.7888	0.7887	0.7886	0.7884
130	0.7883	0.7882	0.7881	0.7880	0.7879	0.7878	0.7877	0.7876	0.7875	0.7873
131	0.7872	0.7871	0.7870	0.7869	0.7868	0.7867	0.7866	0.7865	0.7864	0.7862
132	0.7861	0.7860	0.7859	0.7858	0.7857	0.7856	0.7855	0.7854	0.7853	0.7852
133	0.7850	0.7849	0.7848	0.7847	0.7846	0.7845	0.7844	0.7843	0.7842	0.7841
134	0.7840	0.7838	0.7837	0.7836	0.7835	0.7834	0.7833	0.7832	0.7831	0.7830
135	0.7829	0.7828	0.7827	0.7825	0.7824	0.7823	0.7822	0.7821	0.7820	0.7819
136	0.7818	0.7817	0.7816	0.7815	0.7814	0.7813	0.7812	0.7811	0.7809	0.7808
137	0.7807	0.7806	0.7805	0.7804	0.7803	0.7802	0.7801	0.7800	0.7799	0.7798
138	0.7797	0.7796	0.7795	0.7794	0.7793	0.7792	0.7791	0.7790	0.7789	0.7787
139	0.7786	0.7785	0.7784	0.7783	0.7782	0.7781	0.7780	0.7779	0.7778	0.7777
140	0.7776	0.7775	0.7774	0.7773	0.7772	0.7771	0.7770	0.7769	0.7768	0.7767
141	0.7766	0.7765	0.7764	0.7763	0.7762	0.7761	0.7760	0.7759	0.7759	0.7758
142	0.7757	0.7756	0.7755	0.7754	0.7753	0.7752	0.7751	0.7750	0.7749	0.7748
143	0.7747	0.7746	0.7745	0.7744	0.7744	0.7743	0.7742	0.7741	0.7740	0.7739
144	0.7738	0.7737	0.7736	0.7736	0.7735	0.7734	0.7733	0.7732	0.7731	0.7730
145	0.7730	0.7729	0.7728	0.7727	0.7726	0.7725	0.7725	0.7724	0.7723	0.7722
146	0.7721	0.7721	0.7720	0.7719	0.7718	0.7717	0.7717	0.7716	0.7715	0.7714
147	0.7714	0.7713	0.7712	0.7712	0.7711	0.7710	0.7709	0.7709	0.7708	0.7707
148	0.7707	0.7706	0.7705	0.7705	0.7704	0.7703	0.7703	0.7702	0.7702	0.7701
149	0.7700	0.7700	0.7699	0.7699	0.7698	0.7698	0.7697	0.7696	0.7696	0.7695
150	0.7695	0.7694	0.7694	0.7693	0.7693	0.7692	0.7692	0.7691	0.7691	0.7691

APPENDIX #7: PRILEPIN CHART

It is surprising to note that many coaches are unaware of the existence of the Prilepin chart, an essential tool in the planning of strength training. It was developed by **Alexander Prilepin**, a Soviet weightlifting coach, between 1975 and 1985, after analyzing the training books of over a thousand national and international weightlifting champions. The athletes he followed won a total of 85 medals (including 5 Olympic gold medals) and set 27 world records. Prilepin created the following table from his data, showing the intensity with which an athlete should train and the number of reps and sets to complete per workout without placing too much stress on the nervous system.

Percentage (1RM)	Number of repetitions per set	Total number of repetitions	Total number of repetitions (optimal)
55-65	3-6	18-30	24
70-80	3-6	12-24	18
80-90	2-4	10-20	15
90+	1-2	4-10	4

Here is how to read the Prilepin chart:
1. The **percentage (1RM) column** represents the percentage to use according to your maximum (1RM).
2. The **number of repetitions per set column** represents the number of reps you should do per set.
3. The **total number of repetitions column** represents the minimum and maximum number of reps you should do per workout. It also determines the number of sets to be completed. For example, at 85% for sets of 4 reps, you could do between 3 and 5 sets (12 and 20 reps total).
4. The **total number of repetitions (optimal)** column represents the optimal number of reps to perform for a workout. For example, at 85%, 5 sets of 3 repetitions would be optimal (15 reps in total).

APPENDIX #8: DROPSET CLUSTER CHART

Dropset cluster (100-150 kg)

100%	100		103		105		108	
95%	95.0	20 + 10 + 5 + 2.5	97.5	20 + 10 + 1.25 + 5 + 2.5	100.0	20 + 10 + 5 + 5	102.5	20 + 10 + 5 + 2.5 + 1.25 + 2.5
90%	90.0	20 + 10 + 5	92.4	20 + 10 + 1.25 + 5	94.7	20 + 10 + 5 + 2.5	97.1	20 + 10 + 5 + 2.5 + 1.25
85%	85.0	20 + 10 + 2.5	87.2	20 + 10 + 1.25 + 2.5	89.5	20 + 10 + 5	91.7	20 + 10 + 5
80%	80.0	20 + 10	82.1	20 + 10 + 1.25	84.2	20 + 10 + 2.5	86.3	20 + 10 + 2.5

100%	111		113		116		118	
95%	105.0	20 + 15 + 5 + 2.5	107.5	20 + 15 + 5 + 1.25 + 2.5	110.0	20 + 15 + 5 + 5	112.5	20 + 15 + 5 + 5 + 1.25
90%	99.5	20 + 15 + 5	101.8	20 + 15 + 5 + 1.25	104.2	20 + 15 + 5 + 2.5	106.6	20 + 15 + 5 + 2.5
85%	93.9	20 + 15 + 2.5	96.2	20 + 15 + 2.5	98.4	20 + 15 + 5	100.7	20 + 15 + 5
80%	88.4	20 + 15	90.5	20 + 15	92.6	20 + 15 + 1.25	94.7	20 + 15 + 2.5

100%	121		124		126		129	
95%	115.0	20 + 15 + 2.5 + 5 + 5	117.5	20 + 20 + 5 + 2.5 + 1.25	120.0	20 + 20 + 2.5 + 5 + 2.5	122.5	20 + 20 + 1.25 + 2.5 + 5 + 2.5
90%	108.9	20 + 15 + 2.5 + 5 + 1.25	111.3	20 + 20 + 5	113.7	20 + 20 + 2.5 + 5	116.1	20 + 20 + 1.25 + 2.5 + 5
85%	102.9	20 + 15 + 2.5 + 2.5	105.1	20 + 20 + 2.5	107.4	20 + 20 + 2.5 + 1.25	109.6	20 + 20 + 1.25 + 2.5 + 1.25
80%	96.8	20 + 15 + 2.5 + 1.25	98.9	20 + 20	101.1	20 + 20	103.2	20 + 20 + 1.25

100%	132		134		137		139	
95%	125.0	20 + 20 + 5 + 2.5 + 5	127.5	20 + 20 + 2.5 + 10 + 1.25	130.0	20 + 20 + 5 + 2.5 + 5 + 2.5	132.5	20 + 20 + 5 + 5 + 5 + 1.25
90%	118.4	20 + 20 + 5 + 2.5 + 1.25	120.8	20 + 20 + 2.5 + 10	123.2	20 + 20 + 5 + 2.5 + 5	125.5	20 + 20 + 5 + 5 + 2.5
85%	111.8	20 + 20 + 5	114.1	20 + 20 + 2.5 + 5	116.3	20 + 20 + 5 + 2.5	118.6	20 + 20 + 5 + 5
80%	105.3	20 + 20 + 2.5	107.4	20 + 20 + 2.5 + 1.25	109.5	20 + 20 + 5	111.6	20 + 20 + 5

100%	142		145		147		150	
95%	135.0	20 + 20 + 5 + 5 + 2.5 + 5	137.5	20 + 20 + 5 + 5 + 5 + 2.5 + 1.25	140.0	20 + 20 + 5 + 10 + 5	142.5	20 + 20 + 10 + 10 + 1.25
90%	127.9	20 + 20 + 5 + 5 + 2.5 + 1.25	130.3	20 + 20 + 5 + 5 + 5	132.6	20 + 20 + 5 + 10 + 1.25	135.0	20 + 20 + 10 + 2.5 + 5
85%	120.8	20 + 20 + 5 + 5	123.0	20 + 20 + 5 + 5 + 1.25	125.3	20 + 20 + 5 + 2.5 + 5	127.5	20 + 20 + 10 + 2.5 + 1.25
80%	113.7	20 + 20 + 5 + 1.25	115.8	20 + 20 + 5 + 2.5	117.9	20 + 20 + 5 + 2.5 + 1.25	120.0	20 + 20 + 10

The sequences shown are the different iron plate discs (in kg) to be placed on each side of a 20 kg bar.

(continued)

Dropset cluster (150-200 kg)

100%	150		153		155		158	
95%	142.5	20 + 20 + 10 + 10 + 1.25	145.0	20 + 20 + 10 + 5 + 2.5 + 5	147.5	20 + 20 + 10 + 10 + 2.5 + 1.25	150.0	20 + 20 + 10 + 10 + 5
90%	135.0	20 + 20 + 10 + 2.5 + 5	137.4	20 + 20 + 10 + 5 + 2.5 + 1.25	139.7	20 + 20 + 10 + 10	142.1	20 + 20 + 10 + 10 + 1.25
85%	127.5	20 + 20 + 10 + 2.5 + 1.25	129.7	20 + 20 + 10 + 5	132.0	20 + 20 + 10 + 5 + 1.25	134.2	20 + 20 + 10 + 2.5 + 5
80%	120.0	20 + 20 + 10	122.1	20 + 20 + 10 + 1.25	124.2	20 + 20 + 10 + 2.5	126.3	20 + 20 + 10 + 2.5

100%	161		163		166		168	
95%	152.5	20 + 20 + 10 + 2.5 + 10 + 2.5 + 1.25	155.0	20 + 20 + 10 + 10 + 2.5 + 5	157.5	20 + 20 + 10 + 5 + 10 + 2.5 + 1.25	160.0	20 + 20 + 10 + 5 + 10 + 5
90%	144.5	20 + 20 + 10 + 2.5 + 10	146.8	20 + 20 + 10 + 10 + 2.5 + 1.25	149.2	20 + 20 + 10 + 5 + 10	151.6	20 + 20 + 10 + 5 + 10
85%	136.4	20 + 20 + 10 + 2.5 + 5	138.7	20 + 20 + 10 + 10	140.9	20 + 20 + 10 + 5 + 5	143.2	20 + 20 + 10 + 5 + 5 + 1.25
80%	128.4	20 + 20 + 10 + 2.5 + 1.25	130.5	20 + 20 + 10 + 5	132.6	20 + 20 + 10 + 5 + 1.25	134.7	20 + 20 + 10 + 5 + 2.5

100%	171		174		176		179	
95%	162.5	20 + 20 + 10 + 2.5 + 10 + 5 + 2.5 + 1.25	165.0	20 + 20 + 10 + 5 + 2.5 + 1.25 + 10 + 2.5 + 1.25	167.5	20 + 20 + 20 + 10 + 2.5 + 1.25	170.0	20 + 20 + 20 + 1.25 + 10 + 2.5 + 1.25
90%	153.9	20 + 20 + 10 + 2.5 + 10 + 5	156.3	20 + 20 + 10 + 5 + 2.5 + 1.25 + 10	158.7	20 + 20 + 20 + 10	161.1	20 + 20 + 20 + 1.25 + 10
85%	145.4	20 + 20 + 10 + 2.5 + 10	147.6	20 + 20 + 10 + 5 + 2.5 + 1.25 + 5	149.9	20 + 20 + 20 + 5	152.1	20 + 20 + 20 + 1.25 + 5
80%	136.8	20 + 20 + 10 + 2.5 + 5 + 1.25	138.9	20 + 20 + 10 + 5 + 2.5 + 1.25	141.1	20 + 20 + 20	143.2	20 + 20 + 20 + 1.25

100%	182		184		187		189	
95%	172.5	20 + 20 + 20 + 2.5 + 10 + 2.5 + 1.25	175.0	20 + 20 + 20 + 2.5 + 1.25 + 10 + 2.5 + 1.25	177.5	20 + 20 + 20 + 10 + 5 + 2.5 + 1.25	180.0	20 + 20 + 20 + 10 + 10
90%	163.4	20 + 20 + 20 + 2.5 + 10	165.8	20 + 20 + 20 + 2.5 + 1.25 + 10	168.2	20 + 20 + 20 + 10 + 5	170.5	20 + 20 + 20 + 10 + 5
85%	154.3	20 + 20 + 20 + 2.5 + 5	156.6	20 + 20 + 20 + 2.5 + 1.25 + 5	158.8	20 + 20 + 20 + 10	161.1	20 + 20 + 20 + 10
80%	145.3	20 + 20 + 20 + 2.5	147.4	20 + 20 + 20 + 2.5 + 1.25	149.5	20 + 20 + 20 + 5	151.6	20 + 20 + 20 + 5 + 1.25

100%	192		195		197		200	
95%	182.5	20 + 20 + 20 + 1.25 + 10 + 10	185.0	20 + 20 + 20 + 5 + 2.5 + 10 + 5	187.5	20 + 20 + 20 + 5 + 2.5 + 1.25 + 10 + 5	190.0	20 + 20 + 20 + 10 + 10 + 5
90%	172.9	20 + 20 + 20 + 1.25 + 10 + 5	175.3	20 + 20 + 20 + 5 + 2.5 + 10	177.6	20 + 20 + 20 + 5 + 2.5 + 1.25 + 10	180.0	20 + 20 + 20 + 10 + 10
85%	163.3	20 + 20 + 20 + 1.25 + 10	165.5	20 + 20 + 20 + 5 + 2.5 + 5	167.8	20 + 20 + 20 + 5 + 2.5 + 1.25 + 5	170.0	20 + 20 + 20 + 10 + 5
80%	153.7	20 + 20 + 20 + 1.25 + 5	155.8	20 + 20 + 20 + 5 + 2.5	157.9	20 + 20 + 20 + 5 + 2.5 + 1.25	160.0	20 + 20 + 20 + 10

The sequences shown are the different iron plate discs (in kg) to be placed on each side of a 20 kg bar.

APPENDIX #9: CLASSIFICATION OF TRAINING TECHNIQUES BASED ON EXPERIENCE

LEVEL 1 [<1 year]

Accumulation methods			
Maximal aerobic speed (MAS)	Postactivation	Burn set	5-10-20 triset
Limited aerobic endurance	Triset	Forced set	4-rep system
Long-term aerobic endurance	Pre-post-fatigue	Cheat set	Speed-set training
Full-body split	Mechanical dropset	Super-pump set long version	Power circuit training
Lower- and upper-body split	The 21	Super-pump set regressive version	Small-angle training
Push–pull split	Giant organic set 1	Double progression method	Bookend training
3-day split	Giant organic set 2	Maximum contraction	Elastics training
Push–pull–isolation training	Maximal fatigue	Constant tension	Variable resistance training
4-day split	Postfatigue isometric	Descending sets 1	Machine muscle
Unilateral split	Rest-pause	Descending sets 2	Posing
5-day split	Extended 7's	Descending sets 3	Maximum duration isometric
Submaximal set	Alternating rest-pause	German volume phase 1	Timed sets
Failure set	Super slow reps 5 5	German volume phase 2	Isometric with perturbations
Hypertrophy 12RM-10RM-8RM-6RM	Super slow reps 10-4	Regressive concentric–isometric	Quasi-isometric eccentric
Agonist superset	Negative reps	Eccentric–concentric contrast	Iso-max eccentric
Antagonist superset	Super slow eccentric reps	Eccentric–isometric contrast 1	General standards 13RM-30RM
Complementary superset	Regressive eccentric reps	Eccentric–isometric contrast 2	Stages 20RM-20RM-20RM-30RM-30RM
Dropset	Double contraction	Concentric static-dynamic	Stages 20RM-15RM-12RM-20RM
Double dropset	4 × 10 per minute	Tempo contrast	Circuit
Holistic set	Overload in big waves	6 × 6 × 6	Minicircuit
Prefatigue	Stage 10RM-6RM	5 × 6	100 repetitions
Postfatigue	Stage 6RM-10RM	1-rep to 1-set method	70 repetitions
Metabolic training	Internal pyramid method	Density training	Strength intervals (cardioacceleration)
Metabolic prefatigue	External pyramid method	Unilateral exercises	Short internals at 60%
Metabolic postfatigue	Rack pyramid method	ECO training method	Long intervals at 60%
Preactivation	Pure concentric	Nubret pro-set	Continuous work at 40%
2-day split	Tabata method	Powerwalking	16-week evolution
Uniangular triset	Super-pump set short version	4-minute muscle	Rest period 15RM
Intensification methods			
Explosive static-dynamic	Ballistic exercises	5 × 5	1-minute intervals at 85%
Olympic weightlifting variations	Sport-specific movement with overload	5 × 5 higher strength	Squat-bench-deadlift split
Traditional exercises with max power	Metabolic training	Ballistic isometric	

(continued)

LEVEL 2 (1-2 years)

Accumulation methods

Back-to-back training	Giant organic set 5	German volume phase 3
Twice-a-day training	Full giant organic set	Anaerobic lactic capacity
Prepotentiation	Super negative reps	Dropset with progressive reps
Postpotentiation	Hypertrophy circuit	Overreaching method
Giant organic set 3	Breathing squat	HSS-100
Giant organic set 4	Muscular chaos	Isometric strength
Continuous plyometric circuit	Intermittent strength-speed	5 × 10
German volume phase 4		

Intensification methods

Anaerobic alactic power	Interset decreasing loads	Depth jump
Anaerobic alactic capacity	Grouping	Overspeed eccentric
Acceleration	Grouping dropset	Drop and catch
Maximum speed (velocity)	1-minute intervals at 90%	Drop, catch, and lift
Speed endurance	Wendler method	Plyometrics with or without load
Sprints with sled, tire, or parachute	5-3-2 split	Complex training
Contrast sprints with sled, tire, or parachute	Westside method	Variable resistance with bands
Assisted overspeed with band	Heavy lifting and manual isometrics	Repeated jumps, impulses, and throws
Contrast sprints with a partner	Kulesza method	Canadian ascending–descending training
Climbing acceleration	Bulgarian method	Russian complex training
Climbing maximal speed	Overload in small waves	Russian complex training (emphasis on strength)
Contrast climbing maximal speed	5 × 10	Russian complex training (emphasis on speed)
Maximum downhill speed	Max effort with variable resistance	Bulgarian complex training
Contrast maximum downhill speed	Isometric strength	Big Kahuna
Acceleration with changes of direction	Extended 5's cluster	Big Kahuna regression
Change of direction cone drills	Classic cluster	Big Kahuna progression
Anaerobic lactic power	Antagonist cluster	Intermittent plyometric circuit
Anaerobic lactic capacity	Mentzer cluster	Continuous plyometric circuit
General standards 1RM-5RM	Maximum intensity isometric	Intermittent strength-speed
Strength in multiple splits	Electrostimulation	45-second circuit
Maximum weight 1	2/1 technique	Landmine circuit
Maximum weight 2	2-movements technique	Antagonist Russian complex
Stage 5RM-3RM	Depth landing	Potentiation + metabolic
Partial reps with max effort	Starting strength	Maximum contraction cluster

LEVEL 3 (>2 years)

Accumulation methods

	The layer system	

Intensification methods

Super-Pletnev	Functional isometric cluster	Supramaximal cluster
The inch program	Overshoot (with weight releasers)	Contrast with weight releasers
Dropset cluster	The layer system	120/80 method
Accentuated eccentric cluster	Pure eccentric (maximal and supramaximal)	

Perceived effort

☐ ☐ ☐ ☐ ☐

Effect on
hypertrophy

☐ ☐ ☐ ☐ ☐

Effect on strength
and power

☐ ☐ ☐ ☐ ☐

Effect on muscular
endurance

☐ ☐ ☐ ☐ ☐

Experience required

☐ ☐ ☐

☐ Accumulation
method

☐ Intensification
method

YOUR TIPS

NAME OF YOUR TECHNIQUE

HOW DOES IT WORK?

ADVANTAGES

DISADVANTAGES

PRESCRIPTION TABLE

Load	Number of repetitions per set	Number of sets per exercise	Number of exercises per muscle group	Rest between sets

VISUAL OF YOUR TECHNIQUE

From K. Arseneault, *The Complete Guide to Strength Training Methods* (Champaign, IL: Human Kinetics, 2024).

APPENDIXES | 333

TECHNIQUES INDEX

P = Training plan; S = Training strategy

Technique name	#	Chapter	Plan or strategy	Page
Continuous work at 40%	219	8	S	270
Contrast climbing maximal speed	12	1	S	32
Contrast maximum downhill speed	14	1	S	34
Contrast sprints with a partner	9	1	S	29
Contrast sprints with sled, tire, or parachute	7	1	S	27
Contrast with weight releasers	180	5	S	217
Density training	146	3	S	175
Depth jump	175	5	S	212
Depth landing	174	5	S	211
Descending sets 1	128	3	S	157
Descending sets 2	129	3	S	158
Descending sets 3	130	3	S	159
Double contraction	108	3	S	137
Double dropset	75	3	S	104
Double progression method	124	3	S	153
Drop and catch	177	5	S	214
Drop, catch, and lift	178	5	S	215
Dropset	74	3	S	103
Dropset cluster	53	2	S	78
Dropset with progressive reps	137	3	S	166
Eccentric–concentric contrast	138	3	S	167
Eccentric–isometric contrast 1	139	3	S	168
Eccentric–isometric contrast 2	140	3	S	169
ECO training method	148	3	S	177
Elastics training	158	3	S	187
Electrostimulation	170	4	S	203
Explosive static-dynamic	182	6	S	224
Extended 5's cluster	49	2	S	74
Extended 7's	100	3	S	129

Technique name	#	Chapter	Plan or strategy	Page
External pyramid method	115	3	S	144
Failure set	69	3	S	98
Forced set	119	3	S	148
Full-body split	57	3	P	86
Full giant organic set	96	3	S	125
Functional isometric cluster	55	2	S	80
General standards 1RM-5RM	22	2	S	46
General standards 13RM-30RM	209	8	S	260
German volume phase 1	132	3	S	161
German volume phase 2	133	3	S	162
German volume phase 3	134	3	S	163
German volume phase 4	135	3	S	164
Giant organic set 1	91	3	S	120
Giant organic set 2	92	3	S	121
Giant organic set 3	93	3	S	122
Giant organic set 4	94	3	S	123
Giant organic set 5	95	3	S	124
Grouping	33	2	S	57
Grouping dropset	32	2	S	56
Heavy lifting and manual isometrics	37	2	S	62
Holistic set	76	3	S	105
HSS-100	161	3	P	190
Hypertrophy 12RM-10RM-8RM-6RM	70	3	S	99
Hypertrophy circuit	109	3	S	138
The inch program	44	2	P	69
Intermittent plyometric circuit	201	7	S	248
Intermittent strength-speed	203	7	S	250
Internal pyramid method	114	3	S	143
Interset decreasing loads	31	2	S	55
Isolated active stretching	226	9	S	282
Iso-max eccentric	169	4	S	202

P = Training plan; S = Training strategy

Technique name	#	Chapter	Plan or strategy	Page
Isometric strength	43	2	S	68
Isometric with perturbations	167	4	S	200
Kulesza method	38	2	S	63
Landmine circuit	205	7	S	252
The layer system	162	3	P	191
Limited aerobic endurance	20	1	S	40
Long intervals at 60%	218	8	S	269
Long-term aerobic endurance	21	1	S	41
Lower- and upper-body split	59	3	P	88
Machine muscle	160	3	S	189
Max effort with variable resistance	42	2	S	67
Maximal fatigue	97	3	S	126
Maximum aerobic speed (MAS)	19	1	S	39
Maximum contraction	126	3	S	155
Maximum contraction cluster	56	2	S	81
Maximum downhill speed	13	1	S	33
Maximum duration isometric	164	4	S	197
Maximum intensity isometric	165	4	S	198
Maximum speed (velocity)	4	1	S	24
Maximum weight 1	25	2	S	49
Maximum weight 2	26	2	S	50
Mechanical dropset	88	3	S	117
Mentzer cluster	52	2	S	77
Metabolic postfatigue	81	3	S	110
Metabolic prefatigue	80	3	S	109
Metabolic training	207	7	S	254
Minicircuit	213	8	S	264
Muscular chaos	125	3	P	154
Negative reps	104	3	S	133

Technique name	#	Chapter	Plan or strategy	Page
Nubret pro-set	150	3	S	179
Olympic weightlifting variations	183	6	S	225
Overload in big waves	111	3	S	140
Overload in small waves	40	2	S	65
Overreaching method	149	3	P	178
Overshoot (with weight releasers)	191	6	S	234
Overspeed eccentric	176	5	S	213
Partial reps with max effort	30	2	S	54
Passive static stretching	223	9	S	279
Plyometrics with or without load	184	6	S	226
PNF, agonistic reversal	236	9	S	292
PNF, contract–relax	233	9	S	289
PNF, hold–relax	234	9	S	290
PNF, repeated contractions	237	9	S	293
PNF, rhythmic initiation	229	9	S	285
PNF, rhythmic stabilization	232	9	S	288
PNF, slow reversal	230	9	S	286
PNF, slow reversal–hold	231	9	S	287
PNF, slow reversal–hold–relax	235	9	S	291
Posing	163	4	S	196
Postactivation	83	3	S	112
Postfatigue	78	3	S	107
Postfatigue isometric	98	3	S	127
Postpotentiation	85	3	S	114
Potentiation + metabolic	208	7	S	255
Power circuit training	155	3	S	184
Powerwalking	222	8	S	273
Preactivation	82	3	S	111
Prefatigue	77	3	S	106
Pre-post-fatigue	87	3	S	116

P = Training plan; S = Training strategy

P = Training plan; S = Training strategy

REFERENCES

Scientific Studies

1. Adams K., O'Shea J. P., O'Shea K. L., Climstein M. "The Effect of Six Weeks of Squat, Plyometric and Squat-Plyometric Training on Power Production," *Journal of Applied Sports Science Research*, 1992, 6(1): 36-41.

2. Doss W. S., Karpovich P. V. "A Comparison of Concentric, Eccentric, and Isometric Strength of Elbow Flexors," *Journal of Applied Physiology*, 1965, 20: 351-353.

3. Douglas J., Pearson S., Ross A., McGuigan M. "Chronic Adaptations to Eccentric Training: A Systematic Review," *Sports Med*, 2017, 47(5): 917-941.

4. Drinkwater E. J., Lawton T. W., Lindsell R. P., Pyne D. B., Hunt P. H., McKenna M. J. "Training Leading to Repetition Failure Enhances Bench Press Strength Gains in Elite Junior Athletes," *J Strength Cond Res*, 2005, 19(2): 382-388.

5. Farthing J. P., Chilibeck P. D. "The Effects of Eccentric and Concentric Training at Different Velocities on Muscle Hypertrophy," *Eur J Appl Physiol*, 2003 Aug, 89(6): 578-586.

6. Gołaś A., Maszczyk A., Zajac A., Mikołajec K., Stastny P. "Optimizing Post Activation Potentiation for Explosive Activities in Competitive Sports." *J Hum Kinet*, 2016, 52: 95-106.

7. Goto K., Nagasawa M., Yanagisawa O., Kizuka T., Ishii N., Takamatsu K. "Muscular Adaptations to Combinations of High- and Low-Intensity Resistance Exercises," *J Strength Cond Res*, 2004, 18(4): 730-737.

8. Güllich A., Schmidtbleicher D. "MVC-Induced Short-Term Potentiation of Explosive Force," *IAAF*, 1996, 11(4): 67-81.

9. Harris N. K., Cronin J. B., Hopkins W. G. "Power Outputs of a Machine Squat-Jump Across a Spectrum of Loads," *J Strength Cond Res*, 2007 Nov, 21(4): 1260-1264.

10. Hernandez J. P., Nelson-Whalen N. L., Franke W. D., McLean S. P. "Bilateral Index Expressions and iEMG Activity in Older Versus Young Adults," *J Gerontol A Biol Sci Med Sci*, 2003, 58(6): 536-541.

11. Hollander D.B., Kraemer R.R., Kilpatrick M.W., Ramadan Z.G., Reeves G.V., Francois M., Hebert E.P., Tryniecki J.L. "Maximal Eccentric and Concentric Strength Discrepancies Between Young Men and Women for Dynamic Resistance Exercise." *J Strength Cond Res*, 2007 Feb, 21(1): 34-40.

12. Kraemer W. J., Ratamess N. A., Volek J. S., Häkkinen K., Rubin M. R., French D. N., Gómez A. L., McGuigan M. R., Scheett T. P., Newton R. U., Spiering B. A., Izquierdo M., Dioguardi F. S. "The Effects of Amino Acid Supplementation on Hormonal Responses to Resistance Training Overreaching," *Metabolism*, 2006, 55(3): 282-291.

13. Marek S. M., Cramer J. T., Fincher A. L., Massey L. L., Dangelmaier S. M., Purkayastha S., Fitz K. A., Culbertson J. Y. "Acute Effects of Static and Proprioceptive Neuromuscular Facilitation Stretching on Muscle Strength and Power Output," *J Athl Train*, 2005, 40(2): 94-103.

14. Massey C., Maneval M., Moore M., Johnson J. "An Analysis of Full Range of Motion vs. Partial Range of Motion Training in the Development of Strength in Untrained Men." *J Strength Cond Res*, 2004, 18: 518-521.

15. Mookerjee S., Ratamess, N. "Comparison of Strength Differences and Joint Action Durations Between Full and Partial Range-of-Motion Bench Press Exercise," *J Strength Cond Res*, 1999, 13(1): 76-81.

16. Peck E., Chomko G., Gaz D. V., Farrell A. M. "The Effects of Stretching on Performance," *Curr Sports Med Rep*, 2014, 13(3): 179-185.

17. Pennington J., Laubach L., Marco G., Linderman J. "Determining the Optimal Load for Maximal Power Output for the Power Clean and Snatch in Collegiate Male Football Players," *J Exerc Physiol Online*, 2010, 13: 10-19.

18. Roig M., O'Brien K., Kirk G., Murray R., McKinnon P., Shadgan B., Reid W. D. "The Effects of Eccentric Versus Concentric Resistance Training on Muscle Strength and Mass in Healthy Adults: A Systematic Review with Meta-Analysis," *Br J Sports Med*, 2009, 43: 556-568.

19. Schoenfeld B. J., Ogborn D. I., Vigotsky A. D., Franchi M. V., Krieger J. W. "Hypertrophic Effects of Concentric vs. Eccentric Muscle Actions: A Systematic Review and Meta-Analysis," *J Strength Cond Res*, 2017, 31(9): 2599-2608.

20. Siegel J. A., Gilders R. M., Staron R. S., Hagerman F. C. "Human Muscle Power Output During Upper- and Lower-Body Exercises," *J Strength Cond Res*, 2002 May, 16(2): 173-178.

21. Tabata I., Irisawa K., Kouzaki M., Nishimura K., Ogita F., Miyachi M. "Metabolic Profile of High Intensity Intermittent Exercises," *Med Sci Sports Exerc*, 1997, 29(3): 390-295.

22. Tabata I., Nishimura K., Kouzaki M., Hirai Y., Ogita F., Miyachi M., Yamamoto K. "Effects of Moderate-Intensity Endurance and High-Intensity Intermittent Training on Anaerobic Capacity and $\dot{V}O_2$max," *Med Sci Sports Exerc*, 1996, 28(10): 1327-1330.

23. Vanderburgh P. M., Batterham A. M. "Validation of the Wilks Powerlifting Formula," *Med Sci Sports Exerc*, 1999, 31(12): 1869-1875.

24. Yarrow J. F., Borsa P. A., Borst S. E., Sitren H. S., Stevens B. R., White L. J. "Neuroendocrine Responses to an Acute Bout of Eccentric-Enhanced Resistance Exercise," *Med Sci Sports Exerc*, 2007, 39(6): 941-947.

25. Zehr E. P., Sale D. G. "Ballistic Movement: Muscle Activation and Neuromuscular Adaptation," *Can J Appl Physiol*, 1994, 19(4): 363-378.

29. Siff M. C. *Supertraining*, 6th ed., Supertraining Institute, 2003.

30. Simmons L. *The Westside Barbell Book of Methods*, Westside Barbell, 2007.

31. Thibaudeau C. *Theory and application of modern strength and power methods*, F. Lepine Editions, 2008.

32. Thibault G. *Entraînement cardio: sports d'endurance et performance*, Édition Tricycle, 2009.

33. Tsatsouiline P. *Super Joints*, Dragon Door, 2001.

34. Wendler J. 5/3/1. *The Simplest and Most Effective Training System for Raw Strength*, 2009.

35. Wharton J., Wharton P. *The Whartons' Stretch Book: Featuring the Breakthrough Method of Active-Isolated Stretching*, TimesBook (Random House), 1996.

36. Zachazewski J. E. "Flexibility for sports," in *Sports Physical Therapy*, ed. B. Sanders, 201-238, Appleton & Lange, 1988.

37. Zatsiorsky V. M., Kraemer W. J. *Science and Practice of Strength Training*, 2nd edition, Human Kinetics, 2006.

Books

26. Chouinard R., Lacombe N. *Course à pied: le guide d'entraînement et de nutrition*, Guide, Kmag, 2013.

27. Mattes A. L. *Flexibility: Active and Assisted Stretching*, Aaron Mattes Therapy, 1990.

28. Medvedyev, A. S. *A System of Multi-Year Training in Weightlifting*, Sportivny Press, 1989.

Internet

38. T-Nation. "Most Powerful Program Ever?" Retrieved December 2, 2019, from www.t-nation.com/workouts/most-powerful-program-ever

39. T-Nation. "The Layer System." Retrieved December 2, 2019, from www.t-nation.com/workouts/layer-system

RECOMMENDED RESOURCES

Scientific Studies

Ahtiainen J. P., Pakarinen A., Kraemer W. J., Häkkinen K. "Acute Hormonal and Neuromuscular Responses and Recovery to Forced vs. Maximum Repetitions Multiple Resistance Exercises," *Int J Sports Med*, 2003, 24(6): 410-418.

Behm D. G., Blazevich A. J., Kay A. D., McHugh M. "Acute Effects of Muscle Stretching on Physical Performance, Range of Motion, and Injury Incidence in Healthy Active Individuals: A Systematic Review," *Appl Physiol Nutr Metab*, 2016, 41(1): 1-11.

Cini A., de Vasconcelos G. S., Lima C. S. "Acute Effect of Different Time Periods of Passive Static Stretching on the Hamstring Flexibility," *J Back Musculoskelet Rehabil*, 2017, 30(2): 241-246.

Costa P. B., Herda T. J., Herda A. A., Cramer J. T. "Effects of Dynamic Stretching on Strength, Muscle Imbalance, and Muscle Activation," *Med Sci Sports Exerc*, 2014 Mar, 46(3): 586-593.

Lempke L., Wilkinson R., Murray C., Stanek J. "The Effectiveness of PNF Versus Static Stretching on Increasing Hip-Flexion Range of Motion," *J Sport Rehabil*, 2018, 27(3): 289-294.

Medeiros D. M., Cini A., Sbruzzi G., Lima C. S. "Influence of Static Stretching on Hamstring Flexibility in Healthy Young Adults: Systematic Review and Meta-Analysis," *Physiother Theory Pract*, 2016, 32(6): 438-445. Epub July 26 2016.

Milanović Z., Sporiš G., Weston M. "Effectiveness of High-Intensity Interval Training (HIT) and Continuous Endurance Training for $\dot{V}O_2$max Improvements: A Systematic Review and Meta-Analysis of Controlled Trials," *Sports Med*, 2015, 45(10): 1469-1481.

Nóbrega S. R., Libardi C. A. "Is Resistance Training to Muscular Failure Necessary?" *Front Physiol*, 2016, 7: 10.

Odunaiya N. A., Hamzat T. K., Ajayi O. F. "The Effects of Static Stretch Duration on the Flexibility of Hamstring Muscles," *African Journal of Biomedical Research*, 2006, 8(2).

Opplert J., Babault N. "Acute Effects of Dynamic Stretching on Muscle Flexibility and Performance: An Analysis of the Current Literature," *Sports Med*, 2018, 48(2): 299-325.

Robbins D. W., Young W. B., Behm D. G. "The Effect of an Upper-Body Agonist-Antagonist Resistance Training Protocol on Volume Load and Efficiency," *J Strength Cond Res*, 2010, 24(10): 2632-2640.

Robbins D. W., Young W. B., Behm D. G., Payne W. R. "Agonist-Antagonist Paired Set Resistance Training: A Brief Review," *J Strength Cond Res*, 2010, 24(10): 2873-2882.

Sharman M. J., Cresswell A. G., Riek S. "Proprioceptive Neuromuscular Facilitation Stretching: Mechanisms and Clinical Implications," *Sports Med*, 2006, 36(11): 929-939.

Small K., Mc Naughton L., Matthews M. "Systematic Review into the Efficacy of Static Stretching as Part of a Warm-Up for the Prevention of Exercise-Related Injury," *Res Sports Med*, 2008, 16(3): 213-231.

Thacker S. B., Gilchrist J., Stroup D. F., Kimsey C. D. Jr. "The Impact of Stretching on Sports Injury Risk: A Systematic Review of the Literature," *Med Sci Sports Exerc*, 2004, 36(3): 371-378.

Thomas E., Bianco A., Paoli A., Palma A. "The Relation Between Stretching Typology and Stretching Duration: The Effects on Range of Motion," *Int J Sports Med*, 2018, 39(4): 243-254.

Weldon S. M, Hill R. H. "The Efficacy of Stretching for Prevention of Exercise-Related Injury: A Systematic Review of the Literature," *Man Ther*, 2003, 8(3): 141-150.

Books

Alter M. J. *Science of Flexibility*, 3rd edition, Human Kinetics, 2004.

Andrich V. *Sports Supplement Review*, no 4, Mile High Publishing, 2001.

Bompa T. O., Haff G. G. *Periodization: Theory and Methodology of Training*, 5th edition, Human Kinetics, 2009.

Brown L. E., Ferrigno V. A. *Training for Speed, Agility and Quickness*, 2nd edition, Human Kinetics, 2005.

Chu D. A. *Jumping into Plyometrics*, 2nd edition, Human Kinetics, 1998.

Croisetière R. *Musculation*, édition RC, 2004.

Delavier F., Gundill M. *The Strength Training Anatomy Workout*, Human Kinetics, 2011.

Le Gallais D., Millet G. *La Préparation physique: optimisation et limites de la performance sportive*, Éditions Masson, 2007.

Phillips B. *Sports Supplement Review*, no 3, Mile High Publishing, 1997.

Poliquin C. Méthode d'entraînement en force, tiré d'un document de Charles Poliquin.

Shuler L., Cosgrove A. *The New Rules of Lifting*, Penguin Group, 2006.

Simmons L. *Strength Manual for Running*, Westside Barbell, 2017.

Simmons L. *The Rule of Three*, Westside Barbell, 2018.

Tate D. *Elitefts Bench Manual, Elite Fitness Systems*, 2018. Disponible en format e-book au: www.elitefts.com/wp/wp-content/uploads/2018/09/EFSBenchManual.pdf

Thépaut-Mathieu C., Miller C., Quievre J. *Entraînement de la force: spécificité et planification*, INSEP, 1997.

Thibaudeau C. *The black book of training secrets, enhanced edition*, Tony Schwartz, 2007.

Thibaudeau C. *High-threshold muscle building*, Tony Schwartz, 2007.

Veillette R. Méthodes d'entraînement, tiré du cours "Bases scientifiques de la performance au baccalauréat en kinésiologie de l'université Laval," 2007.

Weider J., Reynolds B. *Le Système Weider de musculation*, Éditions Québécor, 1992.

Weineck J. *Manuel d'entraînement*, quatrième édition, éditions Vigot, 1997.

Willey W. *Better Than Steroids,* Trafford, 2007.

Videos

NSCA, "Metabolic Training for Fat Loss—HIT Millennium Style."
Thibaudeau C., "Cluster Training."
Thibaudeau C., "Mechanical Dropset."
Veillette R., "Exercices d'agilité et de renforcement musculaire."

Internet

Nuckols G. "Who's the Most Impressive Powerlifter?" Retrieved December 13, 2019, from www.strongerbyscience.com/whos-the-most-impressive-powerlifter

Westside Barbell. "Cultivators of Strength." Retrieved December 13, 2019, from www.westside-barbell.com

www.crossgymstore.com

www.crossgymstore.com/pro/chains.html

www.crossgymstore.com/pro/elastic-bands.html

www.fitnessentrepot.com

www.roguecanada.ca

www.roguecanada.ca/rogue-chain-kits.php

www.roguefitness.com/rogue-fractional-plates-lbs.php

www.roguefitness.com/rogue-metric-fractional-plates-kgs.php

www.roguecanada.ca/rogue-monster-bands.php

www.roguefitness.com/rogue-weight-releasers

www.theplatemate.com

GLOSSARY

activation—Movement characterized by an unstable environment that is conducive to the recruitment of fast-twitch fibers for stability.

backpedal—Fast sprint backward.

cluster—A set broken into several minisets with short rest periods between them.

CNS—Central nervous system.

MAP—Maximum aerobic power, or the maximum rate at which oxygen can be used during a specified period (usually 2-8 minutes), typically during intense exercise.

MAS—Maximum aerobic speed, the running speed at which your oxygen uptake is at your maximal level.

metabolic—Movement characterized by explosive repetitions lasting 20-60 seconds.

motor unit—A unit composed of a motor neuron and a group of muscle fibers that are innervated by the motor neuron. The number of fibers per motor unit may vary. For example, a motor unit of an eye muscle can contain 5-10 muscle fibers, whereas a motor unit of a quadriceps can contain approximately 150 fibers.

Olympic weightlifting—Weightlifting of a type performed as a competitive event at the Olympic Games (the lifts involved are the snatch and the clean and jerk).

potentiation—Movement performed with great power without deceleration at the end of the concentric phase; it is conducive to the recruitment of fast-twitch fibers (motor units with a high activation threshold) and to the creation of a facilitation effect.

powerlifting—A form of competitive weightlifting in which contestants attempt three types of lifts in a set sequence (squat, deadlift, bench press).

reps—Repetitions.

RM—Repetition maximum.

shuffle—To walk by dragging one's feet along or without lifting them fully off the ground.

Smax—Maximum speed, the fastest speed you can reach in your sport (running, cycling, swimming).

tempo—The speed of effort (e.g., 3-0-1-0). These numbers refer to the eccentric phase (3 seconds), eccentric–concentric transition (0 seconds, fast), concentric phase (1 second), concentric–eccentric transition (0 seconds, fast).

ABOUT THE AUTHOR

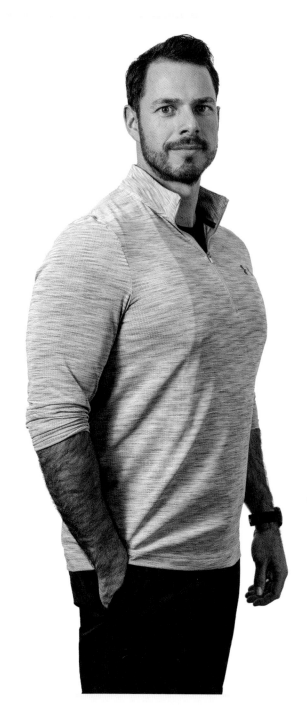

Keven Arseneault, CSCS, is the owner of Keven Arseneault Kinesiologist in Montreal. He is a former co-owner of Maxi-Forme Fitness of Charny and worked at Hardgym Performance, a performance center located in the heart of Québec City, where he was responsible for the training or nutrition of top athletes, including football players (Canadian Football League), hockey players (National Hockey League, Quebec Major Junior Hockey League), strongman athletes on the world circuit, and firefighters competing on the FireFit global circuit. He also specializes in coaching tactical and operational professionals, including firefighters, police officers, ambulance personnel, bodyguards, and military personnel.

Arseneault has competed in five bodybuilding competitions (2004 to 2010) on the Québec and Canadian scene. During those years, he was able to experiment with different nutritional protocols and training to better understand the differences between theory and practice.

He has a master of kinanthropology from Université du Québec à Montréal (UQAM), a bachelor of kinesiology and nutrition from Laval University, and a postgraduate diploma in functional food and health from the same university. He also holds National Strength and Conditioning Association's CSCS certification and has Level 1 certification in weightlifting from the National Coaching Certification Program (NCCP).

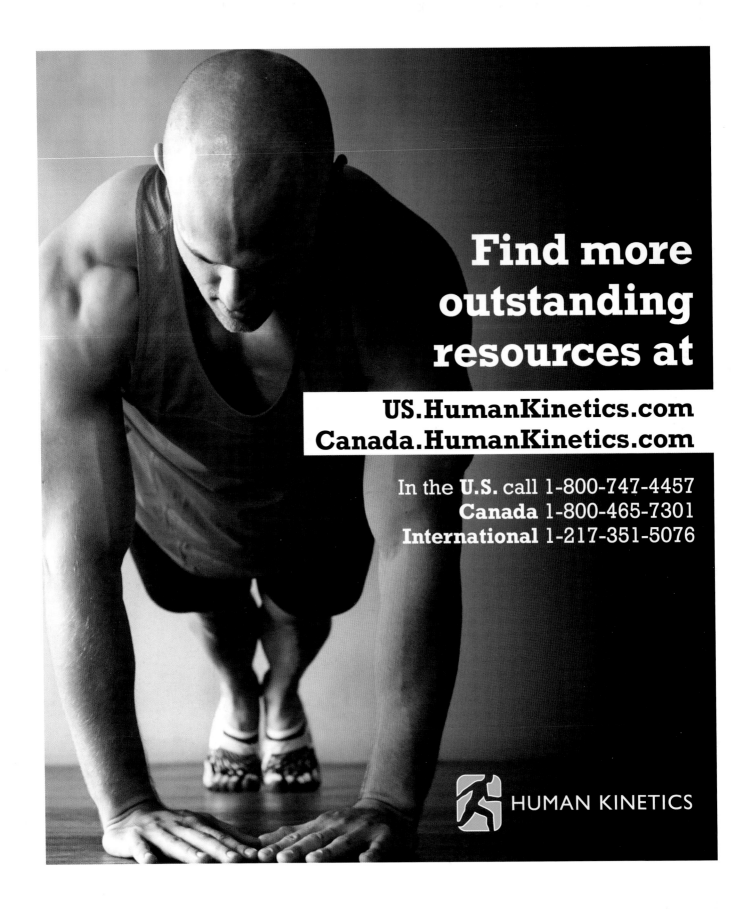